Ethical and Legal Issues in Canadian Nursing

Ethical and Legal Issues in Canadian Nursing

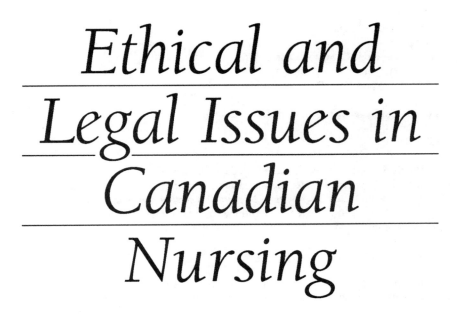

Margaret Keatings, RN, MHSc
Director of Nursing Education & Research
The Toronto Hospital

Assistant Professor of Nursing
University of Toronto

Associate, Centre for Bioethics
University of Toronto

O'Neil B. Smith, BA, LLB
(of the Ontario Bar)
Associate of Stortini Lee-Whiting,
Barristers & Solicitors
Toronto

W.B. SAUNDERS CANADA
a division of
Harcourt Brace & Company, Canada
Toronto Philadelphia London Sydney Tokyo

W.B. Saunders Canada
a division of
Harcourt Brace & Company Canada, Ltd.
55 Horner Avenue
Toronto, Ontario M8Z 4X6

Ethical and Legal Issues in Canadian Nursing

ISBN 0-9205-1317-4

Canadian Cataloguing in Publication Data

Keatings, Margaret
Ethical and legal issues in Canadian nursing

Includes bibliographical references and index.
ISBN 0-9205-1317-4

1. Nursing ethics — Canada. 2. Nursing — Law and legislation — Canada. I. Smith, O'Neil, 1962– II. Title.

RT85.K43 1995   174'.2   C94-932649-6

DESIGN/DESKTOP PUBLISHING: Jack Steiner Graphic Design
EDITING/PRODUCTION COORDINATION: Francine Geraci

Printed in Canada at Webcom.
This book has been bound using the patented Otabind™ process. You can open this book at any page, gently run your finger down the spine, and the pages will lie flat.

Last digit is print number: 9 8 7 6 5 4 3 2 1

Dedicated, with love,
to the life and courage of my mother, Jean.
— MK

To Stephanie, Mom, Dad, and Paul,
for all your love and support.
— OBS

Acknowledgements

The task of writing this book has been a long and, at times, arduous one. During its completion, we relied upon the help, support and encouragement of people too numerous to mention who inspired us to persevere.

In particular, we wish to thank Gerry Mungham at W.B. Saunders Canada for his patience and for the opportunity to write this book, as well as our editor, Francine Geraci, for her tireless efforts in polishing and refining the manuscript and for her always helpful suggestions.

We extend a personal thank you to Robert Boucher, who in spite of his busy schedule as a graduate student took the time to critique the ethics portion of the book and offered much appreciated suggestions for improvement.

We also acknowledge and are deeply indebted to those who reviewed the manuscript and provided helpful comments, constructive criticism and suggestions, especially: Sharon Wilson, RN, MEd, MScN, Faculty of Nursing, Ryerson Polytechnic University, Toronto; Sherry D. Wiebe, BN, LLB, Winnipeg; Barbara Mathur, RN, MScN, MA, College of Nursing, University of Saskatchewan, Saskatoon; Leah Evans Parisi, RN, EdD, JD, Faculty of Nursing, McMaster University, Hamilton; and Patricia A. McLean, RN, BN, LLB, Managing Director, Canadian Nurses Protective Society, Ottawa.

Finally, we would be remiss if we did not acknowledge the patience of the secretaries and staff in the Nursing Education and Research Department of The Toronto Hospital, who tolerated chaos and upheaval particularly during the final stages of the manuscript's development.

Margaret Keatings, RN, MHSc
O'Neil B. Smith, BA, LLB

A Note from the Publisher

Thank you for selecting *Ethical and Legal Issues in Canadian Nursing* by Margaret Keatings and O'Neil B. Smith. The authors and publisher have devoted considerable time to the careful development of this book. We appreciate your recognition of this effort and accomplishment.

We want to hear what you think about this Canadian book. Please take a few minutes to fill out and mail the stamped reader reply card at the back of the book. Your comments and suggestions will be valuable to us as we prepare new editions and other books.

In the last half century, great and rapid advances in medical technology have made it possible for people to live lives that are much longer than those of any previous generation. With this technology, such ethical and legal issues as withdrawal of treatment, euthanasia, and assisted suicide have received increasing attention in the media and among the public.

The questions and dilemmas posed by these issues have not escaped nursing practitioners. Nurses are in the front lines of such dilemmas and are usually the ones who bear the brunt of fashioning new and effective, yet ethical and sensitive, solutions to such problems in their day-to-day practice. To date, few Canadian textbooks have dealt with these matters.

Ethical and Legal Issues in Canadian Nursing is by no means a comprehensive or exhaustive study. This book is intended for nursing students and clinicians as an overview and summary of the more prominent issues faced by nurses in everyday practice. Chapters are arranged to facilitate both class discussion and individual study. Point-form Chapter Objectives guide the reader through the material to come; each chapter Summary reiterates and reinforces the key points.

Part I establishes a conceptual framework. Chapter 1 contains a brief background and introductory discussion. Chapter 2 describes the theory and structure of Canada's legal system. Chapter 3 reviews the laws governing nursing across Canada and summarizes the functions and structures of the various provincial and territorial nursing regulatory bodies. Chapter 4 provides a basic overview of ethical theory as a basis for examining the underpinnings of nursing codes of ethics.

Part II looks at the ethical and legal aspects of various prominent issues facing nurses and health practitioners today, including consent to treatment, substitute decision making, euthanasia, the right to die with dignity, withdrawal of treatment, assisted suicide, caregiver rights and responsibilities, nursing documentation, and patients' rights.

Throughout Part II, some ethical and legal issues are illustrated by means of hypothetical case studies. The chief questions arising from each case are set forth, and possible solutions are suggested and integrated with the applicable principles from ethics and Canadian law. The case studies are meant to encourage discussion and debate among students or practitioners and their colleagues. Readers are encouraged to use the model ethical decision-making framework presented in Chapter 4 (pp. 105–106) in discussing approaches and solutions to the problems raised in the case studies.

The authors' goal throughout has been to explain and discuss ethical and legal concepts in Canadian nursing today in as lucid a style as possible without overburdening the reader with legal jargon and complicated analysis. Such analysis, while beneficial to the lawyer, is of limited use to the nursing practitioner. Where legal concepts are discussed, selected terms are highlighted in bold type and are defined and explained in the Glossary at the back of the book (pp. 260–266).

We regard Ethical and Legal Issues in Canadian Nursing as a work in progress. Many of the issues and concepts discussed are still being debated and fought out in the courts and health care institutions throughout the country. We welcome suggestions, criticism and comments from readers in our continuing effort to improve this work.

Margaret Keatings, RN, MHSc
O'Neil B. Smith, BA, LLB
Toronto, April 1995

CONTENTS

PART

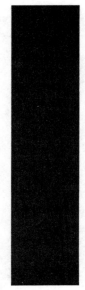

Introduction

CHAPTER One

Nursing, the Law, and Ethics

CHAPTER OBJECTIVES

The purpose of this chapter is to enable the reader to:
- identify the reasons why nurses must be familiar with the law and ethics
- clarify the knowledge required to practise according to ethical and legal standards
- articulate the role of professionals in serving the public interest
- understand how and why the field of ethics has grown over recent years
- appreciate the challenges faced by nurses when dealing with complex legal and ethical issues.

Introduction to Law and Ethics

Nurses must be familiar with the law, ethics, ethical theory, and the workings of Canada's legal system as these pertain to their profession. Nurses, like other professionals, operate within a framework of legal and ethical rules and guidelines. These are aimed at ensuring consistency, quality, competency, and safety to consumers of health services, while preserving respect for individual rights and human dignity.

As part of their professional role, nurses must make and act on decisions that relate to both independent practice and collaborative roles and relationships. For all of these decisions and actions the nurse as a professional is held accountable to individual patients, their families, health care team members, employers, the profession, and society as a whole. This process of decision making and action requires a sound knowledge base, practical and reasoning skills, and a willingness both to take risks and to be accountable. Frequently, our decisions and subsequent actions relate to, or are influenced by, law and ethics. As such, they are guided by a set of rules (the law) and our individual and collective values and beliefs (ethics).

Members of professional groups have an obligation to serve the public interest and the common good because their roles, missions, and ethical foundations focus not only on the individuals they serve, but on society as a whole. Professionals have this authority, and therefore this responsibility, because of their unique body of knowledge, skills, and expertise. Our society has traditionally been dependent on professionals as custodians of such fields as knowledge, health, law, and education. Professionals are therefore placed in a position of respect, and they are accordingly given the power and authority to engage in decisions that influence and shape public policy, law, and societal norms. As technology advances and society becomes more complex, professionals become more specialized and hence acquire new power, and correspondingly greater ethical responsibility.[1]

In recent years, the field of ethics in health care has grown to meet the increasing complexity and volume of ethical dilemmas. This increase is primarily due to the growing sophistication of medical science and advanced technology. This rise in ethical dilemmas has contributed to caregiver stress, poor communication, uncertainty, and value conflict. There is also a growing awareness of patients' rights and a greater emphasis on respect for individual autonomy. Consequently, a growing number of advocacy groups have been created to represent the interests of various patient constituencies.

As medical science and technology advance, traditional norms and values are challenged by questions about what we are doing in health care, how and why we are doing these things, and whether we ought to be doing them in the first place. New technology has made it possible for us to affect various life processes in ways that pose moral and legal problems for health care professionals, patients, and society alike.

Nurses, in particular, have been challenged by this increase in ethical and legal dilemmas and concerns. As they confront and experience each new issue, they may be confused by the often conflicting interplay of ethics and law. They are forced to deal with these dilemmas and conflicts within the context of a health care system strained by limited funds and resources as they continue to face the challenge of providing quality ethical care to patients.

Nurses must therefore have a high level of awareness of the ethical and legal issues they face. More than any other health professional, they are in sustained contact with patients in the home, in the community, and in the institutional setting. Nurses must fulfil the important task of supporting patients and their families, as well as intervening or lobbying on behalf of those patients when necessary. Their role involves professional and trusting relationships with people throughout the life continuum from birth to death, which require knowledge, skill, and sensitivity with regard to health care issues as well as their ethical and legal dimensions.

The situations nurses face as health professionals may involve clear institutional rules and procedures, or straightforward legal rules and statutes. Yet, many situations are more complicated and require us to decide, from many possible alternative courses of action, what is the morally correct thing to do. At times, conflicts may arise in situations where what we believe to be the most morally correct course of action may not necessarily be supported in law.

Since society holds nurses to high standards of professional, moral, and ethical competence, it also affords them certain rights and privileges. The law strives to keep these competing interests in constant balance. It regulates the education and licensing of nurses; the conditions of their employment; their collective bargaining rights; their rights, duties, and responsibilities toward patients, physicians, other health care professionals, the public, and each other; and a host of other matters. Furthermore, the legal system provides a forum for resolving disputes and conflicts which inevitably arise when these divergent interests clash.

Thus, for example, a nurse who is being made to work in conditions that are unsafe or even dangerous has recourse against the employer under occupational health and safety legislation in force in some provinces. Likewise, a patient who has suffered injury or harm as a result of the negligence of a nurse may commence a civil suit in the courts against that nurse and the hospital for damages.

Similarly, a nurse may be working in a situation where the mental competence of a patient is in doubt and that patient's consent is needed for necessary medical treatment. In such a case, the law will usually provide guidelines and procedures for obtaining the required consent from a substitute decision maker.

There are many other reasons why nurses should be familiar with the law and have a basic understanding of Canada's legal system. Firstly, the everyday actions and decisions made by nurses affect the basic rights of their patients. These actions and decisions may involve going beyond the usual consensual barriers. For instance, a patient who needs an injection may readily consent by holding out an arm to the nurse who administers it. However, in cases where a patient is unable to consent owing to physical or mental incapacity, the nurse bears the onus of ensuring that any action undertaken or treatment administered is in the patient's best interests and consistent with that patient's wishes. Failure to do so leaves the nurse open to the risk of a civil suit for damages from the unconsenting patient or the next-of-kin. Furthermore, health care professionals are under a positive duty to ensure that the patient understands the nature of the illness, the need for treatment, and all the attendant risks and benefits of such treatment, if that patient is to give as fully informed a consent as the law requires.

Secondly, the law, the Canadian Nurses Association's *Code of Ethics for Nursing*,[2] and each provincial regulatory body impose certain requirements upon nurses with respect to their level of professional knowledge and skill. Failure to meet these requirements, or undertaking the practice of nursing in a situation where the nurse has not received adequate training, leaves that nurse open to disciplinary action from the nurse's provincial professional governing body and, if the conduct is serious enough, perhaps the courts.

Thirdly, nurses have access to confidential information about individual patients. They have both legal and ethical[3] obligations to keep all such information confidential and not to divulge it without the patient's consent. In cases where that consent cannot be obtained, they may reveal only as much as is absolutely necessary in the interests of the patient. They may disclose information only to persons whose participation in the patient's treatment is necessary. There may be cases where nurses may be required to divulge such information in court in the form of testimony. Knowledge of the workings of the law, of the rules of evidence, ethics, and of the judicial system, provides a framework when determining whether to disclose sensitive and confidential information about a particular patient.

Fourthly, nurses have access to drugs that are heavily regulated by legislation and hospital procedures governing their use, dispensation, and handling. An understanding of the legal system and of the law and rules of negligence underscores the importance of following such procedures and regulations when administering any medication. Not only civil, but also criminal consequences can flow from a breach of such laws.

Fifthly, as stated earlier, the nursing profession is faced with many new ethical dilemmas, such as the patient's right to refuse treatment and the question of euthanasia. An understanding of the present state of the law and how such law is shaped by values is essential in grasping the complexities of these issues and in formulating an ethical and legal course of action when providing care to terminally ill patients. Often, such issues arise before laws can be made to deal with them. Knowledge of the legal system gives the nurse a better appreciation of the fact that the law often is not an exhaustive source of guidance and direction in these issues, and also that it is slow to adapt legal solutions to them. As well, the nurse will see that the law is, not infrequently, out of step with current societal values in these areas. Law is usually perceived as a "black and white" proposition, while ethical situations—such as euthanasia and physician-assisted suicide—are vastly more complicated by shades of grey. Today, the single biggest challenge facing the law and our legal system is the attempt to come to terms with the grey areas and to provide more realistic and practical guidelines for dealing with ethical dilemmas.

Clearly, the impact of the law on the nursing profession is widespread and significant. An understanding of its structures, terminology, and mechanisms is thus a valuable part of the nurse's education and professional development. The authors have tried to lay the basis for such an understanding in the chapters that follow.

Summary

The key points introduced in this chapter include:
- the reasons why nurses must be familiar with the law and ethics
- the knowledge required to practise according to ethical and legal standards
- the role of professionals in serving the public interest
- the reasons why the field of ethics has grown in recent years
- the challenges faced by nurses when dealing with complex legal and ethical issues.

References

1. Jennings, B., Callaghan, D., Wolf, S.M. (1987, February). The professions: Public interest and common good. *Hastings Center Report* (pp. 3–4).
2. Canadian Nurses Association. (1991). *Code of ethics for nursing.* Value v: Competent nursing care, Obligation 1 (p. 9). (See Appendix A, page 233.)
3. Ibid., Value iii (p. 5).

CHAPTER   *Two*

The Canadian Legal System

CHAPTER OBJECTIVES

The purpose of this chapter is to enable the reader to:
- distinguish between the two primary legal systems in Canada—French civil law and English common law—and appreciate their sources
- understand the legislative process
- distinguish between tort law and criminal law
- understand battery and negligence as they relate to nursing practice
- describe the federal structure of Canada, its Constitution and the *Charter of Rights and Freedoms*
- understand the basic structure and functions of the court system.

With the exception of the Province of Quebec, the Canadian legal system is derived from English **common law**. Historically, Canada is a confederation of former British colonies and colonial territories settled largely by English, Scottish, Welsh, and Irish settlers in the eighteenth and nineteenth centuries. These settlers brought with them not only their language and culture, but also the legal structures and principles of the mother country. The Province of Quebec, on the other hand, was initially settled by French settlers and for a large part of its history was ruled by the kings of France under French civil law.

French Civil Law

What is today Quebec was governed exclusively under French **civil law** until the French colonies in North America were ceded by France to Great Britain in 1763 under the Treaty of Paris which concluded the Seven Years' War. French civil law was based upon the Roman civil law system, which is still prevalent in most Western European countries. This is one of the legacies of the ancient Roman Empire, which controlled much of Europe until its collapse in the sixth century A.D.

In Roman civil law systems, legal rules and principles that establish the rights and responsibilities of individuals are formally written or, as lawyers say, **codified** in a single document known as a **civil code.** Lawyers and judges view this code as the chief source of all rules and principles necessary to resolve disputes or legal issues.

English Common Law

Unlike civil law systems, the majority of the common law is not written down or codified as statute law. **Statute law** is a formal written set of rules passed by a parliament or other legislative body to regulate a particular subject matter, such as, for example, Ontario's *Highway Traffic Act,*[1] which regulates motor vehicles, drivers, and the rules of the road.

In the common law system, many of the essential rules and principles that govern day-to-day life, such as the laws of negligence and of contract, are informally contained in a massive and ancient body of precedent developed through centuries of adjudication. **Precedents** are individual sets of judges' written reasons for deciding a particular case. They usually contain the facts of the case, the legal issues to be decided, the legal principles to be applied, and a reasoned discussion of how those principles apply to the case at hand. Precedents are usually published in volume form by category such as the place (e.g., provincial or federal level), subject matter (e.g., criminal cases, family law cases, tort law cases, civil procedure cases) or the level of court that rendered the decisions (e.g., B.C. Court of Appeal, Federal Court of Appeal, Supreme Court of Canada).

Legal principles and rules are distilled and developed from these precedents, then applied to relevant cases by judges. These principles and legal rules are said to be pre-existing, culled from ancient customs and the unwritten common law of England. This body of precedent is called **case law.**

Sources of the Common Law

The two primary sources of law in the common law legal system are case law and statute law. A secondary source of law is found in textbooks and journals written by legal scholars and experts. These writers may address specific topics such as contracts or property law, and the scope may be narrow or broad. Such writings are called **doctrine** in civil law systems. Though invaluable to common law scholarship and legal education, doctrine is not as authoritative or persuasive to common law courts as it is to their civil law counterparts, and it is subordinate to statute and case law.

Custom constitutes another, less prominent source of law in common law systems. Custom, as its name suggests, means that in the absence of specific and applicable legal principles in either case law, statutes, or doctrine, the courts will be guided by the long-standing practices of a particular industry, trade, or other activity.

Table 2-1 lists the four major sources of common law.

TABLE	2-1
Sources of common law (in decreasing order of authority).	

SOURCE AND DEGREE OF AUTHORITY	DEFINITION AND CHARACTERISTICS
Statute law and regulations Most authoritative in a common law court; override case law in a court of law.	Formal written laws and regulations passed by legislature or cabinet that set forth rules and principles governing a particular subject.
Case law (precedents) Very authoritative; depends on the level of court that rendered the particular decision and its relationship to the court considering the precedent.	Individual court decisions constitute body of precedent in which rules, definitions of legal concepts, and legal principles fashioned by judges over centuries are found; for application in future similar-fact situations.
Doctrine Seldom seen as authoritative by common law judges; depends on the stature of, and respect accorded to, the author of the work within the legal community.	Articles, studies, texts, treatises and other materials by leading legal scholars and academics that elucidate a particular area of law. These usually comment on statute and case law and attempt to elaborate upon, and further interpret, legal principles found in these sources.
Custom Least authoritative; there must be a complete absence of guidance from the other sources before the courts will resort to custom.	Principles and rules of a particular trade, upon which courts will draw when statutes and the common law are silent on a particular issue. The courts elevate accepted practice in a particular trade to a rule of law.

Case Law (Precedent)

Case law is a collection or body of judges' decisions rendered over centuries of judicial consideration and refinement. This feature is found in many nations, Canada among them, that have embraced the English common law. Each case expresses a legal principle which is applied by judges to resolve a legal issue arising in a given situation.

For example, there is a legal principle stating that a party (person) suing or claiming negligence against another person must prove that he or she has suffered damages, that the other party owed him or her a **duty of care,** and that the damages were caused by the other's breach or failure to perform that duty. This rule evolved from early cases in which someone was harmed as a result of another person's carelessness. The courts sought to protect people generally from carelessness, yet they did not wish to impose unreasonable restrictions on people. Therefore, they developed the requirement to prove the existence of three elements: duty of care; harm or damages; and cause and effect between the damages and the actions of the person who has the duty of care.

The use of precedent and case law is best illustrated in the example of a lawsuit. Here, each party to the suit, called a **litigant,** cites case law to the court containing facts similar to the case at hand. Each litigant relies on cases containing a principle or rule of law which, if applied in this case, will yield a result favourable to him or her. In our example in the previous paragraph, if the person bringing the suit cannot prove any damages, the case would, following precedent, be dismissed. Case law might be used to establish the amount of the damages, if they are proved.

The court must select from among these precedents those that are most relevant and most authoritative or binding. It applies the principle stated in the precedent to the facts of the case then before it. The court may elaborate or expand upon the principles derived from previous cases, thus further developing the law. In this sense, common law is fashioned by judges, who have to observe established legal rules in doing so. The decision itself then becomes a further precedent, which serves to bolster or destroy a future litigant's case in similar circumstances.

In English common law, unlike Roman civil law systems, **inferior courts** are bound to decide cases in a fashion similar to any applicable existing precedent of a superior court. This is called the doctrine of **stare decisis.** An inferior court (usually a trial court) is judicially subordinate to an appellate (appeal) court in the hierarchical court structure. We say that the lower court is subordinate in that it is bound to follow the decisions and precedents of the higher one. Stare decisis, which, translated from Latin, roughly means "to abide by the decision,"[2] dictates that a court presented with a prior decision containing facts similar to the case then before it, must decide the present case using the same legal principles and rules pronounced in the prior decision. (Jurisprudence is often used in similar ways by lawyers in Quebec; however, the bulk of legal argument that takes place in court usually relies heavily on the many articles and sections of the *Civil Code* itself.)

The application of precedent in the English common law is designed to achieve two primary objectives. First, the law must be consistent. Review of relevant case law is necessary to determine which judicial pronouncements have the force of law and which have been overruled by subsequent higher court decisions. Consistency is achieved by judges and the legal profession applying the same legal principles in the same circumstances in a similar manner over time. Consequently, a degree of certainty is a characteristic of the common law system.

Second, the common law strives to be predictable. Common law philosophy holds that if lower courts were not bound to follow the decisions and precedents of higher ones, then the outcome of a given case would be unpredictable. A court would be free to decide the case on the basis of any principle of its own choosing, regardless of existing legal principles and rules enshrined in case law. This would defeat the requirement of consistency, as we would never know which principles would be applied in a given situation.

In the common law tradition, predictability and consistency of the law are seen as conducive to a well-ordered society in which people know their rights and obligations toward one another. For example, they allow A. to enter into a contract with B., because A. knows that the law will enforce the contract in favour of A. if B. attempts to break it. This certainty follows from a primary legal principle established in case law that people who freely enter into contracts should and will be bound to perform their obligations, unless the contract is contrary to existing law or public policy. Within such a legal framework, a society flourishes both socially and economically, as people can predict the likely legal consequences of their activities. This lends greater stability to their social and economic endeavours.

This body of precedent spans roughly nine centuries and has become quite large and comprehensive. Over time, case law has developed and adapted, albeit slowly, to changing social, moral, and economic conditions and situations.

Statutes and Regulations

Case law is a slow means of altering and fashioning the law to meet changing social and economic conditions. Yet, the impact of court decisions on society is significant and far-reaching.

Courts are by nature conservative institutions. They define their main role as that of interpreting and applying an existing body of laws and regulations rather than creating law from abstract principles. The court, as the impartial arbiter of societal conflicts, is usually loath to infringe upon Parliament's power to make the nation's laws.

Perhaps the best example of this is found in the recent judicial treatment of abortion laws and laws dealing with assisted suicide. Until recently, the courts upheld laws that prohibit abortions except in special cases. The *Criminal Code of Canada* made it an offence for anyone to perform such a procedure unless it was intended to preserve the life of the mother and was deemed necessary by a hospital committee. In a legal challenge of the provision within the *Criminal Code,* the Supreme Court of Canada in *R v. Morgentaler* ruled the law unconstitutional as violating a woman's right to life and personal security.[3] Abortion is therefore regulated by provincial health care legislation, not by the federal criminal power.

With respect to the controversial issue of assisted suicide, the *Criminal Code of Canada* makes it an offence for anyone to assist or counsel a person to take his or her own life.[4] The recent decision of the Supreme Court of Canada in the case of Sue Rodriguez[5] illustrates the court's reluctance to strike down statutory provisions. Parliament will have to amend this provision to change the law.

The Legislative Process

The slower pace of pre-industrial life may have been well suited to the gradual and incremental approach of common law courts. However, today's society demands more rapid response, which our legal institutions are ill suited to provide. For example, the euthanasia issue has been a long-standing concern. Here, the legislative branch of government is called upon to enact new laws in response to such needs.

Canada is a constitutional monarchy with a responsible form of government. This means that government ministers sit in Parliament and are accountable to it for the exercise of governmental power. Its government comprises three branches: the *judicial branch,* or the courts that apply the law impartially to resolve disputes between individuals or an individual and the State; the *executive branch,* or the Queen and her ministers who enforce the law; and the *legislative branch,* which consists of Parliament and the provincial legislatures.

In Canada the power to make law rests with **Parliament** or, in the case of a province, the legislative assembly. Parliament consists of the Queen's representative, the Senate, and the House of Commons. Provincial legislatures in Canada have only one house, usually called the **legislative assembly**. Parliament and the provincial legislatures make statute laws which are also called "Acts" or statutes. These take priority over the common law and may confirm, clarify, alter, limit, or rescind the common law as determined by the courts. Further, Parliament and the legislatures can adopt urgently needed laws more quickly and comprehensively than can the courts if sufficient political will exists and is brought to bear. This may not always happen, however, and the courts will be left with this task. The legislatures may also legislate in new areas upon which the courts have not yet pronounced, thereby pre-empting judicial "lawmaking" that might steer the law in a direction other than that desired by elected lawmakers.

Cabinet ministers, including the prime minister, who is the head of the government, are usually elected members of the House of Commons belonging to a political party holding the majority of the seats in that House. Ministers can also be chosen from the Senate, but this is a rare occurrence. By unwritten *constitutional convention* (a practice that is not a part of the legal written Constitution, yet is followed by tradition) such members are entitled to form a government, since with their majority in Parliament, they are said to command the confidence of the House.

Government ministers and the prime minister are formally appointed and chosen to form a government by the governor general, who is the Queen's representative. Provincial governments are formed in the same way; however, the provincial lieutenant-governor, the Queen's representative in that province, makes the formal appointment.

Before it can become law, a statute must pass the scrutiny of Parliament or, in the case of a provincial law, the legislative assembly. The draft version of a proposed law, called a **bill,** is usually prepared by a legislative committee made up of members of Parliament in order to address a specific area of concern to the government, special interest groups, constituents of a particular geographic region, or the general public. It can deal with any subject within the jurisdiction of the assembly in which it is to be proposed, such as criminal law, taxation and government spending, agricultural policy, health care, education, foreign policy, defence, and a host of other areas of concern to various sectors of society. The subject matter of the proposed legislation will depend on whether it comes within an area of federal or provincial jurisdiction according to the Constitution. (The federal structure of Canada's Constitution is discussed later in this chapter.)

The procedure followed in Parliament[6] and in the provincial legislatures when passing a bill into law is essentially the same, with a few variations across provincial boundaries.

The bill is first introduced in the legislature and given a formal reading. At this stage, the bill is read out in parliament in summary form and may be taken to a vote without any further debate. The bill is then put through a second reading for lengthy debate on its merits. At this stage, no amendments may be introduced to the bill.

If approved in principle, the bill is then taken to a committee of the legislature for detailed study. Public hearings may be held at which witnesses, private individuals, special interest groups, and others may provide information, make submissions suggesting changes or deletions, or advocate for the addition of further provisions deemed desirable. The bill is discussed, refined, and amended, taking into account the recommendations of the participants and the members of the committee studying it. Upon completion, the committee usually prepares a report to the legislature recommending changes to the draft. On second reading, the bill is again taken to a vote, where the legislature may approve it in principle.

The recent hearings of the Ontario legislature's Standing Committee on Administration of Justice on that province's proposed *Advocacy Act* and companion legislation provide an interesting illustration of this process. These hearings were held in early 1992. The eleven-member committee considered several pieces of legislation[7] pertaining to consent to treatment, the appointment of persons to make decisions on behalf of persons incapable of doing so for themselves, advocacy legislation to provide services to vulnerable persons, and other issues. During the hearings, the committee heard from approximately seventy groups and individuals, including physicians, lawyers, hospitals, public health agencies, and charitable groups active on behalf of disabled and mentally ill persons, the elderly, patients' rights, and children's rights. Throughout the hearings, the views and suggestions of these various groups were considered by the committee and, in some instances, specific provisions of the draft legislation were altered as a result of their recommendations. This consultative process gives citizens the opportunity to shape the legislation that affects the lives of all members of society.

The bill is then put to a third reading in which the legislature considers the committee's report. Usually, each of the bill's provisions is debated until it is put to a third and final vote.

If passed, the bill is then submitted to the lieutenant-governor for the Royal Assent in the case of provincial legislation; if it is a bill of the House of Commons of Canada, it is laid before the Senate, where it proceeds in the same fashion. If passed by the Senate, the bill is then submitted to the governor general for the Royal Assent. Royal Assent is given as a matter of course since, again by convention, the Queen's representative must defer to the wishes of the government of the day. This procedure is reversed if the bill originates in the Senate.

A bill becomes law on proclamation or on a specific date after it receives the Royal Assent and becomes an Act of Parliament or of the provincial legislature. In many cases, an Act has the force of law upon proclamation and publication in an official government publication called a *gazette*.

At this point, all citizens are deemed to know the law and to be governed by it. As unreasonable as this may seem, the purpose of this rule is to ensure the efficient and impartial enforcement of the law. Otherwise, anyone could argue ignorance of the law in his or her defence. The law would then be unenforceable, and chaos would ensue. Thus, the rule that "ignorance of the law is no excuse" is fundamental to any society's ability to govern itself and maintain order.

In fact, most governments in Canada do much more to promulgate new laws than merely print them in gazettes. They usually send detailed press releases and communiqués to the media in an effort to make new laws known to as many people as possible. Furthermore, the gazettes, statutes, and regulations themselves are available in law libraries and through government bookstores. Though it may not always be easy, it is always possible to find legislation in these sources.

Parliamentary and provincial statutes usually contain a short title, for example, the *Highway Traffic Act.*[8] It may have a preamble that briefly states why the Act was passed and its purpose. The Act will also contain one or more numbered and detailed sections or clauses setting forth definitions, conditions, prohibitions, and remedies that are sought to be regulated by the Act.

As comprehensive as these provisions may seem, they cannot provide for every situation that the government desires to regulate. Additional legislative details may be set forth in **regulations** passed by Order-in-Council by the cabinet under the specific authority of a particular statute. Details that must be amended from time to time are often governed by way of regulations. It is also significant that regulations are much easier to enact, since they are passed in cabinet away from the scrutiny of the full legislature.

Regulations have the same force of law as statutes, but are inferior to the Act from which they flow. The statute takes priority. In the event that a regulation goes beyond the authority granted in the statute, a court may strike down such a regulation and refuse to enforce it. The government of the day, therefore, must always ensure that any regulations it passes are consistent with the particular Act that gives it the authority to make these regulations.

Since the legislative branch of government has the ultimate power to make law (subject, of course, to any restrictions contained in the Constitution), it follows that statute law will take precedence over the common (i.e., judge-made) law. If there is a conflict or contradiction between a principle of common law and a provision found in a statute of Parliament or of a provincial legislature, then a court is bound to apply the statute. The court presumes that it was the intent of the legislature to alter the common law by enacting the statutory provision.

For example, before the passage of the negligence statutes of the various common law provinces, the common law held that a person suing another for negligence could not recover any damages whatsoever regardless of fault if the person claiming the damages (the **plaintiff**) had in any way, however slight, contributed to the accident or occurrence that caused his or her injury or damage. Thus, even if the **defendant** (the person being sued) was 99% to blame for the plaintiff's injuries, the claim would fail if the plaintiff was just 1% at fault. This was found to be manifestly unjust, yet the courts continued to uphold the common law rule. It took the passage of the various negligence statutes in the provinces early in this century to change it.

Today, a plaintiff who is, say, 20% responsible for his or her own injuries is still entitled to recover 80% of the damages from the defendant (provided the defendant has been found liable to that extent). If there is more than one defendant, the court will apportion liability among the various defendants to the extent to which each is to blame for the occurrence as well as the plaintiff (if he or she is in any way liable).

The Quebec *Civil Code*

Despite its many similarities with common law, Quebec civil law deserves separate discussion. It has many features and characteristics that are unique to civil law countries. While Quebec's legal system is principally derived from the French one, for historical, social, and geographical reasons, it has also been influenced (to some degree) by English common law.

In the Quebec system, the primary source of law is the *Civil Code:* a lengthy, detailed, and comprehensive statute that sets out a variety of legal rules and principles dealing with such matters as contracts, civil wrongs (e.g., trespassing, slander, assault), negligence, family relations, children's rights, marriage, property rights, wills and the laws of inheritance, corporate law, and insurance law. (This list is not exhaustive.)

Quebec's legal system, as in the common law provinces, also has a body of precedents called **jurisprudence.** In the Quebec system, jurisprudence takes a back seat to the Code. Jurisprudence is merely persuasive evidence of how previous courts have treated a particular provision of the Code.

As well, Quebec has a body of statute law, but the *Civil Code* takes precedence unless the statute expressly states otherwise. Ultimately, the court consults the Code as its primary source of law to resolve civil disputes.

Doctrine, that is, the scholarly writings of experts in the law, is another guide that has the force of law for the civilian court. It takes precedence even over the jurisprudence of a higher court in helping a judge to interpret a provision of the *Civil Code* and to apply it in a particular situation. Doctrine may take the form of law review articles, textbooks on a particular topic, or frequently, detailed multi-volumed treatises on various areas of the civil law. The more respected the author, the more respected, relevant, and authoritative that author's works will be in the eyes of the court. By contrast, doctrine in the common law is seldom seen as authoritative, and it is never treated as binding.

While a civilist court is not strictly bound by decisions of a higher court, this does not mean that it can ignore such jurisprudence. A court in Quebec is still required to treat such decisions with utmost respect and must have a sound reason, either in the Code itself, in accepted doctrine, or in subsequent decisions, for departing from a precedent. This is more so in Quebec compared to other civil law countries because of the influence of English common law on Quebec's judicial traditions. An added consequence of the non-binding nature of civil law jurisprudence is that the courts have somewhat greater leeway in applying the Code's various provisions to new situations. Because of this characteristic, civil law has often been said to have greater flexibility and adaptability than the common law.

Table 2-2 lists the three major sources of civil law.

An interesting example that illustrates the court's deliberative process is found in the recent and controversial decision of the Quebec Superior Court in the case of *Nancy B. v. Hôtel-Dieu de Québec.*[9] This case involved a young woman of twenty-five stricken with Guillain-Barré syndrome, a rare and incurable neurological disease which, in its final stages, leaves a person completely paralyzed and dependent on a respirator. A patient such as Nancy B. can survive for years; however, he or she is incapable of physical activity. Nancy B.'s life was limited to lying in bed and watching television. Her mental faculties were keen, yet she felt trapped in a useless body, an existence that she found unbearable. She expressed a wish to die a natural death, and requested that her intravenous feedings be discontinued and her respirator turned off. The physician and hospital involved in her care had difficulty complying with her request and took the matter to a higher authority.

Nancy retained a lawyer and brought an application in the Quebec Superior Court for an injunction (a court order) directing the hospital and physician to

TABLE	2-2
Sources of civil law (in decreasing order of authority).	

SOURCE AND DEGREE OF AUTHORITY	DEFINITION AND CHARACTERISTICS
Civil Code of Quebec, statutes and regulations Code is binding on all courts, as are statutes and regulations; Code is often used as an aid in interpreting a statute and usually takes precedence, unless the statute says otherwise.	The Code embodies rules, definitions, and legal principles regulating many areas of provincial law. Other statutes and regulations supplement the Code and usually regulate a specific area (e.g., highways).
Doctrine Usually given wide deference and seen as very persuasive and authoritative in a civil law court.	Articles, books, treatises, and other written materials by leading legal scholars. These are used by the courts as an aid to interpreting ambiguous provisions of the Code or statutes.
Jurisprudence Persuasive but not binding; accorded less authority in some cases than doctrine. It is seen as evidence of how other courts have interpreted and applied the law in past cases.	Resembles common law case law (see Table 2-1, page 9), but is not strictly binding on civil law courts.

cease all treatment, nourishment, and use of the respirator, so that she might die a natural death. The Court considered a provision of the Civil Code[10] stipulating that no one could be made to undergo medical treatment of any kind without that person's consent. It held that this provision applied to this case, and thus Nancy had the right to refuse further treatment. The court also considered certain doctrine holding that, absent a threat to the rights of others or a threat to public order, the right was effectively absolute. To supplement the Code, the court relied on further doctrine stating that the act of placing a person on a respirator constituted medical treatment and thus fell within the meaning of the provision of the Code.

In dealing with the argument that to remove Nancy from the respirator would entail a violation of the _Criminal Code of Canada_ (insofar as the physician and hospital would be assisting her in committing suicide, or could be committing murder), the court stated that the discontinuation of treatment would merely allow a _natural_ death to occur. It noted, referring as well to American case law, that neither murder nor suicide is the consequence of a natural death. Thus, the removal of the respirator could not be classified as assisted suicide or murder.

The court further reasoned that these particular provisions of the *Criminal Code* could not reasonably be interpreted in such a way as to make removal of the respirator an offence. To do so would hamper the medical profession in that any course of treatment, no matter how ineffective, could never be discontinued once undertaken. This, the court held, could not have been the intent of Parliament in enacting these provisions. It thus ruled that Nancy had the right to withhold consent to this treatment, and accordingly granted her the injunction. After the time for an appeal of the decision had lapsed, the respirator was disconnected, and Nancy died shortly after.

This example demonstrates the civil court's use of doctrine and case law from another jurisdiction in interpreting a crucial provision of the *Civil Code*, and illustrates how the courts of Quebec tend to value doctrine to a far greater extent than do their common law counterparts.

The *Civil Code of Lower Canada* (as Quebec was called before Confederation) was originally enacted in 1866. Since that time, it has undergone numerous changes and additions, yet it remains essentially a nineteenth-century document. In response to massive changes and advances in technology and society since Confederation, the Quebec government commissioned a comprehensive study and review of the existing Code in 1955, with a view to preparing a completely new and revised Code ready to meet the needs of twentieth-century Quebec.

The result of this lengthy undertaking was the passing in 1992 of a completely new Quebec *Civil Code*, which came into force on January 1, 1994. The new Code has added provisions dealing with areas of law unforeseen in the nineteenth century. It makes provision for consent to medical treatment, enshrines the right to refuse treatment, expands children's rights to have a say in their treatment, and enacts a host of other new provisions dealing with mentally incompetent or terminally ill persons, organ donation, substitute decision making, and other areas.

Civil Law as Distinct from Criminal Law

The term "civil law" has several distinct meanings to lawyers and judges. In one sense, it describes a legal system based on Roman law, such as Quebec's, in which legal principles and rules are codified and form the primary source of law.

In another sense, civil law refers to a body of rules and legal principles that govern relations, respective rights, and obligations among individuals, corporations, or other institutions. It is separate and distinct from criminal law, which is chiefly concerned with relations between the individual and the state and the breach of criminal statutes. Civil law includes law related to contracts, property, family, marriage and divorce, tort and negligence, wills and inheritance, the creation and administration of business and non-profit corporations or partnerships, insurance, copyright, trademarks and patents, employment and labour.

To give a simple example of a civil law relationship, suppose that a steel company enters into an agreement with a car manufacturer to supply sheet steel in the construction of automobiles. After a few months, automobile sales plummet, and the manufacturer finds that it no longer needs as much steel as it contracted to buy from the steel company. The car manufacturer's executives determine that it is cheaper to breach the contract with the steel maker by refusing to pay for any more steel than to continue the contract. It notifies the steel company of its intention to terminate the agreement. The steel company would then have several options, one of which is to sue the car manufacturer for damages for breach of contract.

For an example in nursing, suppose that a nurse is called upon one night to administer an antibiotic to a patient suffering acute appendicitis. In error, the nurse administers the wrong antibiotic. Furthermore, it is noted in the chart that this patient is allergic to that particular antibiotic. The patient consequently suffers an anaphylactic reaction resulting in brain damage. He emerges from a coma two weeks later, at which time it is determined that he has suffered partial paralysis of his left side. The brain damage is later shown to be permanent and irreversible. In such a case, the patient and his family would have the right to sue the nurse, and even the hospital, for professional negligence.

These two cases are essentially private disputes between two sets of individuals seeking redress in the courts. In each example, the State (or more specifically, society) is not directly interested in the outcome of the case. It is a mainly private dispute which the court will resolve by drawing upon relevant legal principles and rules. The court's decision may later be applied in similar cases. In this broader context, society is indeed interested in the outcome, which may form the impetus for amending or creating legislation to regulate the particular nursing practice that gave rise to the negligence.

Another distinction within both civil law and criminal law is that between substantive and procedural laws. **Substantive laws** create rights and obligations between individuals—for example, laws governing the creation of a contract, the rights of a spouse within marriage, an employee's rights against an employer's, or the creation and governance of a corporation. **Procedural laws,** on the other hand, regulate how those rights are preserved and enforced in the courts. These would include the rules of court governing how a lawsuit is started, when it may be started, what documents must be filed, and in which court. They may also govern the application of substantive laws in other situations.

Torts

The nursing example discussed above illustrates a situation in tort law. A **tort** is a civil wrong committed by one person against another such as to cause that other some injury or damage, either to person or property. Torts may be intentional or non-intentional. An assault is an example of an intentional tort, in that the person who commits it intends the action that causes harm to the victim. Non-intentional torts generally constitute **negligence**. In our previous example, the nurse did not intend to cause harm to the patient, but was negligent in giving the wrong medication and in failing to notice that the patient was allergic to it.

In civil law, torts (and contractual matters), duties correspond with obligations. Specific provisions of the *Civil Code* define and govern the concept and the elements that must be proved in court for the plaintiff to recover damages. Under civil law, anyone under a duty not to cause harm to another is at fault if he or she fails in that duty by not acting according to the expected standard of care.

Intentional Torts

Battery and assault

Of particular importance to the nursing profession is the concept of battery and assault. Since much of a nurse's work involves the physical touching of patients for the administration of injections, sutures, intravenous lines, and other such intrusive measures, a nurse must understand that such procedures may be instituted only upon a consenting patient. Consent may be expressed and obtained in writing or may be implied and inferred from the patient's conduct.

Battery in the common law is defined as the intentional bringing about of a harmful or offensive and non-consensual contact with the person of another.[11] An example would be one person striking another. The harmful or offensive contact may be either direct, such as a slap in the face, or indirect, such as pulling away a person's chair, causing him to fall to the ground.[12] In either case, there has been an intentional interference with the bodily integrity and security of another. Moreover, these acts are seen as potential inducements to further violence, because the victim may be provoked into retaliation. The chief aim of tort law is to curb violence by making perpetrators of such acts civilly liable to their victims for damages.

The offensive or intrusive conduct need not be violent, as even seemingly insignificant unwanted touching may amount to battery. The perpetrator need not intend any harmful result. Thus, even such conduct as a kiss on the cheek meant as a compliment may amount to battery if it is not consented to by the recipient.

However, certain common, everyday acts will not usually amount to battery. For instance, shaking hands is not considered battery, since it is a western custom in greeting acquaintances. Thus, one need not ask another's permission prior to shaking hands. Since it is a custom, the law would infer consent on the part of the recipient.

Assault is the "intentional creation of the apprehension of imminent harmful or offensive contact."[13] For example, if one person lunges threateningly at another who is close by, but does not actually strike, that person is still liable to damages for assault. A court would likely conclude that the victim was reasonably apprehensive of being harmed in this situation and that the threat was imminent. However, there will be no assault if the victim could not reasonably conclude from the circumstances that the perpetrator was actually able to carry out the threat. The reasonableness of the victim's state of mind is key here. There is no requirement that the perpetrator actually be able to carry out the threat. It is sufficient that the evidence of the circumstances in which the threat was made led to a reasonable conclusion that the defendant was able to carry it out.

Consent

In cases where the aggrieved person has consented to the conduct being visited upon him or her, the perpetrator may escape liability for such conduct in some cases. Consent can be explicit (expressed) or implied by the circumstances or the conduct of the aggrieved person. *Expressed consent* may be given orally or in writing. The written consent is not consent in and of itself, but rather is evidence that the party giving it has consented to an act.

Implied consent is agreement to an act inferred from the actions of the recipient. An example of implied consent in a medical setting might be a patient's holding out an arm to a nurse to have blood pressure checked. The patient cannot then be heard to say that he did not consent to the touching, since a reasonable person would imply from his conduct that he consented. This illustrates another aspect of implied consent, that is, the existence of consent is measured against an objective standard. Such consent is found to exist where the plaintiff's conduct is such that a reasonable person viewing all the surrounding circumstances would conclude that consent had been given.

For consent to be valid in law, the person giving it must be capable of giving consent. In the case of a mentally ill patient, consent to a given treatment may or may not be valid depending on whether the mental illness makes that patient unable to appreciate the nature, quality, and consequences of the proposed treatment. Children under the age of majority (or under sixteen, in some provinces) usually cannot consent to medical treatment, in which case their parents or legal guardians would be called upon to give consent. However, if the child is old enough to understand the nature and risks of the proposed treatment, the caregiver or institution may rely upon that consent.

Consent will also be invalid if it was obtained by force or fraud. For example, an unscrupulous physician might persuade a patient to have sexual relations with him in the belief that doing so will cure her of an ailment.[14] Her consent would thus have been obtained by fraud as to the true nature of the act to which she was agreeing. In law, this is no consent at all. Duress or the use of force also invalidates any consent, because the recipient is obviously not making a decision of his or her own free will. Only a freely given and voluntary consent is valid in law.

In the context of health care, it is important for any professional to remember that no medical treatment, no matter how crucial to the health or survival of the patient, may be administered without that patient's consent, unless the situation is life-threatening and the patient is unconscious or mentally incompetent.[15] Furthermore, only that specific treatment which is consented to may be administered, and in most cases, only those health care professionals specified in the specified in the patient's consent may administer the consented-to treatment. The patient must give an *informed consent*. This means that the nature of the treatment to be administered, its benefits and attendant risks, and any and all material information must be given to the patient for that patient's consent to be valid.

The issue of consent, and its many ethical and legal pitfalls, is as relevant to the nursing profession as it is to physicians. Many fine lines are drawn, and it is not always easy to determine the extent and scope of the consent. Chapters 6 and 8 will elaborate upon this issue.

Non-intentional Torts

Negligence

As previously suggested, in the common law, negligence falls under the non-intentional category of torts. A defendant may still be liable for a tort while not having intended any harm or injury. For a defendant to be liable for **negligence**, three elements must be present.[16] First, the defendant must owe a duty of care in law towards the plaintiff. Second, the defendant must have breached that duty and failed to discharge the standard of care required by the law in the particular situation. Third, the plaintiff must have suffered damage or harm caused by the defendant's breach of the duty of care. Another related legal principle is that if the plaintiff was in any way partly responsible for his or her injuries as a result of negligence, the defendant will be absolved of liability to the extent of the plaintiff's own negligence. This principle is called **contributory negligence**.

To return to our nursing example, it is clear that this nurse owed a duty of care to her patient. In reading the medication labelling incorrectly and failing to notice that the patient was allergic to the medication that he subsequently received, the nurse breached the duty she owed to that patient. As a direct result of that breach, the patient received a harmful substance and suffered a severe allergic reaction. His ensuing brain damage was a direct and foreseeable result of that breach.

Duty of care, standards of care, proximate cause, and contributory negligence are factors that help determine whether or not a defendant will be held **liable** (responsible) in a case of negligence. We will now discuss each of these factors in detail.

Duty of care

To be liable in tort, a defendant must owe a duty of care to the plaintiff, either personally or as a member of a class. The law imposes a duty of care in many but not all situations. If there is no duty of care in law, the defendant will not be liable to the plaintiff, even if the defendant's conduct was the immediate cause of the plaintiff's injuries.

The common law holds that one owes a duty of care to those people who are close to, or closely connected with, one's conduct or activities such that a reasonable person could foresee harm or injury occurring to such persons as a result of negligent acts or conduct. Professionals such as nurses owe a duty of care to those who retain their services to act in a competent and diligent manner according to the standard of the reasonably competent nurse. This includes a responsibility for the nurse, as with any other professional, to keep abreast of current developments and techniques within the profession and to undertake retraining as necessary.

The classic definition of the duty of care can be found in an old case that originated in Scotland in the early 1930s: a person has a duty to avoid any acts or omissions that one could reasonably foresee would be likely to injure his or her neighbour. In the decision in *Donoghue v. Stevenson,* Lord Atkin, one of the Lord Justices of the House of Lords to which the case had been appealed, spoke of the duty thus:

> The rule that you are to love your neighbour becomes in law, you must not injure your neighbour; and the lawyer's question, Who is my neighbour? receives a restricted reply. You must take reasonable care to avoid acts or omissions which you can reasonably foresee would be likely to injure your neighbour. Who, then, in law is my neighbour? The answer seems to be—persons who are so closely and directly affected by my act that I ought reasonably to have them in contemplation as being so affected when I am directing my mind to the acts or omissions which are called in question.[17]

To illustrate, suppose that Neighbour A., a property owner, decides one evening to set off fireworks in her back yard. Her yard is quite small, and her home is located in a heavily populated suburban area. The fireworks she has obtained are large and powerful, the type usually reserved for large public displays. She sets off many fireworks at once and indiscriminately. During the course of the evening, a live cinder descending from the sky lands on the jacket sleeve of a neighbouring boy who had entered A.'s yard, fascinated by the fireworks. The boy's jacket catches fire, and he suffers second- and third-degree burns to 50% of his upper body before another adult smothers the flames. Will A. be liable for the boy's injuries?

The key question is: Was it reasonable to assume that neighbourhood children might stray into A.'s yard to watch the display? In other words, ought A. to have had the boy in mind as a person likely to be injured by the fireworks? Who else might she reasonably have had in mind? Other children? Adults? Her immediate neighbours? These are the questions that courts ask when deciding whether or not a duty of care exists in a particular situation. If it is reasonable to assume that the boy was likely to be harmed by A.'s conduct given the child's close proximity or connection to A., then A. owed a duty of care to the boy. A. will also owe a duty of care to any other person who it is reasonably foreseeable might be injured by her conduct.

A duty of care will be found to exist where one person has placed others in peril as a result of his or her conduct. Furthermore, a person who creates a hazard, even unwittingly and through no negligence of his or her own, may still be held liable if he or she fails to warn others of the hazard and they are injured.

It is both interesting and disturbing to note that under the common law (unlike Quebec[18] and the civil law countries of Europe) there is no general duty to aid someone in peril.[19] This is one illustration of the divergence that can

occur between law and ethics. What may clearly be a moral or ethical imperative may not necessarily be a legal requirement.

For example, a passer-by may observe a man dying of cardiac arrest without
rendering assistance. There is no positive duty to act in such cases.[20] However,
most human beings, acting morally, would likely intervene to save a person in
obvious danger. Where someone does act, the law imposes a duty of care upon
him not to conduct such rescue negligently. A person who fails in a rescue bid
may be civilly liable for any injury or death resulting to the person being res-
cued.[21] Usually, however, to be found liable, the rescuer's conduct must amount
to gross negligence—that is, a substantial and marked departure from the standard of the reasonably competent and skilled rescuer.

Nurses have a special relationship to those whom they serve, and it is thus
desirable to impose on them a duty of care.[22] They have special training and expertise and are required to exercise a very high degree of care in carrying out
their tasks.

Breach of the standard of care

How do courts determine whether or not a defendant's conduct has been negligent? The common law has developed the concept of the **standard of care** as
an objective measure of such conduct. If a defendant's conduct is seen as having
fallen below the standard of what a competent person, acting reasonably and
responsibly in similar circumstances, would have done, a court may find that
defendant's conduct to be negligent.

The particular standard against which any given conduct is judged will vary
depending on the circumstances and people involved. For example, a doctor
will be judged by the standard of the reasonably competent physician.
Similarly, a nurse's conduct in the treatment of a patient who has suffered harm
as a result of his or her acts or omissions will be judged by the standard of the
reasonably competent nurse.

The nurse in our example would not be judged by the standard of the most
highly qualified expert in the field of nursing, but rather by the average standards of the reasonable nurse possessed of reasonable knowledge, skill, and
ability. These would include minimal standards of competence and knowledge
set by the governing body for nurses in the various provinces, and any applicable standards prescribed by the health care institution in which that nurse is
employed.

Such standards also include the requirement to keep up to date with the
latest professional and technological developments. Additional training should
be taken as required to maintain expertise to the appropriate standard. A professional who fails to keep up to date runs the risk of employing methods that
have been discredited or proved harmful by the latest studies and thinking in
that field. If that professional's conduct were ever called into question, such
failure would be evidence of negligence.

Proximate cause and remoteness

The third element of negligence is that a defendant will be liable for harm to a plaintiff if that harm was caused by the defendant's negligent conduct. This seems straightforward and logical. However, can a plaintiff be compensated for all possible harm that may occur as a result of the defendant's negligent act?

To illustrate, we return to our example of Neighbour A. igniting fireworks in her yard. Suppose that during the display, another live cinder from a descending rocket is carried by the wind into a nearby industrial park. Among the many enterprises in this park is a chemical factory that produces highly flammable cleaning solvents. In its yard are stored finished solvents, chemicals used in their manufacture, and several railway tank cars containing hazardous waste chemicals. An employee of this manufacturer has carelessly punctured one of the solvent containers, and solvent has leaked out in and about the yard. The live cinder lands in a pool of solvent and immediately ignites it. The ensuing blaze destroys the facility and causes the toxic waste chemicals to burn. Hazardous fumes and heavy black smoke billow into the air, necessitating the evacuation of much of A.'s suburban neighbourhood. Furthermore, several firefighters are seriously injured by the fumes while dealing with the conflagration. Can A. possibly be held liable for all this damage resulting from her careless fireworks display? Some courts may hold A. liable only for the injury to the boy, while others may extend the scope of A.'s liability to include the fire and injury to the firefighters.

Such a train of events is often referred to as a *chain of causation*. A chain of causation could easily apply in a health care setting, where many health care professionals may be involved in treating a patient with numerous medical problems and complications. The actions of each member of the health care team in treating such a patient would have to be examined to determine how those particular actions influenced the course of the patient's condition and how reasonably foreseeable this could have been.

Negligence law holds that a defendant should be held liable only when his or her acts of negligence are the **proximate cause** of the ensuing harm. A defendant should not be held accountable to the plaintiff for all possible results of negligent conduct, no matter how remote or unforeseeable. The court will ask whether the resulting harm or damage was a reasonably foreseeable consequence of the defendant's act or omission.[23] If it was, the defendant will be held liable for any resulting loss.

The exact manner in which the loss occurs, however, need not be foreseen.[24] If in the example of Neighbour A., it was foreseeable that a live cinder could cause damage through fire, but an explosion was highly unforeseeable, then A. would still be liable, since some sort of damage through fire occurred.[25] If, on the other hand, the risk of fire was seen as remote, then there would be no reasonably foreseeable risk, and A. would be absolved of liability.

Contributory negligence

In earlier times under the common law, if a plaintiff was found to be partly at fault for the harm he or she suffered, the law would deny him or her the right to recover damages from the defendant.[26] Today, in all common law provinces, a plaintiff may still recover even if partly at fault, but the damages awarded will be reduced by the percentage to which he or she was to blame or contributed to the loss.[27] Of course, if the evidence shows that the plaintiff was completely to blame for the harm that befell him or her, the defendant would escape liability entirely.

Returning to our fireworks example, suppose that the solvent manufacturer sued A. for damages resulting from the fire. A. can raise the fact that one of the manufacturer's employees carelessly punctured the solvent drum, and that this caused the solvent to leak and ignite more readily. A. might also claim in her defence that the manufacturer was partly to blame for the damage and harm because of the negligent way in which the various materials in the yard were stored.

The court will apportion the liability among the parties, that is, it will determine as best it can the percentage or proportion to which each party is to blame for the loss. In this respect, the law is basically the same in all common law provinces and the Province of Quebec, where it is known as the principle of *common fault.*[28]

Voluntary assumption of risk

A plaintiff may lose all rights of recovery against a negligent defendant if that plaintiff consented in some way to the defendant's conduct. The plaintiff may then be said to have voluntarily assumed the risk of harm that was likely to result from the defendant's conduct. This defence is known by the Latin maxim, "*Volenti non fit injuria.*" ("He who consents cannot receive an injury."[29]) It is a defence insofar as the onus is on the defendant to prove that the plaintiff voluntarily assumed the risk of injury.[30] There is no onus on the plaintiff in this regard. In most cases, the plaintiff's assumption of the risk is implied by the conduct of the plaintiff in the circumstances; it is rarely specifically expressed.

In our fireworks example, suppose that Neighbour B., an experienced fireworks technician, is watching the spectacle in A.'s yard. Because of her inexperience, A. has been igniting the fireworks far too close to surrounding spectators, including Neighbour B. One of the rockets is pointed at an awkward angle, inadvertently in B.'s general direction. The rocket is fired; B. is hit and badly burned. B. sues A. for damages, alleging that she was negligent in the manner of setting off the rocket. A. could plead, in her defence, that B., as an experienced pyrotechnician, must have been aware of the danger caused by the rocket and the negligent manner in which it was being fired. Despite this, he chose to remain where he was and failed to point out a danger, which would have been evident to him. A. could thus say that B., by remaining silent, and by standing near the fireworks, voluntarily assumed the risk that he would be burned by the rocket.

What Is a Lawsuit?

Thus far, we have dealt with the rights and duties of individuals, and with the mechanics and workings of tort law. This area has perhaps the greatest significance for the nursing profession. Tort law affects the nursing process directly insofar as nurses are professionals whose conduct must meet the appropriate standard of care. (Collective agreements and other employment matters that affect the daily working lives of nurses will be discussed in detail in Chapter 10.) Individual rights are adjudicated and enforced by means of the court action.

In Canada, a lawsuit is not usually the first step in an attempt to resolve a contractual, tortious, or other legal dispute. Informal attempts to resolve the problem may include discussions between the parties, mediation or arbitration, or other complain mechanism. Lawyers may be engaged in the early stages to resolve the dispute without resort to the courts. If this fails, a court action must be started by the aggrieved party.

The process for starting a lawsuit is broadly similar in all provinces. It is controlled by a code usually referred to as the **rules of civil procedure**, or the rules of court, which are detailed regulations passed by the government setting out how a court action is conducted, which documents must be filed in which court and by whom, other detailed provisions governing examinations of parties, summonses to witnesses (subpoenas), the manner of serving notice, and other such matters. It is initiated by filing a **statement of claim**[31] or writ of summons in the appropriate court.[32]

This document, which is usually filed on behalf of the plaintiff by his or her lawyer, is also referred to as an "originating process" because it initiates the action. It sets out, in concise numbered paragraphs, the plaintiff's version of the facts relied on to support the claim made against the defendant or defendants,[33] but it may not set out any of the evidence by which the plaintiff intends to prove his or her case.

The statement of claim is then issued by the court in which it is filed, and a court file is opened at the court office for the action. This file will contain all court documents relevant to this action. Once the claim is issued, the lawsuit officially commences. A copy of the statement of claim must then be served on (given to) the defendant or defendants personally within a specified period of time.[34]

In turn, the defendant has the right to file a **statement of defence** to the plaintiff's claim within a specified time. Failure to file a statement of defence will prevent the defendant from participating in the action. Furthermore, a defendant who fails to file a defence to the action may be deemed by the rules of court of the particular province to have admitted the truth of the allegations contained in the statement of claim.[35]

The statement of defence, like the statement of claim, sets forth in concise, numbered paragraphs those facts upon which the defendant relies in his or her defence to the claim. This statement of defence must, in turn, be served on the plaintiff and filed in the court office where the action was commenced within a specified time. Failure to file in time may mean the defendant will lose all opportunity to defend the action. The statements of claim and defence are collectively known as **pleadings.**

Assuming the defendant has filed a defence, the next step requires all parties to exchange all relevant documentary evidence upon which they intend to rely at the trial. The economy of the rules of civil procedure of all provinces requires that each party to a lawsuit make full **disclosure** to the others of all relevant evidence, both oral and documentary, in that party's possession or control. This policy is designed to eliminate the element of surprise in litigation. It is felt by policy makers that avoiding surprise is less costly in the long run and promotes settlement of cases without the need for expensive trials. If both parties to a lawsuit are fully aware of the strength of the other's case, each can assess the chance of success more realistically.

Thus, a party who realizes that his opponent has the evidence necessary to prove her case will be more willing to settle the matter than risk a loss for a higher sum at the conclusion of the trial. A key provision of the law of costs is a further factor in this equation: the unsuccessful party must not only pay his or her own legal fees, but will usually be ordered to pay those of the victorious opponent at the end of the trial.[36]

Disclosure is achieved through two mechanisms: documentary discovery and the oral examination for discovery. **Documentary discovery** is a process requiring each party to the action to disclose to the other the existence of any documents relevant to the issues raised in the pleadings, and further, to provide actual documents or copies of same upon the request of the other party.[37] The party shows that he or she has disclosed all such documents by swearing an **affidavit** which lists all these documents. Failure to disclose the existence of a document relating to the action means that the party cannot rely upon it at trial.

In an **examination for discovery**, each party, in the presence of his or her own lawyer, is asked a series of questions relevant to any matter raised in the pleadings by the opposing party's lawyer. The questions and answers are recorded either by means of audio tape or by a stenographer at an official examiner's office. The party being examined answers under oath as if giving testimony in open court; however, no judge is present at this stage. An examination is not a trial.

The answers given at the examination enable each party to know the other's position and the kind of testimony that the other is likely to give at trial. They can also be used to test the credibility of a party whose answer at discovery differs from that given at trial.

A party who knows the strengths of the other's case and the weaknesses of his or her own is able to assess the risks of taking the matter to trial. This can promote settlement. For example, a plaintiff may conclude after the examination that the defendant has little evidence with which to prove his or her case. The plaintiff can then bring more pressure to bear upon the defendant to settle the case on as favourable a basis as possible without incurring the expense of a full trial.

If the parties are unable to settle the action at this stage, then the matter proceeds to trial. Each party summons all necessary witnesses and documents to prove his or her case. Meanwhile, a trial date is set.

Before the trial, however, one last effort will be made to encourage the parties to settle by means of the **pre-trial conference**. Here the parties' lawyers, in the presence of a judge, advance (put forth) their clients' respective positions on liability, the amount of the damages, and the prospects of settlement of the case. With limited evidence, the judge then indicates how the matter may be decided. To prevent bias, the pre-trial judge is not the one who will try the case. If a settlement is still not achieved, the parties prepare for trial.

A civil action may be tried by judge alone or by a court consisting of judge and jury, according to the wishes of any one of the parties. However, certain types of actions, because of their nature or complexity, may only be tried by a judge alone.[38] The number of jurors varies from province to province. A civil trial jury is composed of fewer jurors than the twelve required in a criminal trial. For example, Ontario requires no more than six persons,[39] while Newfoundland requires nine jurors.

During the trial, the **burden of proof** is upon the plaintiff. This means that the case must be proven by the plaintiff. A plaintiff must present enough evidence to show that the injury or harm was caused, on a balance of probabilities, by the defendant. If at the end of the trial the plaintiff has failed to prove his or her case, or the evidence is at best inconclusive, the defendant will be found not liable, and the action will be dismissed.

If the plaintiff wins, judgement is granted, which is a court order stating that the defendant is to pay to the plaintiff a certain sum of money as damages. **Damages,** or monetary compensation for the harm incurred by a plaintiff as a result of the defendant's negligence, willful tort, or breach of contract, are one **remedy** the court may award. Damages compensate for losses due to pain and suffering, medical expenses incurred in the case of a personal injury suit, loss of earnings, and loss of future income.

Once having obtained judgement, the plaintiff will then have to enforce it. Most defendants do not pay a judgement once it is obtained. A plaintiff must now expend further sums to recover on the judgement by means of a **judgement debtor examination,** during which a defendant debtor (called a "judgement debtor" because he or she owes money according to a court order) is asked questions about his or her financial resources, property, and ability to pay the judgement.

The plaintiff can have any of the defendant's assets (e.g., the defendant's home, land, bank accounts, securities, automobiles, jewellery, or other such property) seized and sold by the **sheriff** (a court official) at an auction in order to realize the necessary funds to satisfy the judgement. The defendant's wages can also be **garnisheed,** meaning that the defendant's employer (or any other debtor of the defendant) will be required to pay a portion of the defendant's weekly or monthly wages (or the debt itself, in the case of a debt owed to the defendant) to the sheriff for the benefit of the plaintiff and any other creditors of the defendant. Through these mechanisms, the law permits a successful plaintiff to bring considerable pressure to bear on a delinquent debtor.

Criminal Law

Thus far we have been discussing court actions involving one or more individuals asserting private claims. These are classed as civil law. Other cases concern society collectively when they involve a breach of fundamental values and rules that threatens the peace, stability, order, and well-being of all its citizens. This concern is the focus and province of criminal law.

The federal government is charged constitutionally with making criminal law in Canada.[40] This ensures one uniform set of criminal laws for the whole country. The provinces cannot make criminal law, though they may impose fines and short prison terms for breach of provincial laws.[41]

Most criminal law is contained in the *Criminal Code of Canada*,[42] which was originally passed by Parliament in 1892.[43] It is a lengthy statute containing a comprehensive and detailed list of criminal offences as well as a code of procedure governing arrests, laying of charges, release on bail, preliminary hearings, trials, and sentencing. It also contains provisions dealing with appeals from verdicts and sentences, and release pending appeal. The most comprehensive revision in the Code's history took place in 1955[44]; however, it has since been amended many times.

As comprehensive as it is, the Code is not an exhaustive repository of all criminal offences in Canada. Other federal statutes such as the *Narcotic Control Act*,[45] the *Food and Drugs Act*,[46] the *Income Tax Act*,[47] the *Competition Act*,[48] the *Fisheries Act*,[49] and the *Canada Shipping Act*,[50] to name a few, create further criminal offences.

Classes of Criminal Offences

There are three classes of criminal offences under the *Criminal Code*:

(1) indictable offences,
(2) summary conviction offences, and
(3) dual procedure (or hybrid) offences.

Summary conviction offences are generally of a less serious nature. They include such offences as causing a disturbance,[51] discharging a firearm in a public place,[52] loitering,[53] trespassing at night,[54] vagrancy,[55] and so forth.[56] Such offences are tried before a provincial court judge. No jury is employed in such a trial. If the accused is convicted, he or she is liable to a prison term of up to six months, a fine of up to $2000, or both, unless the Code or other statutory provision creating the offence specifies another punishment.[57]

Indictable offences are generally more serious. These include murder (both first- and second-degree),[58] manslaughter,[59] attempted murder,[60] criminal negligence causing death,[61] robbery,[62] theft of property having a value of over $1000,[63] treason,[64] conspiracy to commit an indictable offence,[65] and so on.[66]

Given their more serious nature, the procedure for trying indictable offences is more complex than that for summary conviction offences. After being arrested and charged, an accused person is first brought before a justice of the peace or a provincial court judge. Depending on the type of offence, the accused will be tried by a provincial court judge alone,[67] or may elect (choose) a mode of trial as allowed under the Code for certain indictable offences.[68] If the indictable offence is one that allows the accused to elect, the choices include:

(1) trial by a provincial court judge without a jury and without a preliminary inquiry;
(2) a preliminary inquiry and trial by a judge (other than a provincial court judge) without a jury; or
(3) a preliminary inquiry and trial by a court composed of a judge and jury.

If the accused fails to make an election, the third option is automatically assigned.[69] For those indictable offences listed in section 469 of the Code (treason, etc.), the accused is automatically tried by a court composed of a judge and jury, having first had a preliminary inquiry. The accused is given no choice, although he or she may, if the Crown prosecutor agrees, be tried by a judge without a jury.[70] The jury is composed of twelve Canadian citizens over eighteen years of age.

The purpose of the **preliminary inquiry** is to determine whether the Crown has sufficient evidence such that a reasonable jury, reasonably instructed in the law could (not would) convict the accused of the offence.[71] It is not a trial. If the provincial court judge, after conducting the hearing, concludes that the evidence is deficient, the accused will be discharged. This does not mean, however, that the accused has been found not guilty, since there has been no trial. It means only that there is insufficient evidence to satisfy the *standard* (test) described above, and that the accused should thus not be made to stand trial.

Indictable offences carry much greater penalties ranging from over two years to life imprisonment as well as substantial fines. Such prison sentences are served in penitentiaries administered by the Government of Canada. If the sentence is less than two years' imprisonment, as in the case of summary conviction offences or provincial offences, it is served in a provincially administered correctional institution.

The third class of offence under the Code is that of **dual procedure** or hybrid offences. These are sometimes referred to as "offences triable either way."[72] They are hybrid in that the Crown, in whose name an accused person is prosecuted, may choose to try the accused summarily or indictably.[73] Until the Crown attorney prosecuting the case makes the choice, the offence will be deemed to be indictable.[74] If the Crown elects to proceed summarily, the accused will be tried by a provincial court judge alone. Should the Crown choose to proceed by indictment, the accused will be called upon to elect the mode of trial in accordance with the procedure outlined above.

The Presumption of Innocence

In Canada, as in all western democracies, an accused person is deemed inno-
cent until proven guilty. Not only is this principle enshrined in the *Criminal
Code*,[75] but more significantly, it is also a fundamental right guaranteed in the
Canadian *Charter of Rights and Freedoms*.[76] Section 11(d) of the Charter reads:

> 11. Any person charged with an offence has the right ... (d) to be presumed inno-
> cent until proven guilty according to law in a fair and public hearing by an inde-
> pendent and impartial tribunal.

The *Charter of Rights and Freedoms* has been an integral part of the Canadian
Constitution since 1982. It sets forth the basic legal and democratic rights of
citizens, rights which the State cannot abridge or infringe upon without
breaching the Constitution. (The Constitution and the *Charter of Rights and
Freedoms* will be discussed more fully later in this chapter.)

There are two consequences of the presumption of innocence for both the
Crown and the accused. First, the Crown must prove all the essential elements
of a case to satisfy the standard of proof beyond a reasonable doubt. It is for the
Crown to prove the offence. The burden of proof refers to the degree of proof
that the Crown must attain in order to secure a conviction. Second, while the
accused may refuse to *lead* (present) any evidence, more frequently the focus of
the defence is to establish reasonable doubt.

Rules of Evidence

Evidence is the material with which the Crown builds and proves its case
against the accused. Only evidence that is relevant to an issue in the trial and is
probative (proves something) may be admitted. Hearsay evidence, that is, testimony by a witness that he or she heard a third party make a factual statement
regarding an issue in the trial, generally cannot be offered as proof of the truth
of such facts, although there is a trend to allow some hearsay evidence provided
it does not gravely damage the accused's case (i.e., it is not prejudicial) and
proves something in issue.

For example, suppose A., a witness to a murder trial, states on the witness
stand that he overheard B. (who is not a witness and is not present in court) say
that C., the accused in this trial, had committed the murder. Such a statement
would be ruled inadmissible as hearsay evidence, although it could be allowed
for the sole purpose of proving that the statement was made.

Evidence usually takes the form of oral testimony from witnesses. It may
also consist of written documents, photographs, video or audio tape, or other
physical form, such as finger prints, DNA samples, blood samples, or ballistics
(gunshot evidence). This evidence must be sufficiently probative, that is, it
must have value to convince the judge or jury beyond a reasonable doubt that
the accused committed the offence with which he or she stands charged. If the
Crown's evidence leaves at least a reasonable doubt in the mind of the judge or
jury, the law requires that the accused be acquitted (found not guilty).[77]

The accused need not present any evidence at the trial, since he or she cannot be compelled to give evidence against himself or herself.[78] This means that the accused may choose not to testify. If the Crown has presented enough evidence to secure a conviction, the accused, in turn, should present enough evidence to raise a reasonable doubt in the mind of the judge or jury. If the defence's evidence is enough to raise such a doubt, the accused must be acquitted.

Elements of a Criminal Offence

Most[79] criminal offences have two main elements: a physical element and a mental element. The physical element is known in law by the Latin term **actus reus**. Thus, for example, in the offence of assault, the physical conduct of striking the victim constitutes the actus reus. The mental component, known by the Latin term **mens rea,** is the element of intent. In most cases, a person must intend to commit the act with which he or she is charged. Thus, in an assault, the mens rea is the perpetrator's intention to strike the victim. The perpetrator's willful direction of his or her body to commit the physical act is the actus reus.

The link between these two elements, insofar as proving the offence is concerned, is that a conscious rational person, thinking rationally, would always intend his or her physical conduct. This means that a sane person, acting voluntarily and rationally, who is seen physically striking another, is usually presumed to have intended that result. In other words, such conduct is the product of a conscious mind acting voluntarily. The two elements of the offence must therefore both be present.[80]

For example, suppose a woman suffers a head injury in an automobile accident. She is released from the hospital several days later, seemingly recovered from her injuries. One night she gets out of bed, proceeds to the kitchen, and obtains a carving knife which she uses to stab her sleeping husband repeatedly. The husband dies. The woman discovers the murder the next day and to her horror, concludes from the physical evidence at the scene that she committed the deed.

She has no recollection whatsoever of having done this. She and her husband loved each other. She had no motive nor any wish to see her husband dead, and cannot fathom how she could have done such a thing. Perhaps her head injury caused her to act involuntarily: that is, her actions were not the product of her conscious mind, but merely the automatic movement of her body resulting from the injury to her brain. In such a case, the accused could not be found guilty of murder, as she clearly was not aware of the circumstances, she was not conscious, and she was not acting voluntarily. This defence is known in law as the defence of *non-insane automatism*.[81] It has been accepted in Canadian courts since the Supreme Court of Canada's decision in R v. Rabey.[82]

However, one must not conclude that an accused in such a state is necessarily insane. She may or may not be. If the accused were conscious, she would not have committed the act voluntarily and would be fully capable of knowing the consequences of her actions and of discerning right from wrong. A truly insane person is afflicted with a disease of the mind and is not legally capable of appreciating the nature and quality of his or her actions and their consequences. This would attract a verdict of not guilty by reason of insanity, as provided in sections 16(1) and (2) of the *Criminal Code*:

> 16.(1) No person shall be convicted of an offence in respect of an act or omission on his part while that person was insane.
>
> (2) For the purposes of this section, a person is insane when the person is in a state of natural imbecility or has disease of the mind to an extent that renders the person incapable of appreciating the nature and quality of an act or omission or of knowing that an act or omission is wrong.

We have said that a person's intent can often be discerned or inferred from the circumstances surrounding his or her actions or words. It is through this means that the Crown often proves intent in an offence. This is known as the objective approach to evidence.[83] That is, the court or jury can draw reasonable inferences from the evidence of the accused's conduct or words or the circumstances surrounding the commission of the offence.

The accused who seeks to prove that his or her conduct was not the product of a conscious and voluntary mind bears the burden of presenting psychiatric and other such evidence to prove his or her defence.

Breach of a criminal law through **malfeasance** (doing something that is one's duty to do but doing it badly) or **non-feasance** (failure to act altogether, such as criminal negligence causing death)[84] is also punishable. Here, the accused clearly has not intended to cause death by his or her conduct, but has behaved in a way that departs from the standard of reasonable behaviour expected of members of society. That departure or negligence has resulted in injury to a third party. The injury is so severe (e.g., death) that it ought to be punished, yet the accused did not intend for such injury to result. Can he or she still be convicted?

For example, suppose an accused was driving his car at an excessive speed on a residential street, thereby striking and killing a child. The accused's behaviour is then clearly out of step with the standard of the reasonable driver. His negligent departure from that standard is the mental element required to prove the offence. In other words, he was aware that he was driving at an excessive speed, and he knew or ought to have known that injury could result from his carelessness. The law would thus punish such reckless behaviour in the interest of protecting the public from gross carelessness.

The Canadian Constitution

Canada's **Constitution** was originally passed by the British Parliament in 1867 as the *British North America Act*[85] (now known as the *Constitution Act, 1867*). At that time, and up until well into the twentieth century,[86] Canada was a self-governing colony of the United Kingdom. Unlike the United States and several other countries with colonial histories, Canada became an independent and sovereign nation by evolution, not revolution.

Since Britain possessed ultimate legislative power over Canada, it alone could provide overriding legislation to which all colonial parliaments in British North America, and later the Parliament of Canada, would be subject. Canada has had the power to amend its Constitution since 1982 with the enactment of the *Canada Act, 1982*[87] by the Parliament of the United Kingdom.

It is a fundamental requirement of any democracy that government and its institutions must act legally according to a higher law. The constitution of a country is such a higher law. It is essentially a set of supreme laws that define and regulate the various branches of government. Canada's Constitution includes a *Charter of Rights and Freedoms*,[88] which sets forth the basic legal and democratic rights of Canadians. These are rights the government cannot infringe upon unless it has a justifiable reason. Any governmental action or law that breaches the Constitution is itself illegal and invalid.

The *Charter of Rights and Freedoms*

Canada's *Charter of Rights and Freedoms*[89] is an *entrenched* (integral) part of its Constitution. It codifies as constitutional law many of the fundamental rights and freedoms bestowed upon the Canadian democracy, including freedom of religion and of conscience,[90] freedom of thought and expression,[91] freedom of the press,[92] freedom of peaceful assembly,[93] and freedom of association.[94]

The Charter also guarantees democratic rights such as the right of citizens to vote,[95] the provision that no Parliament or provincial legislature shall continue for more than five years from the date of the last election,[96] and the requirement that Parliament or a legislature must sit at least once every twelve months.[97] As well, Canadian citizens have the right to enter, remain in, and leave Canada, as well as to move and to take up residence in any province to pursue a livelihood (subject to laws providing for reasonable residency requirements in that province).[98] These are called *mobility rights.*

Perhaps the most important rights enshrined in the Charter include the right to life, liberty, and security of the person[99]; to be secure against unreasonable search and seizure[100]; and the right not to be arbitrarily detained or imprisoned.[101]

Any resident who has been arrested or detained has the right to be informed of the reasons for the arrest[102]; to retain and instruct a lawyer without delay, and to be informed of that right[103]; to have the validity of the detention determined by a court, and to be released if the detention is unlawful.[104]

Rights accorded to Canadians during a criminal trial or other proceeding include the right to be informed without delay of the specific offence[105]; to be tried within a reasonable time[106]; not to be compelled to be a witness against oneself[107]; to the presumption of innocence[108]; to reasonable bail[109]; and to be tried by a jury where the punishment for the offence is imprisonment for five years or more.[110]

If tried and acquitted of an offence, a resident of Canada has the right not to be tried for it again. If found guilty and punished, he or she has the right not to be punished a second time for the same offence[111]; not to be subjected to cruel and unusual punishment[112]; not to have evidence given as a witness in a proceeding subsequently used against him or her in another proceeding[113]; and the right to an interpreter if he or she does not understand or speak the language in which the proceedings are being conducted, or is deaf.[114]

Finally, all persons in Canada are equal before the law regardless of race, sex, national or ethnic origin, colour, religion, age, mental or physical disability.[115] This provision is subject to the enactment of laws implementing affirmative action programs for the benefit of disadvantaged groups in society.[116]

While any statute law enacted in Canada is subject to the Charter, it is possible for Parliament or a legislature to forestall this result by invoking the "notwithstanding" clause of the Constitution. This means that a law may continue to apply for up to five years even if it contravenes a provision of the Charter. The five-year limit is designed to ensure that rights are not permanently *infringed* (violated) by a law. After five years, the "notwithstanding" clause expires insofar as it applies to that particular law, unless it is invoked again.

The Charter also contains minority language education rights, and makes French and English the official languages of Canada.[117]

Since the Charter is part of the Canadian Constitution[118] and the Constitution is the supreme law of Canada,[119] any law that is inconsistent with that supreme law has no force or effect. This means that any such law has the same status as if it had never been passed, and any action taken pursuant to it may be declared illegal by the court that rules upon its constitutionality.

Division of Legislative Powers

Canada is a federal state modelled somewhat after the United States' federal system. There are two basic levels of government: federal and provincial. There is also arguably a third level of government at the municipal level. However, municipalities (cities and towns) are created by provincial law and not by the Constitution.[120]

The Constitution assigns power to make law to both levels of government. Thus, the federal Parliament can make law in those areas listed in section 91 of the *Constitution Act, 1867*. These categories include (but are not limited to)[121] the public debt and property, regulation of trade and commerce, unemployment insurance[122]; raising money by any mode or system of taxation; borrowing money on the public credit; the postal service; the census and statistics; national defence; salaries for the civil service; navigation and shipping; marine hospitals and quarantine; coastal and inland fisheries; weights and measures; currency and coinage; the incorporation of banks, banking law and issue of paper money; cheques and negotiable instruments; interest; bankruptcy and insolvency; patents and copyrights; Indians and Indian reserves; immigration and citizenship; marriage and divorce; criminal law (except establishment and administration of the courts), including criminal procedure and penitentiaries; and any subject excepted from the classes of subjects reserved for the provinces.

Similarly, each province may make laws for itself exclusively within those areas listed in section 92 of the *Constitution Act, 1867*. Some of these include: direct taxation to raise revenue; borrowing money on the credit of the province; salaries and establishment of the provincial civil service; provincial prisons, hospitals, and charities; municipal institutions; licences to raise revenue for the province or municipality; local works and undertakings (except certain types reserved for the federal government); incorporations of companies with provincial objects; solemnization of marriage; property and civil rights; administration of justice, including establishment of courts and civil procedure; power to levy fines or punishment by imprisonment for breach of any provincial law; and matters of a local or private nature.

It may appear that there is overlap between the two levels of government. However, in the years since the enactment of our Constitution, the courts have fleshed out these provisions and have built up a detailed body of case law to deal with conflicts between these two levels. These rules ensure that each level knows what areas these categories encompass, and whether its legislation is valid under the powers granted to it by the Constitution.

If there is a conflict between a provincial law and a federal enactment, the courts have determined that the federal law takes precedence. The provincial law will be suspended to the extent that it conflicts with the federal law, even if the provincial law is valid under section 92 of the *Constitution Act, 1867*. Furthermore, any power or area not assigned or mentioned in the Constitution is reserved for the federal Parliament.[123]

Municipalities are created by provincial law. Each province gives its municipalities the power to regulate such matters as garbage collection, road maintenance, maintenance of municipal parks and recreational facilities, traffic by-laws, public health facilities and programs, libraries, and the raising of municipal taxes to fund these activities. The provinces cannot grant municipalities powers that they themselves do not possess under the Constitution.

Of particular significance to nurses is the fact that health care is largely an area of provincial responsibility.[124] (Specific provincial legislation regulating the nursing profession will be discussed in Chapter 3.) Hence the provinces, through their ministries of health, administer and regulate health care industries within their boundaries. This includes such matters as the establishment, administration, and funding of hospitals and clinics; regulations governing the establishment and administration of public hospitals and private health care institutions such as nursing homes, long-term care facilities, and the like; and public health insurance. Regulation of the nursing profession (and other health professions) including the self-governing bodies comes under the province's powers to make laws governing property and civil rights.

In cases where one level of government has overstepped its constitutional authority and enacted legislation that infringes on another level's powers, the courts are called upon to resolve the dispute. Since Confederation, the courts (in particular, the Judicial Committee of the Privy Council, and since 1949, the Supreme Court of Canada) have gradually defined the extent and distribution of powers under the *Constitution Act, 1867*.

For example, the Constitution decrees that the federal Parliament has authority over telegraph lines connecting the provinces.[125] When the Fathers of Confederation drafted the *British North America Act* (as the Constitution was called before 1982), telegraphs constituted the state of the art in communications technology. Future developments in telephone, wireless telegraphy, radio, television, and satellite technology could not have been foreseen at that time. Over the years, the courts have interpreted this particular provision to include such technologies as a logical extension of federal authority over telegraph lines.

The thinking behind such interpretations is that the Constitution is a living document that should be construed in light of current social, economic, and technological conditions, rather than according to the standards and conditions that existed at the time it was enacted. This is a logical extension of the principle that Parliament, which always expresses its will and intent through its legislation, is deemed to be "speaking" in the present at all times. Since the Constitution is a product of Parliament, that legislative body is said to be expressing its will in the present. Therefore, the Constitution should be interpreted as if it had just been written.

The Canadian Court System

The Canadian Constitution also provides for the establishment of a court system to adjudicate upon criminal and civil matters and to interpret the laws.[126] Our court system is organized primarily at the provincial level, where the bulk of litigation occurs. The Constitution gives the provinces the power to establish and maintain provincial civil and criminal courts and to set the rules of civil procedure in these courts. (Recall that criminal procedure is set out in the federal *Criminal Code of Canada*.) The specific court structure varies somewhat from province to province; however, there are fundamental similarities.

Provincial and Superior Courts

Each province has two basic levels of court: a trial level and an appellate (appeals) level. The trial courts vary from province to province in organizational structure and number, but their **jurisdiction** (i.e., matters they can hear and the orders and judgements they can make) is essentially the same. Trial courts are further split into two types: a provincial court and a superior court.

For example, in British Columbia,[127] the provincial court hears summary offence criminal matters and preliminary hearings under the *Criminal Code*, and it operates as a youth court under the *Young Offenders Act*.[128] It also hears civil matters as a small claims court for claims under $10 000.[129] The superior trial court is known as the Supreme Court of British Columbia.[130] The appellate court is a separate court, the British Columbia Court of Appeal.[131]

The difference between the superior courts and provincial courts in the various provinces is that the former are higher in rank and have generally broader powers than the latter. The judges in the superior courts are appointed by the federal government, whereas provincial court judges are appointed by the provinces. Provincial court judges are more restricted in their powers and in the types of matters they may hear.

Similarly, the superior court of a province may be further divided into a trial division and an appeals division, as in Nova Scotia. Sometimes the superior trial court and the appellate court are completely separate, as in Ontario, where trials occur in Ontario Court (General Division) and appeals in the Court of Appeal of Ontario.

In some provinces, some family law matters (except divorce proceedings) are heard in family courts. These may be set up as a division of the provincial court, as in Manitoba,[132] or as a separate court set up by the province, as in Nova Scotia.[133] Either way, provincial family court judges are appointed provincially. Family law matters include custody applications, paternity disputes (the question of whether a named male is the biological father of a particular child), maintenance and support, and criminal matters involving young offenders, that is, children under eighteen who are charged with criminal offences.

Administrative Tribunals

The provinces have also established boards and commissions which, although not courts in the strict sense, nevertheless adjudicate upon the respective rights and obligations of the parties who come before them. Examples of such boards or commissions, known as **administrative tribunals,** include the various provincial human rights commissions, labour boards, energy boards, provincial securities commissions, municipal boards, assessment review boards, and health disciplines boards (which regulate and govern nurses and other health care professionals). The federal government has also created administrative tribunals, such as the National Transportation Agency, the Canadian Radio-television and Telecommunications Commission (CRTC), the Canada Labour Board, the National Energy Board, the Competition Tribunal, and others.

Administrative tribunals are established to administer laws that govern a particular area or sector of the economy. They are given power to grant licences, rule on complaints, set rates or tariffs, and hear grievances against persons or parties coming within their jurisdiction.

For example, the health disciplines boards established by the various provinces establish minimum standards of competence and enforce these standards among various health care professionals. They may have the power to grant permission to practise a given profession or use a professional title (such as RN) within the province and to discipline members who breach the standards or ethical rules of that profession. Thus, they operate like a court in that they have a duty to decide on such matters fairly and impartially and to give the parties before them a full opportunity to be heard and to present their case.

In the event that the board in question has failed to live up to the duty of fairness, its decisions are reviewable by a court. Otherwise, the operations and decisions of these boards are final and cannot be appealed to the courts. In this way, the government seeks to avoid overburdening the courts with highly complex matters best left to a board whose members have the necessary experience and expertise to decide on them.

Roles of Trial Courts and Appellate Courts

A trial court hears matters as a court of **original jurisdiction** or a court of first instance. This means that it is the first court to hear a case. Once a trial court makes a decision or renders a verdict, that decision or verdict may be appealed to an appellate court, which reviews the proceedings of the lower trial court to ensure that no procedural, evidentiary, or other rules of law were breached or misapplied, that the trial court acted within its powers or jurisdiction, and that the accused's constitutional rights were not violated (especially in the case of a criminal trial).

An appeal is not a new trial. There are no witnesses, and new evidence is seldom heard in an appeal. It is simply a review of the trial to ensure that no errors of law were made. Appeals courts review the decisions of trial courts if one or more of the parties to the case contests the decision. At an appeal hearing, lawyers for the parties argue (depending on whether they are the **appellants'** or **respondents'** counsel) that the trial court made a mistake in its interpretation or application of a point of law in some way material to the verdict or finding of liability, or that it erred in the way it calculated the plaintiff's damages, for example. The appellate court then has the power to substitute its own verdict or decision for that made by the trial court, or it may order that a new trial take place. In such a case, the matter is treated as if the first trial never took place, and the whole trial procedure is repeated.

The Federal Court and Supreme Court of Canada

Under the Constitution, the Parliament of Canada may also establish courts for the administration of the laws of Canada. This essentially means laws made by the Parliament of Canada, or matters over which the federal government has constitutional authority (except matters governed by the *Criminal Code*). Under this provision, the federal government has established the Federal Court of Canada,[134] which is divided into a trial and an appellate division.

The trial division of the Federal Court hears a more restricted class of subjects, since most matters are litigated in the provincial courts. It hears matters involving lawsuits against the Queen in right of Canada (i.e., the federal government) and federal employees in their capacity as employees of the government; taxation matters; suits involving Indian or Native land claims and bands; matters relating to members of the Canadian Armed Forces serving outside Canada; claims made against any federal board, commission, or administrative tribunal; suits between a province and the federal government or between two provinces, where the provinces have agreed by legislation that such matter should be heard in the Federal Court; matters involving patents, trademarks, copyrights, and industrial designs; matters involving suits under federal legislation; immigration and citizenship appeals; matters arising out of maritime (shipping) law or admiralty law; aeronautics; bills of exchange and promissory notes where the federal government is a party; and matters involving works or undertakings connecting one province with another.

The Federal Court of Appeal may hear appeals from a decision or judgement of the trial division, or of a federal board, commission, or tribunal, and any appeal which by law may be taken to the Federal Court. By leave of the Supreme Court of Canada, the Federal Court of Appeal decision may be further appealed to the Supreme Court.

The Supreme Court, established in 1875, is today Canada's highest court. Prior to 1949, any case heard by the Supreme Court could be further appealed to the Judicial Committee of the Privy Council in the United Kingdom. This step reflected Canada's slow evolution to a fully independent nation. Because Canada was still legally a colony of Britain, Canadian citizens (who were also British subjects) could appeal to the Privy Council. Privy Council appeals were abolished in 1949, and since that time the Supreme Court has been the final court of appeal for all cases arising out of Canadian courts. The Supreme Court[135] hears appeals from all provincial appellate courts in Canada and from the Federal Court of Canada. It also is the final interpreter of the Constitution. Its decisions cannot be appealed and are final until and unless the law is amended by Parliament or the Constitution is changed to reverse the Court's interpretation of a particular constitutional provision. Furthermore, all decisions of the Supreme Court are binding on all lower courts.

The Supreme Court is made up of nine judges who serve until age seventy-five. They, like all other federally appointed judges, may be removed from office only by resolution of Parliament. They may be removed if they are not of good behaviour, for example, if they have acted in a manner that shows they are not fit to hold office, or have broken the law.

Summary

The key points introduced in this chapter include:
- the two primary legal systems in Canada—French civil law and English common law—and their sources
- the legislative process

- the distinction between tort law and criminal law
- battery and negligence as they relate to nursing practice
- an overview of the federal structure of Canada, its Constitution and the *Charter of Rights and Freedoms*
- the basic structure and functions of the court system.

References

1. RSO 1990, c. H.8, as amended.
2. This translation is from Stuart, D. (1982), *Canadian Criminal Law* (p. 7). Toronto: Carswells.
3. *R v. Morgentaler*, [1988] 1 SCR 30; (1988) 63 OR (2d) 281 (note); 82 NR 1; 26 OAC 1; 62 CR (3d) 1; 44 DLR (4th) 385; 31 CRR 1 (sub. nom *Morgentaler v. R*), 37 CCC (3d) 449, rev'g. in part (1985), 52 OR (2d) 353; 22 DLR (4th) 641; 22 CCC (3d) 353; 48 CR (3d) 1; 17 CRR 223 (CA), rev'g. (1984), 47 OR (2d) 353; 12 DLR (4th) 502; 14 CCC (3d) 258; 41 CR (3d) 193; 11 CRR 116 (HCJ).
4. *Criminal Code of Canada*, RSC 1985, c. C-46, section 241, as amended.
5. *Rodriguez v. British Columbia* (AG), [1993] BCWLD 347; (1992), 18 WCB (2d) 279 (SC), aff'd. (1993), 76 BCLR (2d) 145; 22 BCAC 266; 38 WAC 266; 14 CRR (2d) 34; 79 CCC (3d) 1; [1993] 3 WWR 553, aff'd. [1993] 3 SCR 519.
6. The procedure is well described in Dawson, R. (1970), *The Government of Canada* (5th ed.; Ward, N., Ed.) (pp. 356–357). Toronto: University of Toronto Press.
7. Namely, Bill 110, *Consent and Capacity Statute Law Amendment Act, 1991*; Bill 74, *Advocacy Act*, 1991; Bill 109, *Substitute Decisions Act*, 1991; Bill 109, *Consent to Treatment Act*, 1991; 1st session, 35th Legislature, Ontario, 40 Elizabeth II, 1991.
8. Supra footnote 1.
9. *Nancy B. v. Hôtel-Dieu de Québec et al.*, [1992] RJQ 361; (1992), 86 DLR (4th) 385; (1992), 69 CCC (3d) 450 (SC).
10. Article 19.1, *Civil Code of Lower Canada*.
11. Fleming, J. (1983). *The Law of Torts* (6th ed.)(p. 23). Sydney: The Law Book Co. See also Linden, A. (1993). *Canadian Tort Law* (5th ed.)(p. 40). Toronto: Butterworths.
12. Linden, ibid., pp. 40-41.
13. Ibid., p. 42.
14. This situation is taken from an actual case; see *R v. Harms*, [1944] 2 DLR 61 (Sask. CA).
15. E.g., see Saskatchewan's *Emergency Medical Aid Act*, RSS 1978, c. E-8, sections 2(b) and 3. This statute permits a registered nurse to administer emergency medical treatment to an unconscious person involved in an accident without incurring liability for negligence as a result of an act or omission on her part. It does not, however, excuse the nurse from gross negligence, that is, conduct that drastically departs from the standard of the reasonably competent nurse.
16. Linden, supra footnote 11, p. 92.
17. *Donoghue v. Stevenson*, [1932] AC 562, at p. 580; 101 LJPC 119, at p. 127; 147 LT 281 (HL); see also Linden, supra footnote 11, p. 258; see also *Heaven v. Pender* (1883), 11 QBD 503.
18. See, e.g., *Gaudreault v. Drapeau* (1987), 45 CCLT 202 (Que. SC), and *Quebec Charter of Human Rights and Freedoms*, RSQ 1977, c. C-12, articles 1, 2, 4, 5, 7, 8, and 49. Article 2 of the Quebec Charter of Rights creates a duty to rescue any person in peril. Such a person has the right, under article 2 of this statute, to aid and rescue and may bring an action for damages against anyone who fails to aid the plaintiff where the defendant's life or that of others is not imperilled by such rescue.
19. Linden, supra footnote 11, p. 266.
20. There are a few exceptions found in criminal legislation as well that require persons to act; see, e.g., *Criminal Code of Canada*, RSC 1985, c. C-46, section 215 (failing to provide necessaries of life to a child), section 218 (abandoning a child), section 216 (duty of persons under-

taking acts dangerous to life to use reasonable skill and care in so doing), and section 217, which reads: "Every one who undertakes to do an act is under a legal duty to do so if an omission to do the act is or may be dangerous to life."

21. Linden, supra footnote 11, pp. 279–281.

22. Ibid., pp. 270–272.

23. *Overseas Tankship (UK) Ltd. v. Mort's Dock Engineering Co. Ltd., The Wagon Mound (No. 1),* [1961] AC 388; [1961] 1 All ER 404 (PC); see also *R v. Cote* (1974), 51 DLR (3d) 244 (SCC); *Abbott et al. v. Kasza,* [1975] 3 WWR 163 (Alta. DC), varied [1976] 4 WWR 20 (Alta. CA); and see Linden, supra footnote 11, pp. 308–309.

24. *Hughes v. Lord Advocate,* [1963] AC 837; [1963] 1 All ER 705 (HL).

25. *Overseas Tankship (UK) Ltd., The Wagon Mound (No. 2) v. The Miller Steamship Co. Pty. Ltd.,* [1967] 1 AC 617; [1966] 2 All ER 709 (PC).

26. See *Butterfield v. Forrester* (1809), 11 East. 60; 103 ER 926.

27. See: Alberta: *Contributory Negligence Act,* RSA 1980, c. C-23, as amended; British Columbia: *Negligence Act,* RSBC 1979, c. 298, as amended; Manitoba: *Tortfeasor's and Contributory Negligence Act,* RSM 1987, c. T90, as amended; New Brunswick: *Contributory Negligence Act,* RSNB 1973, c. C-19, as amended; Newfoundland: *Contributory Negligence Act,* RSN 1990, c. C-33, as amended; Northwest Territories: *Contributory Negligence Act,* RSNWT 1988, c. C-18, as amended; Nova Scotia: *Contributory Negligence Act,* RSNS 1989, c. 95, as amended; Ontario: *Negligence Act,* RSO 1990, c. N.1, as amended; Prince Edward Island: *Contributory Negligence Act,* RSPEI 1988, c. C-21, as amended; Saskatchewan: *Contributory Negligence Act,* RSS 1978, c. C-31, as amended; and Yukon Territory: *Contributory Negligence Act,* RSYT 1986, c.31, as amended.

28. *Quebec Civil Code,* article 1478; and see Linden, supra footnote 11, pp. 440-441.

29. *Black's Law Dictionary* (4th ed.), p. 1746. St. Paul: West Publishing, 1968.

30. Linden, supra footnote 11, p. 457.

31. The document that starts the action is usually referred to as a statement of claim in Ontario and several other provinces. In some provinces, it may instead be referred to as a writ of summons.

32. The appropriate court will be the court that has jurisdiction (i.e., is authorized by law to hear the particular matter). This is discussed in greater detail below.

33. See, e.g., rule 25.06(1) of the Ontario Rules of Civil Procedure (herein referred to as ORCP).

34. This time limit varies from province to province, depending on the provincial rules of civil procedure. In Ontario, for example, the statement of claim must be served within six months of its issue; see rule 14.08(1), ORCP. In British Columbia, a writ of summons must be served within twelve months; see rule 9(1), British Columbia Supreme Court Rules.

35. E.g., rule 19.02(1)(a), ORCP.

36. See, e.g., Ontario's *Courts of Justice Act,* RSO 1990, c. C.43, section 131(1) re: court's general discretion to award costs in a proceeding.

37. E.g., rule 30.02(1), ORCP.

38. These matters include actions where the plaintiff asks for an injunction, the sale of land, a children's or family law matter, the dissolution of a partnership, foreclosure on a mortgage, and other such matters; see, e.g., Ontario *Courts of Justice Act,* supra footnote 37.

39. E.g., Ontario *Courts of Justice Act,* ibid., subsection 108(4).

40. *Constitution Act, 1867,* UK 30 & 31 Vict., c. 3, subsection 91(27).

41. For example, the highway traffic legislation of each province provides for fines and, in some cases, prison terms for breach of its provisions. The provinces have constitutional authority to make laws governing roads and use of motor vehicles. They need to be able to enforce these laws; therefore, they are permitted by subsection 92(15) of the *Constitution Act, 1867* to enact penalties for breach of such legislation.

42. *Criminal Code of Canada,* RSC 1985, c. C-46, as amended.

43. SC 1892, c. 29.

44. *Criminal Code,* SC 1953–54, c. 51. This revision came into force on April 1, 1955. See, generally, Mewett, A. (1993), The *Canadian Criminal Code,* 1892–1992, 72 *Can. Bar Rev.* 1.

45. RSC 1985, c. N-1, as amended.

46. RSC 1985, c. F-27, as amended.

47. RSC 1952, c. 148, as amended.
48. RSC 1985, c. C-32 (formerly known as the *Combines Investigation Act*).
49. RSC 1985, c. F-14, as amended.
50. RSC 1985, c. S-9, as amended.
51. *Criminal Code*, section 175(1)(a).
52. *Criminal Code*, section 175(1)(d).
53. *Criminal Code*, section 175(1)(c).
54. *Criminal Code*, section 177.
55. *Criminal Code*, section 179.
56. This list is not exhaustive.
57. *Criminal Code*, section 787(1).
58. *Criminal Code*, section 235(1). Murder is first-degree murder if the accused has deliberately planned the act. Murder that is not planned and deliberate but, for example, committed in the heat of passion, is second-degree murder. Murder is first-degree murder regardless of planning and deliberation when the victim is a police officer, prison guard, or prison employee, or where the murder occurred as a result of a kidnapping, sexual assault, aircraft hijacking, or hostage taking. See section 231.
59. *Criminal Code*, section 236.
60. *Criminal Code*, section 239.
61. *Criminal Code*, section 221.
62. *Criminal Code*, section 344.
63. *Criminal Code*, section 334(a).
64. *Criminal Code*, section 47.
65. *Criminal Code*, section 465(1)(c).
66. This list is not exhaustive.
67. I.e., for offences such as theft or possession of stolen property of a value under $1000, counselling such an offence, keeping a gaming or betting house, betting, bookmaking, placing bets, lotteries and games of chance (unless held under a government licence), keeping a common bawdy house, cheating at play, fraud in relation to fares, and driving while disqualified (see section 553).
68. I.e., those not listed in *Criminal Code* section 553 and those not contained in section 469. Section 469 offences include treason, alarming Her Majesty, intimidating Parliament or a legislature, inciting to mutiny, seditious offences, piracy, piratical acts, murder, being an accessory after the fact to high treason, treason, or murder, bribery of a judicial office holder, attempting to commit any of these offences, or conspiring to commit any of these offences (see section 554).
69. *Criminal Code*, section 536(2).
70. *Criminal Code*, section 473(1).
71. *United States of America v. Sheppard*, [1977] 2 SCR 1067; (1976), 30 CCC (2d) 424; 34 CRNS 207; 9 NR 215; 70 DLR (3d) 136.
72. Marrocco, F.(1989–90). "The classification of offences and trial jurisdiction." Law Society of Upper Canada Bar Admission Course lecture notes, pp. 1–3.
73. An example is found in section 266, which reads: "Every one who commits an assault is guilty of (a) an indictable offence and liable to imprisonment for a term not exceeding five years; or (b) an offence punishable on summary conviction."
74. This is so by virtue of section 34(1)(a) of the *Interpretation Act*, RSC 1985, c. I-21.
75. *Criminal Code*, section 6(1)(a).
76. Section 11(d) of the *Canadian Charter of Rights and Freedoms*, Part 1 of the *Constitution Act, 1982*, being Schedule B of the *Canada Act 1982* (UK), 1982, c. 11 (herein referred to as "the Charter").
77. This principle has been affirmed in the seminal English decision in *Woolmington v. Director of Public Prosecutions*, [1935] AC 462, at p. 481; (1936) 25 Cr. App. R. 72 (HL); for further discussion of the principle, see Stuart, supra footnote 2, at pp. 32–39. *Woolmington* has been adopted by the Supreme Court of Canada in *R v. Manchuk*, [1938] SCR 341, at p. 349.
78. *Charter of Rights*, section 11(c).

79. Some offences, known as absolute liability offences, merely require proof that the prohibited conduct took place without the requirement that the accused actually intended to commit the offence. For a fuller and classic discussion of absolute liability, strict liability, and mens rea offences, see *R v. Sault Ste. Marie,* [1978] 2 SCR 1299; (1978), 3 CR (3d) 30; 40 CCC (2d) 353; 85 DLR (3d) 161; 21 NR 292.

80. *Fowler v. Padget* (1798), 7 TR 509; 4 RR 511; 101 ER 1103 (KB); but see *R v. Bernard* (1961), 130 CCC 165; 47 MPR 10 (NB CA).

81. See Stuart, supra footnote 2, pp. 77–91.

82. [1980] 2 SCR 513; (1981) 54 CCC (2d) 1; 15 CR (3d) 225; 114 DLR (3d) 193; 32 NR 451. In *R v. Rabey,* the accused was convicted at trial of assaulting a woman with whom he was infatuated and who had rebuffed him. He had no recollection of having done so. The Supreme Court of Canada recognized (in a split decision) that a person might suffer a psychological blow that could cause him to act unconsciously.

83. Stuart, supra footnote 2, pp. 120–123.

84. *Criminal Code,* section 220.

85. UK, 30 & 31 Vict., c. 3.

86. It can be argued that Canada did not legally become fully independent from Britain until April 17, 1982, when the *Canada Act, 1982* was proclaimed by Queen Elizabeth II. This Act irrevocably gave Canada the power to amend (or change) its Constitution through its own legislative action. Prior to this, the Canadian government had to request the British Parliament to pass any amendments to the Constitution, since it was an Act of the British Parliament and only that Parliament could legally amend it. The hallmark of a truly sovereign nation is that all legal and constitutional authority resides within the country itself, including the power to amend its constitution, and that the country is not subject to another country's legislative power.

87. UK (1982), c. 11.

88. Supra footnote 76.

89. Ibid.

90. Charter section 2(a).

91. Ibid., section 2(b).

92. Ibid.

93. Ibid., section 2(c).

94. Ibid., section 2(d).

95. Ibid., section 3.

96. Ibid., section 4(1).

97. Ibid., section 5.

98. Ibid., section 6.

99. Ibid., section 7.

100. Ibid., section 8.

101. Ibid., section 9.

102. Ibid., section 10(a).

103. Ibid., section 10(b).

104. Ibid., section 10(c). This is known as the right to a writ of habeas corpus, which is an ancient type of court order dating back to medieval England. It was granted to those who were detained by the authorities without charge and for no lawful reason, and it is designed to protect citizens against arbitrary detention without charge or trial.

105. Ibid., section 11(a).

106. Ibid., section 11(b).

107. Ibid., section 11(c).

108. Ibid., section 11(d).

109. Ibid., section 11(e).

110. Ibid., section 11(f).

111. Ibid., section 11(h).

112. Ibid., section 12.

113. Ibid., section 13.

114. Ibid., section 14.
115. Ibid., section 15(1).
116. Ibid., section 15(2).
117. Ibid., section 16(1).
118. Ibid., section 52(2).
119. Ibid., section 52(1).
120. *Constitution Act, 1867*, supra footnote 85, section 92(8).
121. This list is not exhaustive.
122. This provision was added in 1940. There was no such scheme in Canada before that time and it was felt that the Parliament of Canada should expressly be given the power in the Constitution to legislate such a scheme.
123. *Constitution Act, 1867*, supra footnote 85, section 91(29).
124. Ibid., section 92(7). The federal government does play an active role in health care, however, through its funding activities, transfer payments to the provinces, and federal/provincial arrangements. In this way, it can influence health care policy in Canada.
125. *Constitution Act, 1867*, supra footnote 87, sections 91(29) and 92(10)(a).
126. Ibid., sections 92(14) and 96 through 101.
127. *Provincial Court Act*, RSBC 1979, c. 341, as amended.
128. RSC 1985, c. Y-1, as amended.
129. *Small Claims Act*, SBC 1989, c. 38.
130. *Supreme Court Act*, SBC 1989, c. 40.
131. *Court of Appeal Act*, SBC 1982, c. 7, Index c. 74.1.
132. *Provincial Court Act*, CCSM c. 275.
133. *Family Court Act*, RSNS 1989, c. 159, as amended by SNS 1992, c. 16 (not yet in force).
134. *Federal Court Act*, RSC 1985, c. F-7. This court was known as the Exchequer Court of Canada before 1971.
135. *Supreme Court Act*, RSC 1985, c. S-26, as amended.

CHAPTER Three

Regulation of the Nursing Profession in Canada

CHAPTER OBJECTIVES

The purpose of this chapter is to enable the reader to:
- understand the scope of laws regulating the nursing profession across Canada
- clarify the role, function, and responsibility of nursing governing bodies
- clarify some of the rules and standards regulating the nursing profession
- articulate the processes and procedures used by governing bodies relating to registration, complaints, discipline, and quality assurance.

As with all self-governing professions in Canada, the nursing profession is regulated provincially. Each province has passed statutes and regulations respecting the governance of nursing, including the nature of the governing body to regulate nurses. It also sets out their powers to establish educational requirements; prerequisites for entry into the practice of nursing; fees; complaints and disciplinary procedures; and professional practice standards, to name but a few.

These regulatory bodies must be distinguished from nurses' unions such as, for example, the Ontario Nurses Association. The latter exist as collective bargaining agents and act solely in the interests of members as employees of various health care institutions. (Labour issues as they relate to nurses are discussed more fully in Chapter 10.)

As Canadians become increasingly aware of their legal rights, they are also questioning the efficacy of health professionals to regulate themselves for the public interest. Thus, the nursing governing bodies and health discipline must set practice standards and codes of ethics that protect the public and provide the benchmarks against which professional practice may be measured. This is of prime importance, as all such bodies are given a mandate to protect the public from incompetent, unskilled, unqualified, or unethical practitioners. Thus, the primary purpose of each governing body is to serve as a watchdog and to promote the welfare of the public in relation to its profession.

In this chapter, we will outline the laws governing the nursing profession in the various provinces and territories of Canada, including organizational structures, methods of regulation, licensing systems, establishment of educational standards, evaluation of the qualifications and skills of nurses, and management of complaints and disciplinary procedures.

Provinces and Territories (Other Than Quebec and Ontario)

The laws regulating nursing in the provinces and territories of Canada (other than Ontario and Quebec) are fairly uniform. They are essentially single-tiered systems, excluding the ultimate governmental authority of their respective ministers of health. In none of these jurisdictions is there an all-encompassing regulatory body for all health professions, although both Alberta[1] and British Columbia[2] have health disciplines boards[3] that regulate a number of health professions. Each provincial nursing regulatory body is responsible directly to the provincial or territorial government and, ultimately, to the public.

Regulatory Bodies across Canada

In British Columbia, there are three professional nursing groups: registered nurses, licensed practical nurses, and registered psychiatric nurses. Registered nurses are governed by the Registered Nurses Association of British Columbia, which is incorporated by the *Nurses (Registered) Act.*[4] Licensed practical nurses do not have their own association per se, but are governed by the Council of Licensed Practical Nurses, whose members are appointed by the provincial cabinet.[5] Registered psychiatric nurses are governed by their own professional body, called the Psychiatric Nurses Association of British Columbia, which is created under the *Nurses (Registered Psychiatric) Act.*[6] The Registered Nurses Association of British Columbia is administered and governed by a board of directors. There are four categories of membership in the B.C. Association: registered nurses, licensed graduate nurses, student members, and honorary members.[7] Further classes of members may be established by the by-laws of the Association as required.

Similarly, in Alberta, registered nurses are self-governed by the Alberta Association of Registered Nurses, which is incorporated under the *Nursing Profession Act.*[8] Licensed practical nurses, psychiatric nurses, and mental deficiency nurses are governed and licensed separately under Alberta's *Health Disciplines Act.*[9] The remaining provinces and both territories also have provincially (or territorially) incorporated associations that self-govern and regulate nursing in their respective jurisdictions.[10]

Objectives of the Associations

The objectives of the various associations are to regulate education, entry into the profession, and standards of practice of members of the profession in the public interest, as well as providing for discipline of members not in compliance.[11] The British Columbia Association's objectives also include the establishment and enforcement of standards of professional ethics among members, as well as the establishment of a patient relations program to prevent professional misconduct of a sexual nature. This provision appears to have been enacted in response to recent findings of widespread sexual abuse of patients by physicians in Canada.[12] In each province, it is the duty of the professional association, as a servant and protector of the public, to regulate the nursing profession and to discharge its responsibilities consistent with the public interest, while balancing the need for autonomy in the functioning of its professionals.

Boards or Council Role

Each association is headed by a board of directors or a council (depending on the province), which governs the day-to-day affairs of the association, as well as providing the mechanism to establish entry criteria and standards of practice. As the primary rule-making body, the council or board enacts rules and by-laws respecting nursing practice standards; standards for admission to nursing schools; the curricula and teaching standards of such schools, although the provinces also have a say in this; student membership; continuing education; reinstatement and renewal of membership; licensing, membership, and other fees; rules governing types of duties and activities that may be carried out by licensed graduate nurses, and so forth. In British Columbia,[13] Alberta,[14] the Yukon,[15] Saskatchewan,[16] Manitoba,[17] New Brunswick,[18] Nova Scotia,[19] and Prince Edward Island,[20] the provincial association's board or council also hears appeals from decisions of its discipline or professional conduct committees.

The councils or boards of the provincial associations may also, in some cases, hear appeals from decisions of the registration committees, or the association's Registrar (as the case may be). In the case of British Columbia,[21] its Council also hears appeals from decisions of the Association's Board of Examiners. The British Columbia, Prince Edward Island, and Newfoundland nursing associations each have a Board of Examiners whose duty is to arrange, set, and mark examinations administered to applicants for registration as registered nurses.[22] The exam administered to applicants is the Canadian Nurses Association Test Standards exam. It is a national exam designed to enable registration of students from one province into the nursing body of another. An appeal from the Board might, for example, involve the Board's decision to refuse an applicant permission to write the registration examination on the grounds that he or she had not met pre-examination requirements.

Registration and Licensing of Nurses

The registration and licensing schemes of the remaining provinces and territories are similar but more traditional. All provincial and territorial laws require applicants for membership in their respective provincial or territorial association to have graduated from an approved school of nursing, and to have passed the requisite nursing registration examination, before they may be admitted as members of the association.

Where applicants have received their training in a province other than the one in which they are applying, the education and training received must be either equivalent to that association's education standards, or it must have been obtained from a Board-approved institution.[23]

In some provinces, applicants who are already registered and licensed to practise nursing in another province, who demonstrate that they are competent, and who are not currently the subject of disciplinary or competency proceedings in any other jurisdiction, will be entitled to registration in the province in which they are then applying.

Some provinces, notably British Columbia, Alberta, Saskatchewan, and Nova Scotia, have instituted licensed (or certified) graduate nursing categories. In British Columbia, Alberta, and Saskatchewan,[24] this is a temporary provision for applicants who have graduated from an approved school or course of nursing and have been employed for a period of time, but have not yet passed the national nursing registration examinations required by the association. This authorizes such nurses to continue to practise under certain terms and conditions pending their passing such examinations. Other provinces and both territories achieve the same result by granting temporary permits to such applicants.

In many provinces and territories, special classes of membership have been established, such as associate membership or (in the case of the Newfoundland Association) honorary membership. The purpose of these separate classes is to provide for those who do not practise in the particular province. The association will want to ensure that the member is still competent, keeping in mind each provincial association's obligation to the public to ensure that members are subject to its discipline and competency requirements.

Unauthorized Practice and Use of Titles

All provinces and both territories restrict the practice of nursing and the use of the title "registered nurse," and the initials "RN" or "RegN," to members of the particular provincial or territorial nursing association who hold a registration certificate or licence, and are members in good standing (i.e., they have paid all membership fees, have not been suspended, nor have they had their membership or licences revoked). Moreover, the provinces of Saskatchewan, New Brunswick, and Prince Edward Island have gone as far as restricting the use of the title "nurse."[25] Any person who represents himself or herself as a registered nurse, provides or offers to provide nursing services, or engages in the practice of nursing, or who uses the term "nurse," or the initials "RN," or any variation thereof, without being a member in good standing of a provincial or territorial association and holding a valid registration certificate, commits an offence. Penalties for such an offence vary from as little as a fifty-dollar fine up to one month in jail (or both) in Newfoundland to as much as several thousand dollars and up to six months' imprisonment in Alberta.[26]

Similarly, a member of an association who is under suspension or whose certificate of registration has been revoked or suspended may be deemed, for the duration of such suspension or revocation, not to be a member of the provincial or territorial association. Such a person then ceases to be a registered nurse and is not entitled to practise nursing, or to represent that he or she is licensed to practise nursing, in the province or territory. If the nurse nevertheless continues to practise, he or she may be charged with unauthorized practice and may be subject to the penalties mentioned above. In addition, continuing practice while under suspension constitutes professional misconduct under some provincial laws.[27]

It is thus important for the registered nurse to make sure that all membership fees are paid on time, as many provincial laws provide that a member's privileges and right to practise are suspended on failure to pay such fees when due. Most (if not all) provinces send notice advising the member that fees are due.[28] But this is not necessarily the case in all jurisdictions, and the practice varies from province to province.

Exemptions

Certain health professions and persons are exempted from registration and licensing requirements under many of the nursing laws across the country. For example, physicians and surgeons, dentists and dental surgeons attending to their patients, registered nursing assistants or licensed practical nurses (who are regulated under another law specifically dealing with RNAs or LPNs), persons rendering emergency first aid to people involved in an accident, and nursing students need not apply for registration and licensing before they may engage in these activities. In all cases, these other health care professionals are already authorized or licensed by their own regulatory bodies to perform such treatments. It would be redundant in these cases to require dual registration.

In the case of persons administering first aid, the law's policy is to encourage "good Samaritans." It is felt that there should be no regulatory prohibitions preventing one person from giving first aid to another in desperate need of it. People should be free to render first aid without fear of prosecution because they are not licensed health care professionals. The acts undertaken, however, should be reasonable and fall reasonably within the competence of the person who undertakes them.

There is an interesting provision respecting registered nurses in the Northwest Territories. In that jurisdiction, a nurse who does anything for which a licence would normally be required under the *Dental Profession Act,* the *Medical Profession Act,* the *Pharmacy Act,* or the *Veterinary Profession Act* in the course of rendering emergency first aid or treatment or alleviating the pain or suffering of a person or animal, is not restricted from acting by any of those statutes. Thus, for example, if a nurse is required, in an emergency, to perform a surgical procedure on a person, and no competent or qualified surgeon is available, he or she may proceed without fear of committing an offence. Similarly, if the treatment is provided to an animal to relieve its suffering, the nurse is permitted to continue without requiring a veterinarian's licence.[29]

Temporary in Another Jurisdiction

The laws of some provinces and the Yukon Territory do not restrict the right to practise of nurses who are duly licensed and qualified to practise in another province, territory, state, or country. For example, suppose Nurse A. is a registered nurse qualified to practise in Alberta. She is accompanying an ill patient from that province on a two-week trip to visit the patient's relatives in Newfoundland, and she is not a member of the Newfoundland Association. Nurse A. will nevertheless be permitted to continue providing nursing services to her patient while they are in Newfoundland, provided the stay is temporary and she does not represent to others that she is licensed or authorized to practise nursing in Newfoundland.[30]

Disciplinary and Competency Matters

Disciplinary and competency matters are investigated by an investigator. If criteria are met, the matter is referred to the professional conduct or disciplinary committee of the provincial or territorial association. Committee members are usually appointed by the board of directors or council of that association, and include lay persons. The procedures for disciplinary hearings and the findings and penalties that can be assessed by the committee are similar to those in Ontario and Quebec.

Step 1: Complaint in Writing

In most cases, a complaint relating to alleged professional misconduct will be filed by the person making the complaint with the Registrar or executive director of the provincial or territorial association to which the member belongs. The complaint must be in writing, must be signed and dated by the person making the complaint, and should name the health care professional who is alleged to have acted in an unprofessional manner. (However, failure to name him or her will not necessarily invalidate the complaint.) Further, it must outline the facts and particulars of the alleged misconduct. A complaint that is not in writing and that is made anonymously is usually ignored.

It is the ethical (and, in Alberta and New Brunswick, the legal) duty of each nurse to report any other nurse who has acted in an unprofessional manner or whose lack of skill, knowledge, or judgement poses a threat to the safety of patients in the nurse's care or who is, by reason of addiction to alcohol or drugs, or mental or physical illness, unable to discharge his or her nursing duties competently or safely. In Alberta, New Brunswick, and many other provinces,

failure to report such conduct or situation will constitute professional misconduct on the part of the nurse whose duty it was to disclose it.

The duty to disclose unprofessional conduct or incompetence is accompanied by a potentially conflicting duty to observe the nurse–client/patient
relationship and to keep confidential any information disclosed by the patient
to the nurse in the course of treatment and the provision of nursing care. If, in
the course of providing treatment to a patient, a nurse gained knowledge from
that patient that another nurse was acting in an unskilled manner, that nurse
may not be entirely free to disclose such information, if to do so would in any
way compromise the confidentiality of the conversation.

It will usually be possible to disclose the information without divulging the
identity of the patient, or other details that would readily identify that patient.
The patient who feels strongly about the professional's conduct may choose to
waive his or her privacy rights and authorize full disclosure. For example,
Ontario's legislation allows (and indeed requires) nurses and other health care
professionals to report knowledge of such allegations obtained in the course of
practising nursing without naming the patient involved, unless the patient consents in writing to having his or her name disclosed in the report.[31] Nevertheless,
this seems to apply only to situations involving sexual abuse, and may not necessarily protect the reporting nurse if the allegations relate to incompetence or
other non-sexual misconduct. Manitoba's legislation, on the other hand, exempts
the disclosure of information obtained, which is confidential by reason of the
nurse–client relationship.[32] Yet even in Manitoba, a nurse, with the patient's
written and freely given consent, could disclose such information to the
Manitoba Association's investigators and disciplinary committee.

Step 2: Investigation

In usual cases, a complaint will be investigated in a preliminary way by a complaints committee, an investigator, or the Registrar of the association in order
to ascertain whether it is well founded or merely frivolous or malicious (e.g.,
where it is brought deliberately to injure a person's reputation).[33] In
Newfoundland, complaints may be investigated and reviewed either by the
Council of the Association itself or by a special committee appointed by the
Council for that purpose.[34]

By statute, members whose conduct or competency is the subject of such
an investigation must be notified immediately upon receipt of a written complaint by their provincial or territorial association. They may also[35] be entitled
to make submissions to the committee or individual conducting a preliminary
investigation. At this stage the complaint may be dismissed if it is unwarranted
or unsupported by the results of the investigation.

In British Columbia, the Yukon, and Manitoba, in a preliminary investigation, inspectors appointed by the board of directors or the committee
investigating the complaint have wide powers to attend, inspect, observe, or inquire into a member's records, place of practice, equipment, and the
supervision of the practice, without a court order. This inspection must comply
with the provincial statute in this regard.[36] Such inspector may copy any

records required in the investigation and must report any findings to the committee. In British Columbia, if authorized by the committee, such investigator may apply for a court order allowing him or her (or another so delegated) to enter the premises or land of anyone named in the order for the purpose of conducting an inspection, examination, or analysis, or to require the production of any record, property, or other items. The order may authorize such a person to inspect or analyze anything seized and to remove any such items for further inspection or analysis. It is essential, for the purposes of fairness and natural justice, that such a person be independent of the disciplinary committee or other tribunal hearing the matter. Otherwise, it may be alleged by the professional under investigation that the committee was biassed and directed the investigation against that professional.

It is important for nurses to realize that they are under a legal duty to cooperate with an inspector and to allow him or her to make examinations without interference. But patient confidentiality must be protected. A lawyer's advice and assistance should always be sought without delay. Legal counsel will be able to apply to an appropriate court for a ruling on whether such a search or seizure is lawful and made according to the procedural safeguards contained in the legislation.

Step 3: Interim Investigation

If it is well founded, the complaint may be referred to a disciplinary committee or a professional conduct committee (depending on the province or territory) for further investigation and then to a hearing, if necessary. If the allegations are of such nature as to show that the nurse being investigated poses a threat to the safety or security of patients, the committee usually has the power to order that the nurse's right to practise be suspended or restricted pending the conclusion of the disciplinary proceedings. This effectively halts the nurse's practice for the duration of the matter, and may be a source of financial or other hardship to the nurse.

A nurse, when faced with an interim suspension or restriction, will in most cases appeal the decision to a court. The nurse may ask that the court lift the disciplinary committee's order on the grounds that the suspension was harsh, unreasonable, or excessive, or that the circumstances do not warrant suspension from practice in that no threat is posed to the public's safety. The granting of such an order is in the court's sole discretion and is not an automatic right.

Step 4: Disciplinary Committee

Before a hearing is scheduled to consider the matter, the committee must first notify the nurse against whom the complaint was brought. The date and time of the hearing will usually be co-ordinated with the nurse's legal counsel, if any. The notice usually specifies the nature of the conduct being reviewed, and the date, place, and time of the hearing by the committee.

The committee will usually hear evidence under oath and record it for the purpose of preparing a transcript for use at a possible appeal. Both the committee or board of directors (as the case may be), and the member whose conduct is being investigated, are entitled to have lawyers present and to submit evidence.

In cases where physical, sexual, or other abuse of a patient by the nurse is alleged, the patient may also be present and be represented by a lawyer. The patient may be the complainant, and if so, will be given an opportunity to relate the facts and basis for his or her complaint. We have previously discussed the use of a victim impact statement, in which the patient explains the impact and effect of the complained-of behaviour on him or her.

The committee, after hearing the evidence, will consider its decision. Depending upon the provincial law, among the possible findings it may make are: that the nurse is innocent of any wrongdoing; or, that the nurse involved is incompetent, unskilled, or otherwise lacking in essential knowledge; or, that he or she is guilty of professional misconduct; or, that the nurse is habitually impaired by the use of alcohol or drugs such that he or she is unable to discharge nursing duties and obligations safely. Many of the provincial statutes specify acts that constitute professional misconduct. Such definitions are not meant to be exclusive, but serve to identify many common situations.

A nurse convicted of an indictable offence under the *Criminal Code,* or an offence under the *Narcotic Control Act* or the *Food and Drugs Act,* may, in British Columbia, Manitoba, Saskatchewan, New Brunswick, and the Northwest Territories, be liable to suspension from nursing practice—in some cases, without any hearing. However, the *Charter of Rights and Freedoms,* as well as principles of natural justice, make it doubtful whether such legislation providing for permanent suspension without a hearing would pass constitutional scrutiny. It is likely that some form of hearing would have to be held, especially if the nurse runs the risk of permanent suspension and, hence, his or her livelihood. However, the particular legislation under which such a suspension would be initiated by a provincial association will require, in some cases, that the nature of the offence be such as would affect the member's nursing practice.

A recent British Columbia court decision involving a licensed practical nurse illustrates how provincial human rights laws may intervene to protect an applicant's right to membership despite that person's prior criminal record.[37] Although the case involved specific legislation applying not to registered nurses, but to practical nurses, the principle is equally applicable to RNs. In this case, a woman had applied for a licence as an LPN after having worked unlicensed as such for a number of years. The Council of Licensed Practical Nurses of British Columbia refused her application on the grounds that she had a prior criminal record consisting of a conviction for shoplifting in the early 1970s. The B.C. *Human Rights Act*[38] prohibits discrimination in employment based on a person's past criminal record unless such a record is related to the person's intended occupation. The practical nurse took her complaint to the B.C. Human Rights Council, claiming that the Licensed Practical Nurses' Council had illegally discriminated against her on this basis. The Human Rights Council found in the nurse's favour and ordered the LPN Council to grant the nurse a licence.

The LPN Council appealed, and the case ultimately found its way to the B.C. Court of Appeal, which upheld the Human Rights Council's decision and confirmed its view that the *Human Rights Act* superseded the statute granting the LPN authority to deny a licence to applicants who are not deemed fit to be licensed. The Court further stated that the Human Rights Council was correct in asserting that the prior criminal record, in this case, was unrelated to the applicant's intended occupation as a licensed practical nurse, and that the discrimination was therefore unlawful.

It is arguable that such a ruling could apply to other provinces, since most provincial human rights laws contain similar provisions with respect to discrimination on the basis of a criminal record. Of course, other prohibited grounds of discrimination apply to bar refusal of a licence or registration on the basis of race, creed, ethnic origin, sex, religion, marital status, physical or mental disability, and, in some provinces, sexual orientation.

Penalties

The penalties awarded to the nurse who has been found guilty of professional misconduct, or who has been found incompetent, include: censure or reprimand before the committee or in writing; conditions placed on the nurse's right to practise, including a requirement that he or she take additional courses or education and pass further examinations; suspension from practice for a specified period of time (e.g., for the completion of such additional training or education); or, in more serious cases, permanent revocation of the nurse's right to practise and expulsion from the nursing association. This, in some provinces, may be accompanied by a further order that the nurse pay the association's legal costs and fees incurred in conducting the investigation and hearing, or pay a fine, or repay to the patient any monies received from the patient for treatment services.

Appeals

The decision of the professional conduct committee as to the finding of guilt, or the penalty awarded, or both, may be appealed to the board of directors or the council of the association by notifying it in writing within a specified time (usually within fifteen or up to thirty days of the decision's being rendered).[39] If the decision on the appeal is still unfavourable, the nurse may appeal, in most provinces, to the provincial superior court (in Alberta, to the Alberta Court of Appeal, which may order a new hearing before the Alberta Court of Queen's Bench). Prince Edward Island, Nova Scotia, and the Yukon Territory do not appear to allow further appeals to the courts, although an application for judicial review can always be brought to challenge the decision on the basis of the denial of natural justice, fraud, or the committee's having exceeded its jurisdiction. In the Northwest Territories and Newfoundland, the decision of the Trial Division of the Supreme Court on an appeal from a disciplinary committee's decision is final and may not be appealed further to their respective Courts of Appeal.

Many of the structures and procedures outlined above are equally applicable to registered nursing assistants (or licensed/registered practical nurses, as they are called in some provinces), as well as registered psychiatric nurses (specifically in British Columbia, Alberta, Saskatchewan, and Manitoba) pursuant to the statutes that regulate those professions.

Quebec and Ontario

Ontario and Quebec have somewhat different and more complex legislation regulating the nursing profession. Each province's laws, in particular Ontario's, is more highly detailed and structured compared with those of the remaining provinces and territories. Thus, the schemes of these two provinces will be looked at in more detail.

In both provinces, the nursing profession is regulated by a two-tiered system: at the higher level, a central administrative body established to govern all professions (as in Quebec) or all health professions (as in Ontario); and under this, the various professional organizations.

The Nursing Profession in Quebec

Office des professions du Québec

In Quebec, a central administrative agency, the Office des professions du Québec, has been established to regulate all professions including lawyers, notaries, chartered accountants, engineers, and architects, as well as physicians, dentists, chiropractors, nurses, and nursing assistants.[40] In short, all the professions that Quebec has decided should be regulated are included in the jurisdiction of the Office. The Office itself and its powers and functions are created and set forth in Quebec's *Professional Code*.[41] This statute also sets out the powers and procedures of the various Bureaus, that is, the rule- and policy-making councils of the various professional corporations that govern the members of each profession. These corporations are akin to the various colleges that regulate the health professions in Ontario.

The Office is primarily engaged in supervisory functions over the many professions under its jurisdiction. Its main task is to ensure that each self-governing profession acts with the protection of the public as its main priority.[42] It oversees the activities of the professional corporations, ensures that each corporation adopts a code of ethics, and further, that each adopts various regulations required by the Code. In particular, the Office must ensure that each professional corporation determines the composition, membership, and procedures of its professional inspection committee, and that each adopts regulations governing quorums at general meetings; dates and procedures for election of the president and directors of the corporation; standards for the equivalence of diplomas issued by educational institutions outside Quebec, and so forth.[43]

In addition, the Office has the power to suggest amendments to any of the regulations made by a corporation. In the event that a corporation fails to make a regulation required by the Code or suggested by the Office, the Office has the power to make the regulation for the corporation, subject to government approval. Finally, the Office is required to make an annual report of its activities to the appropriate minister who, in turn, is required to present the report to the National Assembly.[44] In this way, the legislature maintains a watchful eye over the Office, and policy matters that may arise out of the Office's activities are brought up for debate in a public forum.

Corporation professionelle des infirmières et infirmiers du Québec

Like similar legislation in other provinces, Quebec's *Nurses Act*[45] defines the practice of nursing as an activity whose object is to identify the health needs of people, to contribute to the methods of diagnosing illness, to provide and control nursing care needed to promote health, to prevent illness, to treat and rehabilitate, and to provide care according to medical prescription. This definition is less detailed than that of other provinces, but is fairly succinct and allows greater flexibility of interpretation. It is worded broadly enough to encompass many daily activities and tasks undertaken by modern nursing professionals. Of course, it is not exhaustive of all aspects of nursing; in particular, it does not address directly or explicitly the ethical concerns of nursing.[46]

The definition also serves a legal purpose: it helps in delimiting what acts constitute the practice of nursing for the purpose of identifying possible unauthorized practice. A legal definition of nursing thus assists a court or other administrative tribunal in determining whether a particular act by an individual constitutes nursing practice. In Quebec, the practice of nursing, as in other provinces and territories, is restricted. No one may practise nursing unless he or she is a registered nurse and a member of the Corporation professionelle (or Ordre) des infirmières et infirmiers du Québec, or is otherwise permitted to do so by law. A breach of this provision leaves a person liable to the penalties set out in the *Professional Code*.

In Quebec, each professional corporation is governed by a Bureau whose size varies with the size of the membership in the particular profession. Most of the members of the Bureau are elected from among the membership. The nursing profession is governed by the Order.[47] Its Bureau consists of a president and twenty-eight directors, including a vice-president and a treasurer.[48] The elected directors are chosen at a general meeting by votes of delegates who represent the various sections of the corporation.[49] The Order of Nurses also has a secretary chosen from among the membership for an indefinite term who acts as secretary of the Order, the Bureau, and the Bureau's executive committee, and has custody and control of all records of the Order.[50]

Certain duties of the Bureau are established in the Nurses Act.[51] Specifically, the Bureau must establish the procedures for entry of members on the membership roll; advise the Minister of Health and Social Services on the state and quality of nursing care in the province and of ways to improve the quality of that care; determine the date and place of the annual meeting of the Order; maintain the register of nursing students, and procedures for entry in that register; require annual reports from the various sections; determine those sections that, because of their insolvency or poor use of funds, are to be dissolved or placed under trusteeship, or order inquiries into the affairs of such sections.

In addition, the Bureau must carry out those duties assigned to it by the *Professional Code*.[52] These include, among others, the obligation to appoint committees and determine their powers; issue specialist certificates; hold refresher courses or training periods for members; fix the amount of the annual assessment to be levied of members; strike members off the roll who fail to pay dues, and so forth.[53] The Bureau is also required to set the amounts required to defray the cost of a group professional liability insurance plan, and to designate a provisional custodian who temporarily holds and disposes of the professional records, books, equipment, etc. of a nurse who has ceased to practise. The Bureau has passed a regulation requiring that its members furnish proof of professional liability coverage of at least $500 000. A member must file a certificate that indicates, among other things, the period of insurance coverage and the dollar limits of the policy.[54]

The Bureau must also pass a code of ethics to govern its members, and the *Professional Code*[55] sets out the minimum requirements that must be contained in it. Pursuant to this, the Bureau of the Order of Nurses of Quebec passed its code of ethics in 1976.[56] A new draft code was published in 1992; however, it had not been passed into law as of the date of writing. The existing code defines the duties and obligations of the nurse toward the public and toward clients (i.e., persons who are receiving care from a nursing professional), as well as duties owed to the profession. In particular, it requires that the nurse be reasonably available and diligent, and that he or she subordinate personal interest to that of the client, respect the privacy of the client, and refrain from disclosing confidential information.[57]

Although many nurses are employed in the public sector, some are employed as private nurses and, in some cases, render their accounts directly to their patients. Consequently, the Bureau must establish a conciliation and arbitration procedure for disputes arising between patients and private nurses in connection with nurses' accounts. These procedures provide a streamlined mechanism for settling disputes over accounts, thus avoiding the more costly process of litigation.

Nursing students must be registered with the Order and, once registered, are issued a certificate of registration by the secretary of the Order. Any person possessing a high school certificate or diploma recognized by the Bureau, and who has observed specific formalities set by it, is entitled to registration.[58]

Sections of the Corporation

The Order is further divided into sections based on geographical regions of the province. By law, there must be at least eleven such sections, although the exact number and precise boundaries of each are set by regulations passed by the

Bureau.[59] There are currently thirteen such sections in Quebec.[60] Each constitutes a separate corporation; thus, an attempt has been made to achieve a greater degree of decentralization and regionalization in the governance of the profession.

These sections are not altogether independent, however, since the *Nurses Act* gives the Bureau the power to dissolve or place a particular section under trusteeship if it is determined that the section is insolvent or has failed to make beneficial use of the funds at its disposal.[61] Each section is administered by a council made up of a president, a vice-president, and up to eight councillors.[62] To the extent that these regional sections are autonomous, they are free to determine the rules and procedures for elections of members of the council of the section, the length of their terms, and the exact number of councillors (not to exceed eight); set the date for the election; designate the returning officer for the election; and pass by-laws for the management of the council and administration of its property.[63] In this way, the regional regulation of the profession is encouraged, and each member is given more input into the running of his or her local section. Yet, the degree of autonomy actually enjoyed by these sections must not be overstated, as the Bureau also has the power to disallow any by-law passed by a section if such a by-law conflicts with its own regulations or is "inconsistent with … the general interest of the Order."[64] As well, each section is required to choose auditors at its annual general meeting and to have its books of account audited every year.[65]

The Professional Inspection Committee

The Bureau must have a professional inspection committee[66] to inspect the individual practices of the members of the Order. Its procedure and make-up are determined by regulations passed by the Bureau. The committee may inspect the records, books, registers, medications, poisons, products, substances, and equipment relating to a particular member's practice. It may also, at the Bureau's request, inquire into the professional competence of any member. Members must co-operate with any investigation conducted by the committee, as it is an offence under the *Professional Code* to hinder an investigator retained by the committee or any committee member in the performance of his or her duties.[67] Conviction for an offence under the Code carries with it a fine ranging from $500 to $5000.[68]

The Disciplinary Committee

Each Bureau also has a disciplinary committee responsible for investigating and conducting hearings on disciplinary matters involving members. The chair of such committee must be a lawyer with at least ten years' experience, appointed by the Government of Quebec from among a list of names submitted by the Quebec Bar. This requirement is unique to Quebec. Although the majority of the members of such disciplinary committee are themselves members of the professional corporation, it is felt that the complex procedural rules and regulations respecting the investigation and hearing of disciplinary matters require the expertise of a lawyer. Hence, the chair of the committee is entrusted to a lawyer skilled in civil procedure, the rules of evidence, and basic procedural requirements of such hearings.

The consequences of a hearing into a member's professional conduct carry potentially grave penalties, including permanent revocation of the member's licence, and hence the removal of that member's right to practise. This provision warrants ensuring that all procedural rules and requirements are met, and that the member being investigated is given **due process** (i.e., a full opportunity to defend himself or herself), and a chance to make a complete answer to any allegations of professional misconduct.

Furthermore, a nurse who has had an adverse disciplinary decision made against him or her, such as a reprimand, or more seriously, temporary or permanent revocation of his or her right to practise, may appeal the decision of the disciplinary committee to the Professions Tribunal with permission (in most cases) of that tribunal.[69] The Tribunal itself resembles a court. It is made up of eleven judges of the Court of Quebec, chosen by the Chief Judge of that court.[70]

The Disciplinary Process

Disciplinary procedures under the *Professional Code* of Quebec, as in most other provinces and territories, are fairly straightforward. However, the nursing professional, no matter what province or territory in which he or she practises, is always well advised to obtain legal advice from a lawyer (preferably one who specializes in disciplinary matters involving professionals) immediately upon receiving notification that such proceedings have been brought against him or her. In virtually all cases, a professional facing disciplinary proceedings is entitled to be represented by a lawyer. The lawyer is best able to make sense of the procedures and rules of the disciplinary hearings and is well versed in the rules of evidence. He or she will likely have trial experience and will be skilled in the art of presenting a defence case and of cross-examining witnesses.

In a disciplinary matter in Quebec, a person wishing to make a complaint against a nurse must do so in writing under oath or solemn affirmation, stating the date, place, and nature of the offence that is alleged to have been committed.[71] The complaint is filed with the secretary of the disciplinary committee. Complaints may be lodged by an individual or by a syndic or assistant syndic chosen by the **complainant** (the person filing the complaint) or the Bureau.[72] (A syndic's role and duties are like those of complaints investigators in the other provinces.) The complaint may deal with the member's breach of, for example, the code of ethics, the *Professional Code* itself, the *Nurses Act,* or any regulations made under either of those statutes.[73] It may allege abuse of a patient by a nurse, or that a nurse abandoned or stole from a patient.

The Bureau must then appoint a syndic and assistant syndics, who investigate the complaint made against the member[74] and decide whether or not to lodge a formal complaint against him or her with the disciplinary committee. In either event, they must inform the complainant of their decision and, if a complaint is not lodged, of the reasons for that decision. Everything that is disclosed to the syndic or assistant syndics during an investigation is held in strict confidence, and these officials must take an oath not to divulge any such information without being legally authorized to do so.

If the facts of the offence with which a member is charged are of such nature that the continuation of those acts would pose a serious threat to the public, the complainant can request that the committee strike the member off the roll provisionally (i.e., for the time being).[75] This suspends the member's right to practise. A copy of the complaint is served (given) to the member, who then has ten days to file an appearance (a written notice that he or she will appear to answer the complaint).

If a request has been made to have the member struck off the roll provisionally, a hearing must be held on this question within ten days of the complaint's being served on the member. If the committee deems it in the public interest to strike the member from the roll provisionally, it may do so at the conclusion of the hearing, and the order is effective from the time it is served on the member who is the subject of the complaint.[76]

This hearing determines only whether or not the professional's name should be provisionally removed from the Order's roll, and does not deal with the substance of the complaint itself. The question at this stage is whether the member's alleged conduct is of such nature that it poses a danger to the public and further, whether the protection of the public requires that the member be provisionally suspended. The suspension lasts until such time as it is overturned on appeal, or until the disciplinary hearing itself is resolved in favour of the member.

If the member chooses to appear, he or she, or the member's lawyer, must file an appearance with the Order, accompanied by a declaration in which the member either denies or acknowledges the act that is alleged to have been committed. Failure to file such a declaration is taken to mean that the nurse denies the allegations. A written contestation that sets out the member's own version of the facts may then be filed within ten days of filing an appearance.

The hearing itself is conducted by a panel of the disciplinary committee, made up of three of its members including the chairman of the committee. A notice of the date, place, and time of the hearing must be served on the member and the member's lawyer (if any) at least three days before the date set for the hearing. Testimony given during the hearing (called a **deposition**) is recorded, unless the parties agree otherwise. These recorded proceedings will form the record in the event that the member wishes to contest the committee's decision.

During the hearing, the member must be given every opportunity to make a full and complete defence. The committee has the power to subpoena witnesses, and all parties and witnesses must answer all questions put to them. However, any evidence given by a witness (including the member) may not be used against the member in court.[77] All evidence is given under oath, as in a court trial. This means that anyone who lies or misleads the committee in giving testimony is subject to the same penalties for perjury as in a court case.

Only the committee has the power to determine guilt or innocence with respect to an offence under the Code. In the event that the member is found guilty, the reasons for the verdict must be recorded in writing and signed by the committee members. A penalty must be imposed within thirty days of a conviction. The committee also has the power to order the guilty member to pay the costs of the proceedings, other parties' costs, and the costs of recording the proceedings.[78] These penalties include any one or more of the following: a reprimand of the member; temporary or permanent striking of the member's name from the roll; a fine of at least $500 for each offence; the obligation to remit any money the nurse is holding to any person entitled to it; a revocation of the member's permit or specialist's certificate; or a restriction or suspension of the member's right to engage in professional activities. As well, the committee must publish its decision in a regular newspaper or professional publication in the place where the nurse principally practises. This ensures that notice of the disciplinary proceedings and their result is given to the nurse's clients and members of his or her community. The stigma of such publication alone should be enough to deter a breach of the Code and rules of professional conduct and ethics. Often, however, it is not.

In the event that the Bureau is required to pay a sum of money to the client of a member who was ordered to pay it, such payment is made from an indemnity fund set up for that purpose by the Bureau. This is to ensure that there is money available to compensate persons who have been injured or have suffered harm as a result of the member's breach of a provision of the Code or regulations. It is used in the event that the committee recommends that the Bureau make the payment. If the fund pays the injured client on the member's behalf, then the member is automatically struck from the rolls of the Order until such time as he or she repays the money to the professional corporation.[79]

As part of the penalty assessed against an offending nurse, the committee may order that he or she take a refresher course or refresher training and it may suspend or restrict the member's right to practise until such time as that course or training has been completed.[80] A member whose name has been struck from the roll or whose right to practise has been suspended or restricted may request that he or she be reinstated. The disciplinary committee may make a recommendation to the Bureau as to whether that member should be so reinstated before the expiry of the penalty period originally assessed. The Bureau has the final say in the granting of such a reinstatement, but it is up to the committee whether or not a recommendation to reinstate is passed on to the Bureau.[81]

Appeals of any decision of the disciplinary committee must be made to the Professions Tribunal within thirty days of the date of service of the decision of the disciplinary committee on the member. Most decisions may be appealed only with leave (permission) of the Tribunal. Only a decision of the committee to strike a member from the rolls provisionally may be appealed as of right (i.e., automatically, without permission from the Tribunal). A petition for an appeal is filed by the member with the office of the Court of Quebec (because the Tribunal's members are judges from that court), and a copy is served on every party to the proceedings, as well as the secretary of the disciplinary committee. Other parties might include the person who filed the original complaint and any additional parties who may have had similar complaints arising from the member's conduct, plus any other parties who may have been given permission to participate in the disciplinary proceedings. A petition for leave to appeal (in cases where this is required) must also be filed within thirty days of the committee's decision being served on the member. Such petition must, in turn, be served on the parties to the proceedings and the secretary of the committee.[82]

The Tribunal also has certain investigatory powers. In addition, it may receive, in special circumstances, other evidence that was not presented at the hearing before the disciplinary committee. A date for hearing the appeal is then set and is held open to the public unless the Tribunal orders that it be held *in camera* (Latin, "in private"). It has the power to punish for contempt of court anyone who disobeys one of its orders or publishes evidence contrary to a publication ban. Finally, the Tribunal may confirm, alter, or quash (cancel) any decision submitted to it from a disciplinary committee and make the decision that it feels should have been made in the first place. It can also order the parties, or any among them, to pay the costs of the appeal.[83]

The *Professional Code* also imposes other duties upon the disciplinary committee and the Bureau, such as the obligation to publish notices of disciplinary action and decisions taken against specific members. The corporation must notify its members of the fact that a member has been disciplined, and of the penalty meted out, including the fact that the member's right to practise has been suspended or restricted, or that his or her name has been struck from the roll.

The Nursing Profession in Ontario

The Health Professions Board

The regulatory scheme for nursing in Ontario resembles that of Quebec in that it is a two-tiered system. The Health Professions Board, established under the *Regulated Health Professions Act, 1991*[84] (RHPA), is responsible for the overall supervision of health professions in the province and hears disciplinary appeals from the various professional colleges. This Board is roughly equivalent to the Office des professions du Québec. However, the Ontario statute limits the Board's jurisdiction to health professions only.

The Board is made up of twelve to twenty members appointed by the provincial cabinet, with a chair and one or more vice-chairs as designated by the chair. Each member of the Board serves for a maximum three-year term but each may be reappointed for further three-year terms.[85] As well, the Board is given the power to employ people to aid it in carrying out its many functions. It may hire investigators in disciplinary matters before it, and experts to provide the Board with professional advice and information in connection with registration hearings and reviews or reviews of complaints.[86]

The Health Professions Board is essentially a supervisory body. Its various functions and duties are set out and defined in the *Health Professions Procedural Code*,[87] which is enacted as a schedule to the RHPA and is deemed to be a part of each health profession Act. The *Nursing Act, 1991*[88] is such an Act; therefore, the *Procedural Code* is a part of that Act[89] and has the force of law.

The *Health Professions Procedural Code* (HPPC)

The HPPC is the core of Ontario's system for the regulation of health professions, and it is perhaps the most comprehensive such code in the country. It defines in greater detail the powers and responsibilities of not only the upper tier of the system, that is, the Health Professions Board, but also delimits the powers and authority of the professional colleges of all the health professions subsumed under the Act (including the College of Nurses of Ontario). It establishes procedures for hearing complaints against college members; reviews of registrations of members and appeals of those reviews; inquiries into the fitness or capacity of a member to practise the profession; judicial review of decisions of the Board and committees of the colleges; investigations conducted by the Registrar of a college; and the establishment of a quality assurance committee and a patient relations program. Finally, the HPPC establishes procedures for dealing with complaints of sexual misconduct of a member of a college.

Although it is still too early to tell how well this new system will work, the Code and the Ontario system in general are ambitious and, though not without flaws, they look promising. The Code strives to provide for more input from individual consumers of health services. It provides as well for more sensitive recognition of the rights and needs of those consumers.

The College of Nurses of Ontario

Each of the health professions is regulated and administered by its own professional college, such as the professional corporations in Quebec, and each college is set up under a specific Act of the legislature. Apart from the RHPA, nursing in Ontario is regulated under the *Nursing Act, 1991*.[90] This Act incorporates the College of Nurses of Ontario and defines its powers and responsibilities. In addition, the Act contains a legal definition of nursing, which codifies the scope of nursing practice in Ontario:

> The practice of nursing is the promotion of health and the assessment of, the provision of care for and the treatment of health conditions by supportive, preventative, therapeutic, palliative and rehabilitative means in order to attain or maintain optimal function.[91]

The purpose of this legal definition is to describe the nature and scope of nursing practice. The definition delimits those acts and procedures that are part of nursing practice. The purpose of this definition is to provide a framework to determine whether certain actions constitute the practice of nursing. This will allow a distinction to be drawn between nursing and other professional practices. The definition also aids the courts in interpreting other sections of the Act.

Infrastructure

The College of Nurses of Ontario is led by an executive director who also acts as its Registrar.[92] All persons who are authorized to practise nursing or practical nursing in Ontario, are registered with the College, and have met the prerequisites (including fees) are its members. College membership is divided into two classes, namely, registered nurses and practical nurses (formerly known as registered nursing assistants or RNAs).[93] This feature of combining both registered and practical nurses under the jurisdiction of one professional college is unique to Ontario. In all other provinces and territories, licensed practical nurses, certified nursing assistants, and RNAs are governed by a separate body or other governmental agency.

The College's objectives are set out in the HPPC and include:

(1) regulation of nursing practice and governance of its members;
(2) development, establishment, and maintenance of criteria for persons to whom certificates of registration are issued;
(3) standards of practice to ensure quality professional practice;
(4) standards of knowledge and skill, programs to promote continuing competence among members of the profession;
(5) standards of professional ethics for members;
(6) development of programs to assist individuals to exercise their rights under the *Procedural Code* and the RHPA;
(7) administration of the *Nursing Act, 1991,* and the RHPA; and
(8) any other objectives relating to human health care that the Council may consider desirable.[94]

Such a list assists the courts in interpreting the provisions granting the College specific powers and duties. Similarly, it provides legislative guidance to the courts when interpreting regulations made by the Council (see below). It also helps the College interpret the legislation for the purpose of making policy, creating regulations, and performing its duties under the *Procedural Code,* the *Nursing Act, 1991,* and the RHPA. When acting pursuant to these powers, the College must always have service and protection of the public interest foremost in mind.[95]

Council

The College's governing body is the Council or Board of Directors,[96] which is made up of thirty-nine persons. Twenty-one of the Council are elected by the members of the College according to election procedures set by the Council.[97] Of these, fourteen must be registered nurses, and seven practical nurses. The remaining eighteen members are appointed by the provincial cabinet and must neither be members of the College, nor members of any other health profession's college or council. In this way, there is input from lay persons, which will potentially result in greater public input, scrutiny, and accountability not only of nursing, but also of other health care professions.

As self-governing groups are generally regarded with suspicion, lay representatives may demystify professional regulation and make it more accessible and accountable to the public. The professions have expressed the concern that lay involvement will sacrifice self-governance and professional autonomy. The policy thinking behind such governing structure is that professionals retain the ability to govern and enforce professional standards while still allowing the public some influence on decision making. The drawback to this is that increased input from persons who are not sufficiently versed in the procedures and practices of a profession may unduly hamper the College's activities and independence. On the other hand, input from the consumer should greatly assist answering the question: What makes patients happy? The trend toward allowing non-professionals to sit on the governing bodies of professional organizations is desirable, but some would argue that it should not be permitted to suppress professional independence and self-regulation.

The Council has a president and two vice-presidents elected annually from among its members, one vice-president being a registered nurse and one a practical nurse.[98] It also has seven statutory committees: an executive committee, a registration committee, a complaints committee, a discipline committee, a fitness to practise committee, a quality assurance committee, and a patient relations committee.[99]

The Executive Committee

This committee is charged with exercising the powers of the full Council between meetings of Council. It has all the powers of Council (except the power to make or change regulations or by-laws) to deal with any matter that, in its opinion, requires immediate attention.[100] On the surface, this looks like a great deal of delegated power; however, it allows for greater flexibility in that the full Council need not be called to deal with every crisis or urgent matter. Thus, the committee acts as a caretaker between full meetings of the Council, deals with the day-to-day routine of administration, and screens complaints made against particular members respecting competency and fitness to practise.

The Registration Committee

This committee is responsible for processing applications for registration from prospective members.[101] When a registration application is filed with the Registrar of the College together with the registration fee, the applicant will be registered immediately if the Council's prerequisites have been met. If the application does not meet established prerequisites, it is referred by the Registrar to the registration committee.[102]

The College of Nurses of Ontario has four classes of registration certificates for registered nurses:

(1) General,
(2) Temporary,
(3) Special Assignment, and
(4) Provisional.

Identical classes exist for registration as a practical nurse.[103] The Special Assignment class of certificate is intended for special programs such as, for example, exchange programs involving nurses from other provinces or countries. It is valid for up to a maximum of one year, as specified.

The Provisional class applies to those who have a number of criteria outstanding and are therefore not eligible for general registration (for example, graduate nurses who have completed their course of study but have not yet written their CNATs). It will be valid for a maximum of the earlier of three years or a lesser period stated in the certificate. A Provisional member also may not perform a delegated controlled act and may not self-initiate or delegate a controlled act (see Controlled Acts, below).

The General class applies to members fully qualified to practise within the full scope of nursing.

The Temporary class is reserved for those who will practise only for a specific period of time.

It is the role of the registration committee to review those applications for membership that do not fully comply with the detailed registration requirements. Thus, the committee would, for example, review a foreign applicant's educational credentials to determine whether or not they are equivalent to those that an Ontario resident would obtain in an approved nursing program in that province. As part of its review the committee might find that a particular aspect of that applicant's training was deficient and may order him or her to take further courses or practical training. Alternatively, they may require a person to take and to pass further examinations set by the panel of the committee reviewing the particular case.[104] The Registrar or the committee may impose restrictions and conditions on the granting of a certificate of any class to the applicant. It may also recommend that the Registrar grant a certificate to a person who does not meet all the requirements, except where the requirements cannot be exempted. Any terms and conditions imposed on the certificate must be consented to by the applicant.

The HPPC sets out specific procedures for review of an application. Provisions for notice of the proceedings to the applicant, as well as for reasons why the application has not been automatically approved, are outlined.[105] The applicant is given the right to make written submissions to the committee within thirty days of being given such notice by the Registrar. The review is actually undertaken by a panel of at least three members of the committee. Once a certificate with conditions or limitations is issued, the applicant may later request the committee to vary those conditions and limitations. The committee would do so presumably in the event that the applicant has demonstrated that he or she has met the conditions originally imposed, such as, for example, passing an examination or taking further courses or training.

If the applicant is not satisfied with the committee's decision, he or she may appeal it to the Health Professions Board within thirty days of receiving written notice of the committee's decision.[106] The committee is also given notice of the applicant's appeal, and has fifteen days to respond in writing to the Board. If such an appeal is launched, the committee's decision may not be carried out until and unless it is confirmed by the Board upon review or until the expiration of the time for launching an appeal (i.e., thirty days). The review is conducted by a panel of the Board consisting of at least three but no more than five of its members as selected by the chair. Applicants are given opportunity to make their case before the Board. It may confirm or vary the order of the registration committee or may send the decision, together with the Board's recommendations, back to the committee for further consideration.

The Registrar of the College is charged with keeping a complete and timely register of the names of all members of the College. The register includes details of the class of certificate held by each member. In addition, terms and conditions (if any) imposed on a member's certificate, plus information required to be kept on a member by the committees on fitness and discipline, should be noted. Finally, the Registrar may suspend a member for failure to pay required fees upon giving the defaulting member two months' notice.

The Complaints Committee

This committee deals with complaints about a member's conduct or incompetence brought by such member's patients, colleagues, or other persons. A complaint filed with the Registrar of the College is investigated by a panel of three members of the committee selected by the chair.[107] A complaint must be in writing or recorded on tape, film, disk, or other such medium. If it alleges sexual abuse by a member, it may also be referred by the panel to the quality assurance committee after the panel has concluded its investigation.

The committee's role is to screen complaints involving specific allegations concerning a member's conduct or competence, which may then be referred to the discipline committee. However, the committee may choose to take no further action if it finds the complaint unsubstantiated or frivolous; or it may caution the member about his or her conduct; or it may refer the matter to the executive committee for incapacity proceedings if the conduct demonstrates that the member is incapable of safe or proper practice because of a mental or physical problem.

Before the investigation, the member complained of must be given a copy of the complaint. The committee investigates the complaint and on completion, is required to give the complainant and the member a written notice of its decision within 120 days, otherwise the Health Professions Board may investigate the complaint itself. This is meant to ensure the timely disposition of complaints. If the panel decides to take no action, it must give to both the complainant and the member a copy of its reasons and a notice advising them of the right to request a review of the panel's decision by the Health Professions Board within thirty days.[108] A decision to refer the matter to the discipline committee or the executive committee cannot be appealed. In an appeal to the Health Professions Board, both the complainant and the member who is the subject of the complaint are parties to the appeal. Each is entitled to participate in the review.

The Discipline Committee

The discipline committee is responsible for investigating and adjudicating upon matters involving unethical or otherwise unprofessional conduct of members. This includes matters involving sexual misconduct. It is important to stress that the *Health Professions Procedural Code* applies to all health professions stipulated in statute in Ontario. Any member of any health profession who is alleged to have sexually harassed either a patient, a colleague, or a member of another health profession, including nursing, is subject to the same complaints and disciplinary procedures as nurses. Therefore, the procedures for initiating complaints, including those involving allegations of sexual misconduct, may be used by nurses in respect of improper conduct by other health professionals or fellow members of the College of Nurses.

If, as part of an investigation of a complaint against a member, a specific allegation of professional misconduct is found (since not all complaints against health professionals, no matter how justified, will necessarily involve professional misconduct), the executive committee may refer the matter to the discipline committee.[109] In the case of sexual misconduct, the executive committee, in deciding whether to refer the matter to the discipline committee, must consider the reports filed by other health professionals with respect to the member's conduct and, in particular, their opinions as to the likelihood of the member's abusing patients in the future.[110] In the meantime, the member's licence may be suspended or restrictions may be placed on the member's certificate of registration. However, the member must be notified in writing of the committee's intentions before such restrictions or suspension may be imposed.

Where the matter is referred to the discipline committee, a hearing will be held by a panel of at least three but no more than five members of that committee. The professional whose conduct is being investigated has the right to participate in the proceedings and to be represented by a lawyer.[111] The College and the professional against whom allegations have been made will be the parties to the hearing. If another person's conduct, competence, or good character is an issue in the proceedings against the professional, that other person may also be permitted to participate in the hearing to the extent permitted by the panel hearing the matter.

The professional complained of must be given at least ten days' advance opportunity to examine any evidence and a copy of any expert's report to be given at the hearing. He or she must be advised of the identity of any witnesses who will be testifying. If these requirements are not met, the evidence will be inadmissible. However, the panel still has the power to allow the evidence if it ensures that the professional's interests in the case are not harmed thereby, that is, that he or she is not harmed by the lack of notice or opportunity to examine the evidence in advance of the hearing.

The hearing will normally be open to the public; however, where issues of personal privacy or safety or public security outweigh the policy of open proceedings, the hearing may be closed. As well, any evidence disclosed at an in camera hearing must not be disclosed to the public or anyone not involved in the hearing.[112] If a witness will be testifying as to the professional's sexual misconduct (including, but not limited to, sexual abuse), that person's identity must, at the person's request, be kept confidential. All evidence given at the hearing must be recorded, and a transcript made available to any party at that party's request and expense.

The panel is also bound by the rules of evidence. Any evidence that could not be admitted in a civil court cannot be admitted at the hearing. In making its findings, the panel must confine itself to considering the evidence properly before it.[113] In other words, the panel cannot consider anything that its members may have heard or read (e.g., in the news media or in discussions or conversations outside the hearing), nor may it consider any evidence that it has ruled to be inadmissible. As well, it would be ethically improper and illegal for any member of the panel to discuss the matter with other persons outside the confines of the hearing room.

If a member has been found guilty of an offence relevant to his or her suitability to practise, has sexually abused a patient, has been found guilty of professional misconduct in a jurisdiction outside Ontario, or has committed an act of professional misconduct as defined by regulations passed by the College, that panel must find the member guilty of professional misconduct.[114]

The College of Nurses of Ontario has passed extensive definitions of professional misconduct, including thirty-seven specific acts. Examples include contravening a standard of practice of the profession or failing to meet the standard of practice of the profession[115]; improperly discontinuing professional services that are needed unless requested by the client to do so, or unless alternative services are arranged, or the client is given a reasonable opportunity to arrange alternative or replacement services[116]; abusing a client verbally, physically, or emotionally[117]; or failing to keep records as required.[118]

One interesting provision having important consequences for nurses states that it is professional misconduct to do anything to a client for a therapeutic, preventive, palliative, diagnostic, cosmetic, or other health-related purpose where consent is required by law, without first obtaining such consent.[119] This is significant in light of Ontario's *Consent to Treatment Act, 1992*,[120] which deals with a patient's consent to medical treatment. This statute contains provisions for informed consent and disclosure of material risks. It will be discussed further in Chapter 6.

The penalties that may be levied against the guilty professional include revocation or suspension of the certificate of registration; imposition of terms, conditions, or limitations on the certificate for a specified period of time, including criteria that must be satisfied before the restrictions, terms, or conditions may be lifted; a reprimand by the panel; or a fine of up to $35 000.

Where the professional has been found guilty of sexual misconduct, he or she can be ordered to reimburse the College for expenses incurred in providing a program for therapy and counselling for patients who were sexually abused by professionals.[121] The guilty professional may also be reprimanded, or his or her licence may be revoked if the sexual abuse consisted of certain specified acts.[122] In such a case, the patient is allowed to make, and the panel must consider, a statement describing the impact that the abuse has had on him or her.

The panel may also, in an appropriate case, order the guilty professional to pay the College's legal costs, its costs of investigating the matter, and of participating in the hearing. A panel might make such an award where the case against the professional was clear and the evidence against him or her so compelling that the professional should have admitted his or her responsibility, but instead chose to force the matter to a hearing.

The committee may find that the professional is incompetent. If his or her professional care demonstrated a lack of knowledge, skill, or judgement, or exhibited disregard for the welfare of a patient, this behaviour may be deemed incompetent. If the professional's conduct demonstrates that he or she is unfit to continue to practise, or that his or her practice should be restricted, the committee may also find that professional incompetent to practise. This is different from a finding of professional misconduct.

Regardless of the nature of the finding, the panel must render its decision in writing and give it to all parties. The College is required by the HPPC to publish its decisions and the reasons for these, including the member's name if he or she requests it, in its annual report and in any other of its publications. (A member might make such a request, for example, where he or she has been cleared of any wrongdoing and wishes to make this known to colleagues and patients.)

The Fitness to Practise Committee

Situations may arise concerning a member's fitness and capacity to practise. Investigation of such matters is the responsibility of the fitness to practise committee of the College of Nurses. Such an investigation will not necessarily raise questions of professional misconduct, but the member's behaviour may be such that there is doubt as to his or her physical or mental abilities.

Inquiries as to a professional's capacity will usually be commenced by the Registrar, using the extensive investigatory powers granted under the HPPC. If the Registrar has reason to believe that the member in question may be incapacitated, the Registrar must report these findings to the executive committee for further action.[123] If further action is warranted, and it has received the Registrar's report or a referral from a panel of the complaints committee, the fitness to practise committee may appoint a board of inquiry to determine whether the professional is incapacitated. A notice of the inquiry must be given to the professional. Some of the board must be drawn from among the College's general membership. In this way, the professional's fitness to practise is evaluated by his or her peers.

As part of its inquiry, the board may order the member to undergo any physical or psychological examinations conducted or ordered by a health professional (e.g., a physician or psychiatrist). Furthermore, the member's licence may be suspended until he or she agrees to be examined.[124] Upon conclusion of the inquiry, the board is required to submit its report to the executive committee which, in turn, may refer it to the fitness to practise committee if it decides that further proceedings are necessary. The professional's licence may be suspended or restricted in the interim on such terms as that committee may order. In any such decision, however, the professional must be notified in writing of the committee's or the board's intention to suspend or place restrictions on the his or her certificate. The professional has fourteen days in which to make written submissions to the committee or board stating why such suspension or restrictions should not be imposed.

The fitness to practise committee then selects a panel of at least three of its members to hold a hearing into the fitness of the professional to practise nursing. Since a hearing will be held, the professional is again entitled to be represented by legal counsel, as are any witnesses who will testify, including any person who may have suffered harm or have been otherwise affected by the member's conduct. Evidence at the hearing will include testimony by medical or psychiatric experts. However, the professional who is the subject of the hearing must be given a copy of the expert's report or a summary of the evidence before it is presented at the hearing.

Unless the professional requests otherwise, the hearing must be closed. The professional's request for a public hearing may be refused if this would compromise public security, or any person's safety or privacy.[125] If the panel concludes that the professional is incapacitated, his or her certificate of registration may be revoked or suspended, or conditions, terms, or restrictions may be imposed on that certificate. In cases where a certificate has been revoked, the professional may apply to the Registrar to have a new certificate issued, or the suspension removed, no earlier than one year after the suspension or revocation.[126]

If the application is turned down by the committee that originally ordered the suspension or revocation (e.g., discipline, fitness to practise), the professional may not bring another application for reinstatement until six months after the decision on the first application for reinstatement.[127] In an application for reinstatement, the committee may lift the suspension or revocation or order the Registrar to impose terms, conditions, and limitations on the certificate.

Any party to a proceeding before the Health Professions Board concerning a registration hearing or review, or before a panel of the discipline or fitness to practise committees (except a hearing for reinstatement), can appeal a decision of one of these bodies to the Divisional Court of Ontario. However, there is no suspension of the order revoking or suspending the member's certificate pending the outcome of such appeal.[128]

The Quality Assurance Committee

Every health profession's college is required under the RHPA to establish a quality assurance committee whose task is to review and examine individual members' practices to identify incompetency, incapacity, professional misconduct, and in particular, the sexual abuse of patients by health professionals. For example, if either the executive committee, the complaints committee, or the Health Professions Board receives a report from the Registrar following an investigation into a member's conduct involving sexual remarks or behaviour directed toward a patient, it may refer the matter to the quality assurance committee.

The HPPC defines sexual abuse of a patient as "sexual intercourse or other forms of sexual relations between the member and the patient, touching of a sexual nature of the patient by the member, or behaviour or remarks of a sexual nature by the member towards the patient"[129] unless it is touching, behaviour, or remarks of a clinical nature that are appropriate in the context of the treatment being provided by the member.

The quality assurance committee will conduct its own investigation into the professional's practice, not only to identify incompetency or incapacity, but also to pinpoint inadequacies in the professional's overall practice, including its operations and facilities. It may appoint an assessor to enter and inspect the professional's premises and records, obtain any other information on the professional concerning the care of patients, confer with the professional concerning the conduct, or require the professional to participate in a program designed to evaluate his or her skill, knowledge, and judgement. Anyone having control of such premises or records must allow an assessor to inspect them unless that person is a patient or a representative of a patient.

If the quality assurance committee believes that, based on its assessment, the professional may have committed an act of misconduct, or may be incompetent or incapacitated, it may disclose the professional's name to the executive committee and the allegations against him or her. On receipt of such information, the committee would refer the matter to the discipline committee or the fitness to practise committee, as required.[130]

The Patient Relations Program and Committee

In conjunction with the activities of the quality assurance committee with respect to sexual abuse of patients by professionals, the College is also required to establish and implement a patient relations program commencing December 31, 1994.[131] This program is intended to prevent and deal with the sexual abuse of patients by health care professionals governed by the RHPA. It requires each college to adopt educational requirements for its members dealing with sexual abuse, guidelines for the conduct of members with their patients, training for college staff in this area, and the dissemination of information to the public regarding the program. The Council of the College will be required to submit a written report describing its program and any changes after the program is implemented. The role of the patient relations committee is to advise the Council as to the nature and content of such a program. Membership of this committee also consists of members of the College who are not members of its Council.

In addition, the HPPC requires any health professional to report a member of any health profession where the person has reasonable grounds, obtained in the course of practice, to believe that the other has sexually abused a patient.[132] The reporting member must file a complaint in writing with the other professional's college, stating the nature of the allegations, the offender's name, and the reporting member's name within thirty days of becoming aware of the sexual abuse. The patient's name may be disclosed in such report only with the patient's consent. Each college must set up and fund a therapy and counselling program for patients who have been sexually abused by its members. Such programs are administered by the patient relations committee.

Controlled Acts

One of the distinctive features of Ontario's system of regulation of the health professions is that the law specifically defines which medical actions and procedures may be performed, and who may perform and delegate them. The system no longer licenses areas of practice, but focusses on these specific acts.

Thus, being a registered nurse does not grant a blanket authorization to perform controlled procedures that the nurse believes to be a part of the profession. A nurse may perform only those controlled acts that nurses are specifically authorized to perform. Needless to say, any act within the scope of nursing practice may be performed by a registered nurse or practical nurse unless it is specifically designated a controlled act, in which case that act may be performed by the nurse only if he or she is authorized by the RHPA, the HPPC, the *Nursing Act, 1991,* and nursing regulations to perform it.

The RHPA strictly regulates health care controlled acts,[133] and states who may perform or delegate them, to whom and by whom. In addition, the registration committee or the Registrar may impose restrictions or limitations upon a specific nurse's right to practise nursing.

The RHPA sets out thirteen controlled acts, which may be performed only by members of a professional college authorized by the college's particular governing statute and regulations[134] to perform the controlled act.[135] If the particular act is to be delegated, it may be delegated only by a member so authorized and only in conformity with the regulations made under the statute governing the member's profession. For example, if a registered nurse is authorized to administer a particular substance by injection,[136] then he or she may delegate the act to a registered practical nurse, provided that the regulations under the *Nursing Act* allow such delegation, and all procedures for delegation set out in such regulations are followed.

The thirteen **controlled acts** include:

(1) communicating a diagnosis or a disorder or disease to a person or that person's personal representative where it is reasonable to believe the person or the representative would rely on such diagnosis;

(2) performing a procedure below the dermis, surface of the mucous membrane, the cornea, or in or below the surface of the teeth (including scaling teeth);

(3) setting or casting a fracture of a bone or a dislocation of a joint;

(4) moving the joints of the spine beyond a person's normal range of motion using a fast, low-amplitude thrust;

(5) administering a substance by injection or inhalation;

(6) putting an instrument, hand, or finger beyond the external ear canal, the point in the nasal passages where they normally narrow, the larynx, the urethral opening, the labia majora, the anal verge, or into an artificial opening into the body;

(7) applying or ordering the application of a form of energy controlled and authorized by law (e.g., radiation);

(8) prescribing, dispensing, or selling drugs (e.g., controlled drugs);

(9) prescribing or dispensing contact lenses or eye glasses other than simple magnifiers;

(10) prescribing hearing aids;

(11) fitting or prescribing a dental prosthesis or periodontal appliance or

device used inside the mouth to protect teeth from abnormal function;
(12) managing labour or delivery of a baby; and
(13) allergy testing.[137]

It is readily apparent that some of these acts would never, under normal circumstances, be performed by a registered nurse or registered practical nurse. Of these thirteen, registered nurses and practical nurses (in certain circumstances) are authorized to perform three, namely items 2 (only those specific procedures below the dermis or mucous membranes, as allowed in the regulations made by the College), 5 (administering a substance by injection or inhalation), and 6 (intrusions by finger, hand, or instrument, as outlined in the regulations made by the College).[138]

Interestingly enough, people falling into certain categories are authorized to perform a great many of these acts regardless of whether or not they are members of a health profession. The RHPA allows anyone to perform any such act if it is done when rendering first aid or temporary assistance in an emergency.[139] This is designed to encourage people to give aid and render assistance in emergencies without fear of contravening the law.

A person is allowed to perform these acts if they are done to fulfil the requirements to become a member of a health profession and the acts are within the scope of practice of that profession and are supervised by a member of that profession,[140] or if the person performs such an act when treating a member of the person's household.[141] In this latter case, however, only those acts numbered 1, 5, or 6 in the above list may be performed.

Exemptions

A person may also perform the acts set out in items 5 and 6 if he or she is assisting someone with that person's routine activities of daily living. This would apply, for example, in the case of a home care worker or friend who was assisting a handicapped person in certain daily tasks which that person could not do unassisted. There has been some concern with this particular exemption. It is felt that persons involved in providing attendant care to the disabled will fall outside the regulatory scheme of the RHPA, thereby defeating the purpose of regulation. On the other hand, advocates for the disabled argued, prior to passage of this legislation, that they did not wish for activities of daily life of the disabled to be subject to governmental regulation and potential interference. This would have occurred had this exemption not been included.

If such an act is done in the context of treating a person by spiritual means in accordance with the tenets of the religion of the person giving the treatment, this is permitted.[142] It is difficult, however, to envisage a situation in which some of these enumerated acts would be performed in a spiritual or religious ceremony, especially procedures below the dermis, or the administration of substances by injection or inhalation. Certain specific acts, such as religious circumcision, are expressly permitted.[143]

The Act also exempts certain communication when it is made in the course of counselling a person about emotional, social, educational, or spiritual matters, provided that the communication is not one that a health profession Act autho-rizes a member to make.[144] Equally significant, the RHPA does not apply to aboriginal healers or midwives when they are providing their services to mem-bers of an aboriginal community.[145] This would, for example, exempt aboriginal healers providing services to residents of an Indian reserve or members of an Indian band. However, if the aboriginal healer is a member of a college, he or she is still subject to its jurisdiction, regulations, and by-laws.

The fact that persons are permitted to perform acts 1, 5, or 6 in the context of treating a member of their household raises some interesting situations. For example, suppose a registered nurse in charge of and responsible for the care of a terminally ill patient is asked by a member of that patient's family to permit a family member to administer morphine by injection to the patient to control pain. The RHPA would allow this provided that the nurse, having delegated a controlled act, ensured that the family member had been adequately instructed in the administration of injections, and that all necessary procedures had been followed.

Use of titles

Apart from regulating the performance and delegation of controlled acts, the RHPA also controls and restricts the use of certain professional titles such as "doctor,"[146] "nurse," "registered nurse," "registered practical nurse," or "regis-tered nursing assistant."[147] In addition, no person may represent to anyone that he or she is qualified to practise nursing in Ontario as an RN or an RPN or as a specialist in nursing unless that person in a member of the College.[148] Anyone violating these provisions is guilty of an offence and is liable to a fine of up to $5000 for a first offence, and up to $10 000 for each subsequent offence.[149]

Other offences

Both the RHPA and the *Nursing Act, 1991* set out other offences. These include obtaining employment for an individual knowing that that person is not com-petent to perform the duties of that position without contravening a provision of the RHPA.[150]

A distinction should be drawn here. "Competent" is used in the sense that the professional has the necessary skills, experience, and knowledge to carry out the duties of the particular provision. This is quite different from being "registered" or "authorized" to perform those duties. The latter expressions convey the idea that an official regulatory agency has assessed and passed judgement upon that person's skills and knowledge and has found these to meet the requirements of regulations. For example, suppose an employment agency found a position for a private nurse who was not a member or was not properly qualified in Ontario, knowing full well that that person was unable to perform any of the controlled acts that nurses are permitted to perform.

Other offences include: obtaining a registration certificate from any one of the colleges by false pretences or knowingly assisting a person to do this[151]; ob-structing an investigator appointed by the Registrar of the College in an investigation into professional misconduct, incompetency, or incapacity of a member[152]; disclosing any information revealed at a hearing or inquiry that is closed to the public[153]; failing to permit an assessor of the quality assurance committee of a college to inspect a member's records or premises[154]; and failing to report a member (of the same or any other college) when there are reasonable grounds to believe that that member has sexually abused a patient.[155]

Finally, no professional may treat a person where it is reasonably foreseeable that serious physical harm may result from the treatment or advice or from an omission from such treatment or advice.[156] Therefore, if serious physical harm is likely to result from a particular treatment or advice given to a patient, that treatment must not be undertaken, nor the advice given. Counselling about emotional, social, educational, or spiritual matters is excepted. These might result in psychological harm to the person, but this is not prohibited by the RHPA. Despite this, it would certainly be unethical to counsel someone such that psychological harm might foreseeably come to that person. Perhaps including "psychological" or "mental" harm in this prohibition would have placed too onerous a burden on health professionals as the mind, its workings, and the genesis of mental disorders are still imperfectly understood. Others would argue that this gap in the law is a further example that what is legal is not necessarily ethical.

Summary

The key points introduced in this chapter include:
- the scope of laws regulating the nursing profession across Canada
- the role, function, and responsibility of nursing governing bodies
- some of the rules and standards regulating the nursing profession
- the processes and procedures used by governing bodies relating to registration, complaints, discipline, and quality assurance.

References

1. *Health Disciplines Act*, RSA 1980, c. H-3.5, as amended.
2. *Health Professions Act*, SBC 1990, c. 50, amended by SBC 1993, c. 48 and c. 50.
3. Properly referred to as the "Health Professions Council" in British Columbia.
4. RSBC 1979, c. 302, as amended.
5. *Nurses (Licensed Practical) Act*, RSBC 1979, c. 300, section 3(1).
6. RSBC 1979, c. 301, as amended.
7. Supra footnote 4, section 3.1(1), amended by SBC 1988, c. 51, section 7.
8. RSA 1980, c. N-14.5, as amended.
9. Supra footnote 1.
10. See British Columbia: *Nurses (Registered) Act*, supra footnote 4, section 2; Alberta: *Nursing Profession Act*, supra footnote 8, section 8(1); Yukon Territory: *Registered Nurses Profession Act*, SY 1992, c. 11, section 2; Northwest Territories: *Nursing Profession Act*, RSNWT 1990, c. N-4, section 2(1); Saskatchewan: *The Registered Nurses Act*, 1988, SS 1988, c. R-12.2, section 3; Manitoba: *The Registered Nurses Act*, CCSM, c. R40, section 2, SM 1989–90, c. 91, section 9; New

Brunswick: *Nurses Act*, SNB 1984, c. 71, section 3; Nova Scotia: *Registered Nurses' Association Act*, RSNS 1989, c. 391, section 3; Prince Edward Island: *Nurses Act*, RSPEI 1988, c. N-4, section 2; Newfoundland: *Registered Nurses Act*, RSN 1990, c. R-9, section 3(1).

11. See Northwest Territories: *Nursing Profession Act*, supra footnote 10, section 3; Yukon Territory: *Registered Nurses Profession Act*, supra footnote 10, section 3; British Columbia: *Nurses (Registered) Act*, supra footnote 4, section 2.1, added by SBC 1993, c. 50, section 38; Prince Edward Island: *Nurses Act*, supra footnote 10, section 9; Newfoundland: *Registered Nurses Act*, supra footnote 10, section 5.

12. See the discussion of Ontario's *Health Professions Procedural Code*, below.

13. British Columbia Act, supra footnote 4, section 28(1).

14. Alberta Act, supra footnote 8, sections 82 and 83. The appeal is heard by an Appeals Committee of the Council of the Association.

15. Yukon Act, supra footnote 10, section 52(1). The appeal is heard by an Appeals Committee of the Board.

16. Saskatchewan Act, supra footnote 10, section 34(1).

17. Manitoba Act, supra footnote 10, section 38(1).

18. New Brunswick Act, supra footnote 10, section 34(1).

19. Nova Scotia Act, supra footnote 10, section 47.

20. Prince Edward Island Act, supra footnote 10, section 27(1).

21. British Columbia Act, supra footnote 4, sections 8(1) and 28(1).

22. Ibid., sections 8 and 9; Prince Edward Island Act, supra footnote 10, sections 12 and 13; and Newfoundland Act, supra footnote 10, section 12.

23. British Columbia Act, supra footnote 4, sections 1 and 12(1); Alberta Act, supra footnote 8, sections 14 and 15 and Alta. Reg. 453/83, sections 3 and 4; Saskatchewan Act, supra footnote 10, section 19; Manitoba Act, supra footnote 10, section 7 and Man. Reg. 459/88, sections 1 and 2; Nova Scotia Act, supra footnote 10, section 7 and NS Reg. 112/86, regulations 2 and 3; Prince Edward Island Act, supra footnote 10, sections 13 through 16 and PEI Reg. EC583/86, sections 2, 3, and 4; Newfoundland Act, supra footnote 10, section 8.

24. British Columbia Act, supra footnote 4, section 13.1; Alberta Act, supra footnote 8, sections 38 and 39; Saskatchewan Act, supra footnote 10, section 20.

25. Saskatchewan Act, supra footnote 10, section 23(1); New Brunswick Act, supra footnote 10, sections 12(1) and 12(14); and Prince Edward Island Act, supra footnote 10, section 17.

26. British Columbia Act, supra footnote 4, sections 15 and 37; Alberta Act, supra footnote 8, sections 3(1), 5, and 107(1); Saskatchewan Act, supra footnote 10, sections 23, 24, and 42(1); Yukon Act, supra footnote 10, sections 14 and 15; Northwest Territories Act, supra footnote 10, sections 30 and 31; Manitoba Act, supra footnote 10, sections 8(1), 10(2) and 50(1) and (2); New Brunswick Act, supra footnote 10, sections 19 and 21; Nova Scotia Act, supra footnote 10, sections 13, 14, and 21; Prince Edward Island Act, supra footnote 10, sections 15, 17, and 28; Newfoundland Act, supra footnote 10, sections 16(1), 18, 23, and 25.

27. See, e.g., Saskatchewan Act, supra footnote 10, section 26(2)(q).

28. See, e.g., Alberta Act, supra footnote 8, section 27(2).

29. Northwest Territories Act, supra footnote 10, section 29.

30. Newfoundland Act, supra footnote 10, section 22(a).

31. *Health Professions Procedural Code*, infra footnote 87, sections 85.1(1) and 85.3(4), added by SO 1993, c. 37, section 23.

32. Manitoba Act, supra footnote 10, section 46(2).

33. Nova Scotia Act, supra footnote 10, section 22; Manitoba Act, supra footnote 10, section 22; Yukon Act, supra footnote 10, section 24; New Brunswick Act, supra footnote 10, section 29.

34. Newfoundland Act, supra footnote 10, sections 21(1) and (1.1), added by SN 1992, c. 28, section 1(1).

35. British Columbia Act, supra footnote 4, section 23.2, added by SBC 1993, c. 50, section 40; Yukon Act, supra footnote 10, section 24(4); Manitoba Act, supra footnote 10, sections 28, 29, and 30.

36. See, e.g., Saskatchewan Act, supra footnote 10, section 26(2); and Northwest Territories Act, supra footnote 10, section 22 (improper conduct).

37. *Mans v. Council of Licensed Practical Nurses* (1990), 14 CHRR D/221; aff'd. (1993), 77 BCLR (2d) 47 (CA).
38. SBC 1984, c. 22.
39. British Columbia Act, supra footnote 4, section 28, as amended by SBC 1988, c. 51, section 29.
40. This list is not exhaustive. There are many other professions regulated by this Act.
41. RSQ, c. C-26, as amended.
42. Ibid., section 12, as amended.
43. Ibid.
44. Ibid., section 16, as amended.
45. RSQ, c. I-8, section 36.
46. However, the *Professional Code,* section 87, requires the Bureau of the Corporation professionelle des infirmières et infirmiers to make a code of ethics.
47. Supra footnote 45, section 2, as amended.
48. Ibid., section 5, as amended.
49. Ibid., sections 16 and 17, as amended.
50. Ibid., sections 18 and 19, as amended.
51. Supra footnote 45.
52. Supra footnote 41, sections 87 through 93, as amended.
53. Ibid., section 86, as amended.
54. Supra footnote 46, regulation 3.
55. Supra footnote 41, section 87, as amended.
56. Supra footnote 46, regulation 4.
57. Ibid., sections 3.03.01 through 3.06.06.
58. Supra footnote 46, sections 33 and 34, as amended.
59. Ibid., section 21.
60. RRQ 1981, c. I-8, regulation 14.
61. Supra footnote 46, section 14, as amended.
62. Ibid., section 24, as amended.
63. Ibid., sections 24, 25, and 28, as amended.
64. Ibid., section 31.
65. Ibid., sections 31.2 and 31.3, added by SQ 1989, c. 32, section 10.
66. Supra footnote 41, section 90, as amended.
67. Ibid., section 114, as amended.
68. Ibid., section 188, as amended.
69. Ibid., section 164, as amended.
70. Ibid., section 162, as amended.
71. Ibid., sections 127 and 129. A solemn affirmation is given in place of an oath (which is usually sworn before God on a Bible or other holy book) in cases where a witness feels that his or her conscience would not be bound by swearing an oath to God (e.g., when a person who does not believe in God is making a complaint or giving testimony).
72. Ibid., section 128.
73. Ibid., section 116.
74. Ibid., sections 121 and 122.
75. Ibid., section 130.
76. Ibid., sections 132 through 134, as amended.
77. Ibid., sections 144 and 149.
78. Ibid., sections 150, 151, 152, and 154, as amended.
79. Ibid., section 159, as amended.
80. Ibid., section 160, as amended.
81. Ibid., section 161, as amended.
82. Ibid., section 164, as amended.
83. Ibid., sections 173 and 175, as amended.
84. SO 1991, c. 18, section 18.
85. Ibid., sections 18, 19, and 20.

86. Ibid., section 24.
87. Ibid., Schedule 2 (herein referred to as "HPPC").
88. SO 1991, c. 32.
89. Ibid., section 2(1).
90. Ibid.
91. Ibid., section 3.
92. Ibid., section 7.
93. Ibid., section 8.
94. HPPC, supra footnote 87, section 3(1).
95. Ibid., section 3(2).
96. Ibid., section 4.
97. Nursing Act, 1991, supra footnote 88, section 9(1)(a).
98. Ibid., section 10.
99. HPPC, supra footnote 87, section 10(1).
100. Ibid., section 12(1).
101. O. Reg. 653/93, section 3.
102. HPPC, supra footnote 87, section 15(1).
103. O. Reg. 868/93, sections 1 and 2.
104. HPPC, supra footnote 87, section 18(2).
105. Ibid., section 15(3).
106. Ibid., sections 21(1) and (2).
107. HPPC, supra footnote 87, section 25.
108. Ibid., sections 26, 27, and 29.
109. Ibid., section 36(1), as amended by SO 1993, c. 37, section 9.
110. Ibid., section 36(2), enacted by SO 1993, c. 37, section 9.
111. Statutory Powers and Procedure Act, RSO 1990, c. S.22, section 10.
112. HPPC, supra footnote 87, section 45.
113. Ibid., section 49.
114. Ibid., section 51(1), as amended by SO 1993, c. 37, section 14(1).
115. O. Reg. 799/93, section 1, paragraph 1.
116. Ibid., paragraph 5.
117. Ibid., paragraph 7.
118. Ibid., paragraph 13. There are many more acts deemed "professional misconduct" contained in this regulation, which should be carefully consulted by the nursing professional.
119. Ibid., paragraph 9.
120. SO 1992, c. 31. This legislation, while not yet proclaimed into law at the time of writing, is expected to come into force in April 1995.
121. HPPC, supra footnote 87, section 51(2), paragraphs 5 and 5.1, as repealed and re-enacted by SO 1993, c. 37, section 14(2).
122. Ibid., section 51(5), enacted by SO 1993, c. 37, section 14(3).
123. Ibid., section 57.
124. Ibid., section 59.
125. Ibid., section 68.
126. Ibid., section 72(1).
127. Ibid., section 72(2).
128. Ibid., sections 70 and 71.
129. Ibid., section 1(3), enacted by SO 1993, c. 37, section 4.
130. Ibid., sections 80 through 83.
131. Ibid., section 84. This section of the HPPC came into force on December 31, 1994, that is, one year after the RHPA came into force.
132. Ibid., section 85.1(1), enacted by SO 1993, c. 37, section 23.
133. RHPA, supra footnote 84, section 27.
134. See Nursing Act, 1991, supra footnote 88, section 4, paragraph 2.
135. Ibid., section 27(1)(a).
136. This is a controlled act under section 27(2), paragraph 5 of the RHPA.

137. Ibid., section 27(2).
138. The regulations with respect to which controlled acts could lawfully be self-initiated or delegated by members, and how, had not yet been passed and were still being negotiated between the Council of College of Nurses of Ontario and the Minister of Health of Ontario at the time of writing.
139. RHPA, supra footnote 84, section 29(1)(a).
140. Ibid., section 29(1)(b).
141. Ibid., section 29(1)(d).
142. Ibid., section 29(1)(c).
143. O. Reg. 887/93, section 2.
144. Supra footnote 84, section 29(2).
145. Ibid., section 35(1).
146. RHPA, supra footnote 84, section 33, Only chiropractors, optometrists, physicians and surgeons, psychologists, and dentists or dental surgeons may use this title.
147. Nursing Act, 1991, supra footnote 88, section 11. The title "registered nursing assistant" and these other titles may be used only by members of the College. Since RNAs will now be called "registered practical nurses," the title "registered nursing assistant" may be used only for a further period of three years from the day the Act came into force, i.e., December 31, 1993. Thereafter, such members may be referred to only as "nurses" or "registered practical nurses." Despite these restrictions, Christian Science nurses may continue to use that title even though they may not be members of the College (section 11(2)).
148. Ibid., section 11(5).
149. RHPA, supra footnote 84, section 40(2); Nursing Act, 1991, supra footnote 88, section 13.
150. RHPA, supra footnote 84, section 41.
151. HPPC, supra footnote 87, section 92.
152. Ibid., section 93(2).
153. Ibid., section 93(1).
154. Ibid., section 93(3).
155. Ibid., section 93(4), added by so 1993, c. 37, section 26(2).
156. RHPA, supra footnote 84, section 30(1).

Ethical Theoretical Perspectives

CHAPTER OBJECTIVES

The purpose of this chapter is to enable the reader to:
- appreciate the complexity of ethical choices nurses make
- understand the influence of values on ethical decision making
- realize the relevance of a solid understanding of ethical theory
- develop a basic understanding of ethical theory and principles
- use the *Code of Ethics* of the Canadian Nurses Association as a guide to ethical practice
- utilize tools and process to assist in identifying, understanding, and working through ethical challenges
- know when and how to utilize hospital ethics committees.

Nurses enjoy a position of extraordinary responsibility in our society. The decisions we make every day influence the quality of life and death of sick, vulnerable people who hold us in their trust. We must believe that our choices are the best we can make. As professionals we must clarify, and justify, our position and opinions to patients, colleagues, our profession, the organizations in which we are employed, and society as a whole.

The nature of our responsibilities forces us at times to make difficult decisions about complex issues. Often, we must choose our course of action from among several alternatives. The relative merit of these choices may be unclear, and we may have to choose the least wrong (or only slighter better) option. How, then, do we make choices that ensure optimal patient care? How do we determine whether the decisions we make are ethical? How can we identify ethical dilemmas and violations? When are ethical violations the result of poor communication and substandard patient care processes? In this chapter, we will show that the process of making and supporting ethical choices can be facilitated through a solid understanding of ethical theory and principles.

Nurses function within a health care team and must relate to many other health professionals. Each member of the team may have a different perspective on an ethical issue, or may share a similar position; but similarities, as well as differences, must be clarified. Without discussion and clarification, on occasion some decisions and actions undertaken by members of the team may be interpreted by others as wrong. If the reasons behind these decisions and actions are explained, they may more readily be understood and respected by others. Within health care, the choices are not easy; it may be difficult to determine, from among many alternative courses of action, which is the best.

Consider, for example, a situation in which the medical team may be aggressively treating a terminally ill patient in the Intensive Care Unit. Some nurses involved may consider this approach wrong because they believe that this plan will only diminish the quality of the dying patient's remaining life. If the medical staff were to clarify their position, the dissenting nurses might discover that the team's actions were based on a belief in the sanctity of life, and the view that the role of the physician is to preserve life at all costs. Possibly, on an earlier occasion, the patient may have asked the doctor to try anything that could preserve life. Though the views of some nurses may not change, they may come to a better understanding of the reasons behind the physicians' actions. This would reduce the moral conflict and distress experienced by some nurses, and ensure better relationships among members of the team.

It is imperative that physicians, nurses, and other team members discuss these kinds of issues together, and attempt to reach consensus on a course of action. Since most ethical dilemmas do not have clear-cut answers, collaboration and effective communication enhance the decision-making process. The communication that is necessary to clarify and justify our moral actions and choices to our professional colleagues is improved through a shared language grounded in a solid foundation of ethical theory. The entire process is enhanced through respect for each others' values and beliefs.

This chapter provides an overview of ethical theory and principles, and discusses the *Code of Ethics for Nursing* of the Canadian Nurses Association (CNA).[1] The CNA's *Code of Ethics* provides a framework to guide the ethical choices and actions of nurses. It makes explicit the rules of ethical conduct that guide Canadian nurses. Each provincial professional organization has its own code, but since the values and principles that guide each provincial code are consistent with those of the CNA, only that Code will be discussed. Thus, the CNA Code serves as a useful template to guide the ethical choices and actions of nurses in Canada.

This chapter will conclude with a framework to guide ethical discussion and decision making.

Ethical Theory

Ethics, the philosophical study of morality, is the systematic exploration of questions about what is morally right and morally wrong. It enables us to evaluate the variables that influence our moral decisions. Some of the factors that help us to determine right and wrong include the norms and beliefs of society, the context of the particular situation, previous experiences with similar situations, the potential outcomes or consequences of actions, the relationship of the individuals involved, and professional and individual values and beliefs. The field of *biomedical ethics* explores ethical questions and moral issues associated with health care. *Nursing ethics* focusses on the moral questions within the sphere of nursing practice and the nurse–patient relationship.

Nurses face ethical choices every day in their practice. The issues faced do not always make headlines. They may deal with important choices in the areas of pain control, patient comfort, restraints, patient choice, and family involvement in care. Ethics is involved when nurses decide how to allocate time and nursing care to patients. Ethics is involved when nurses decide whose needs are met first. Ethics is involved when we show respect for our patients, their families, ourselves, and each other.

Nurses are involved not only in the ethical context of the individual nurse–patient relationship. They are also affected by, and are in a position to influence, the wider context of health and the health care system. A rapidly changing environment influences the number and content of the issues they face. Ethical issues arise as new technology is introduced.

For example, advances in the area of transplantation and reproductive technology force questions about how we allocate these scarce resources, and indeed, whether we should be providing this technology at all. The growth of the consumer movement, the proliferation of special interest groups, and the occupational issues that arise out of collective bargaining and unionization all influence the context of health care today, and hence our ethical choices. The role of the nurse is expanding: nurses are being given more autonomy and with that, more authority and responsibility.

Ethical Issues Nurses Face

Nurses have the opportunity to defend and protect patient rights, to promote compassionate care, and to enhance the dignity and autonomy of patients. As stated earlier in this chapter, often nurses are required to choose from among a number of good or least wrong alternatives, and assess and defend the correctness of choices or actions taken. Many health care questions have no clear-cut answers; thus, how do we decide what is the right thing to do?

Within the context of a health care system strained by limited funds and resources, we frequently face the challenge of providing high-quality and ethical nursing care to our patients. The following scenarios are not uncommon.

An infant in a paediatric centre has been diagnosed with a malignant cerebral tumour. The infant is comatose and non-responsive, and on life support systems. There is nothing the team can do to halt the progress of this terminal disease. They believe it would be in the child's best interest to discontinue life support and to allow the child to die a natural death. The parents disagree and want all measures taken to save their child's life.

Who decides the best interests of this child? Do patients or families have the right to expensive, futile health care? How do the nurses support the parents through this crisis and their ultimate loss?

Joe, a twenty-year-old man diagnosed with schizophrenia since the age of sixteen, is admitted to the psychiatric unit of a community hospital. He is agitated and expresses a wish to "end all this pain." He refuses all medications to deal with his symptoms.

What rights does Joe have in this situation? Is there meaning behind Joe's wish to "end all this pain," or is this merely a symptom of his disease process?

A man with end-stage cancer of the liver is at home receiving palliative care. His wife and children, with minimal support from home care and community nurses, are his primary caregivers. As his condition deteriorates, his symptoms become more difficult to manage. As his family tires, they question whether he might be better in hospital. The patient, however, prefers to die at home.

How does the community nurse manage the conflicting interests of the patient and his family? What is society's role in ensuring adequate resources to address the needs of the dying patient at home?

An elderly patient in a geriatric unit is confused and agitated. The use of physical restraints is considered.

How do we balance the risks and benefits of this option and still respect the patient's wishes?

It is the middle of an evening shift on a busy medical unit. A patient is dying; family and friends are not around.

Do we let this patient die alone?

These are only a few of the complex and difficult issues that nurses face on a regular basis. Furthermore, it is common to confront a number of ethical issues and questions simultaneously. Limited understanding of ethical theory, the lack of knowledge and skill required to address these issues, and lack of appropriate system supports often lead to an avoidance of the issues. Nurses must be able to identify ethical issues and dilemmas, and be able to act toward their resolution, in order to ensure that the appropriate and most ethical care is provided to our patients.

Ethical dilemmas arise when the best course of action is not entirely clear, when we must choose between what is the most right or the least wrong. We rarely face these challenges alone, but as members of a health care team, we must be able to communicate about ethical issues with our colleagues, physicians, multidisciplinary team members, and the patients and families entrusted to our care. Ethical theories provide a framework of principles and rules to help identify ethical issues and reconcile ethical dilemmas or conflicts.

Values

Before we describe the more common ethical theories that are available to assist nurses in their ethical decision making, it is important to clarify the influence of values, not only with respect to ethical theory but to the norms, rules, and laws of our society. Further, since Canada comprises a mosaic of cultural and religious perspectives, nurses care for patients and families whose basic value systems and hence beliefs, rituals, and customs may differ from their own. An understanding of the role of values helps to ensure respect for these differences.

For example, cultural values may influence the beliefs a particular group or society may have about the body after death. These beliefs may then influence the rituals and behaviours associated with death and dying. Nurses who understand these values and differences can then clarify their own roles and enrich their relationship with their patients.

Dealing with differences can be stressful for nurses. Enhanced understanding minimizes this stress and contributes to role clarity and satisfaction. Further, when our behaviours are not congruent with our own values, internal conflicts can arise. It is therefore important for us to understand and respect the values that ground our own ethical perspectives. The *Code of Ethics* of the Canadian Nurses Association, described later in this chapter, articulates value statements to guide the ethical behaviour of nurses and the profession.

Influence on Ethical Decision Making

Our individual values influence how we respond to ethical issues and the decisions we make. A *value* is an ideal that has significant meaning or importance to an individual, a group, or a society. For example, in Canadian society we value individual freedom, health, fairness, honesty, and integrity. We see evidence of these values in our laws, our country's *Charter of Rights and Freedoms*, and our individual and collective actions and behaviours. The structure of the Canadian health care system demonstrates how we value equality, individual rights, health and well-being, quality of life, and human dignity. This is evident in the principle of *universality,* that is, the attempt to provide equal access to health and illness care to all Canadians regardless of where they live and their socio-economic status.

Values influence our beliefs, how we view others, and our opinions in such areas as literature, art, objectives, and ideals. Our behaviours, rituals, symbols, structures, rules, and laws represent the collective values and beliefs of our society. As nurses, we work with and care for others who may have values that differ from our own. In Canadian society, our patients represent a broad spectrum of cultural and religious perspectives. Thus, we must strive to clarify our own values, and respect and learn to understand the values of others.

Values may shift over time within a culture. For example, in recent years our society has become more sensitive to the meaning and quality of life versus prolonging life at all costs. This is evident in the current debates over euthanasia and physician-assisted suicide. Health care practices in the area of palliative care reinforce this growing concern for the quality and dignity of the dying process. Respect for individual rights and freedom is a modern concept that has emerged only over the past couple of centuries and still is more prevalent in western societies.

We develop our values through our life experiences. They emerge through our associations with other people: our families, classmates, friends, teachers, colleagues, personal relationships, religious experiences, and the environment we live in. In recent times, the media and television have also had a strong influence on value development.

Gender is also said to affect the development of values in individuals and groups.[2] Though changing, the nursing profession has been and continues to be dominated by women. As members of a primarily female profession, nurses have traditionally related to physicians, a male-dominated group whose values may have developed differently from our own. Our respective values may influence the perspectives that nurses and physicians bring to the ethical issues and dilemmas we share.

Professional values are an expansion and reflection of our personal values. These values emerge as we are socialized into the nursing profession. Sometimes there is a struggle between personal beliefs and professional responsibilities. As health care professionals, nurses face life-and-death situations, joy, pain, and sorrow that may alter our perspective and reshape and reorder our values. As a result, our combined professional and personal values emerge.

Value conflicts arise in situations where our actions conflict with our beliefs, and this results in stress for health professionals. Value conflict is evident when we hold different views of how a particular ethical dispute should be managed (e.g., withdrawal of treatment, abortion, euthanasia, patient restraint). Our duty as professionals and as members of a health care team requires that we understand and respect the values of other members of that team. Since conflict in values can result in moral distress for health care professionals, it is imperative that we understand our own values, articulate and clarify them to each other, and establish processes whereby this can be done.

Value Clarification

Value clarification facilitates mutual understanding. It is a process through which individuals come to understand what values they hold and the importance of these values relative to others. The values clarification process requires open discussion, communication, active listening, understanding, and mutual respect. The process is enhanced if we share the same language and terminology in relation to ethical issues. A focus on specific situations and case studies helps nurses to identify values, evaluate various responses to specific situations, and hence come to understand the respective perspectives on the issues.

Frequently, the demands of high workload in health care restrict the time available to health professionals to have these discussions. However, structuring our time to allow such dialogue is a worthwhile investment. The rewards include improved communication and collaboration among professional groups, a reduction in moral distress, and subsequent improvement in patient care as ethical problems are addressed and action plans identified.

Normative Ethical Theories

There are many ethical theories to assist nurses in making difficult moral decisions. Knowledge of ethical theory can guide deliberation and improve communication and understanding—among care team members, and with patients and families.

Different ethical theories offer different approaches to the analysis of a particular issue. The following review is not intended as an exhaustive presentation of ethical theories; only a few of the better known theoretical perspectives are presented. Nurses may choose to adopt an approach consistent with their values or beliefs, or select a theory of combination of theories more appropriate to the situation they face.

Ethical theories can be used to develop decision-making tools that can be applied in the clinical setting. One example of such a tool is described at the end of the chapter.

Background

Normative ethical theories provide frameworks and rules to guide decisions about what is right and wrong with respect to our actions and behaviours. Two well-known categories of ethical theory are *deontology* (derived from the Greek *deontor*, "duty") and *teleology* (derived from the Greek *teleo*, "end").[3] *Deontological theories* make explicit those duties and principles that should guide our actions, whereas *teleological theories* focus on the ends or outcomes and consequences of what we do.

In the discipline of philosophy, decisions about what is right and wrong have traditionally required a reasoning process based on an ethical theory or the principles and rules derived from those theories. Opinions without arguments or reasons to support them were discouraged. Emotive responses were devalued, although (as will be seen later in this chapter) our emotional reactions are today considered an important indicator of our ethical perspectives.

Theories are meant to assist in this reasoning process. It is important for nurses to be familiar with the fundamentals of the major ethical theories and the principles and frameworks that can guide and help to communicate ethical decisions.

Deontological Theory

In deontological theory, morals or rules are established to determine what is right or wrong based on one's obligations and duties. These rules are based on unchanging or absolute principles derived from universally shared values. The best-known theory based on duty is that formulated by Immanuel Kant (1724–1804).

Kant believed that right actions should follow from obligations, rules, and duties. He said that one should act on the basis of duty and not from inclination, whim, or emotion. An act in accordance with one's duty is therefore right. If an act or one's motivation is right, then it is intrinsically good; that is, it is good in and of itself. If an act is intrinsically good, then it has moral value and is not dependent on the results, outcomes, or consequences of that action.[4] Therefore, Kant argued that principles, rules, and duties, rather than consequences, should guide our actions. Kant's theory focussed on how these principles and rules should be determined.

Kant believed that valid moral and ethical principles were based on an abstract "a priori" foundation, that is, independent of our empirical reality. Hence, he argued, morality is objectively and universally binding; it is absolute. If it is right it is always right, and not dependent on circumstance or outcome.[5] For example, if telling the truth is morally correct, then that correctness stands regardless of the circumstances or context of the situation.

Moral knowledge, according to Kant, is the knowledge of how we *ought* to behave (what is right), not necessarily how we *actually* behave. That is, how we act as individuals, or the common practices within our society, are not necessarily morally correct, or what we ought to do.[6] For example, abortion is widespread and acceptable within our society. There is no law banning abortion at this time in Canada. Applying Kant's theory, the moral justification of abortion would not be based on the fact that it is not illegal and is practised widely within our society.

Kant believed that through reasoning we isolate these a priori, or absolute, elements that base morality. He claimed that the universal basis of morality lies in an individual's rational nature rather than in human desires and inclinations, because rationality, he argued, is the same for everyone.[7]

To be moral, an individual must demonstrate good will or good intention. Kant argued that good intention is the effort of a rational being to do what he or she ought to do, rather than to act from inclination or self-interest.[8]

Again, good will or intention is intrinsically good; it is not based on results. That is, it is not good merely as a means to something else; it is good in and of itself. A good will (one's motive or intentions) is one that acts for the sake of duty. The duty or obligation of the moral person is to do what is right.[9]

Actions based on inclination or self-interest may be worthy of praise. They may happen to be in accordance with duty, but they do not have "moral" value, since actions, according to Kant, have moral worth only if they are driven by this duty.[10] For example, a rich benefactor may donate a million dollars to a health care agency in order to have the agency renamed in his honour. This act, then, might be praiseworthy and in accordance with duty, but it would not have moral value. Alternatively, an individual recently unemployed who continues to contribute weekly to his church is acting out of duty, and hence his actions have moral worth or value. Actions with true moral worth, when evaluated, stand alone, or independent of another motive. An act performed out of duty, then, has moral worth because of the principle guiding that act; the worth does not spring from the results or outcomes of that act.

The Kantian approach thus emphasizes the concept of duty, which Kant described as the prominent feature of moral consciousness. Duty is derived from a sense of moral obligation. Good will is manifest in acting from a sense of duty, which is different from acting out of mere inclination or desire. Duty is acting in accordance with moral law. The essential characteristic of this law is universality.[11]

Kant set out some ground rules, or *maxims,* for determining rules of conduct. He stated that an act is morally right if and only if its maxim is universalizable. "We must be able to will that the maxim of our action should become a universal law. ... Since you would not want others to behave in the way you propose to behave, you should not behave in that way."[12]

For Kant, the supreme principle that a law of morality must follow is the *categorical imperative.* This is fundamental to Kant's theory on how we identify the rules or principles that guide our actions and moral decisions. "I am never to act otherwise than so that I could also will that my maxim should become a universal law."[13]

According to Kant, we must determine the implications of universalizing the rules that guide our actions. For example, would we be able to establish a rule that lying is morally correct? Could we establish a rule that only doctors may decide on treatment options for patients? What if it were okay to cross an intersection on a red light? A rule must undergo such scrutiny. If it can be applied universally, then it is what we "ought" to do.

One formulation of the categorical imperative requires us to treat each human being or person as an end, never as a means to any other end. This is based in Kant's view that the existence of humanity has in itself absolute worth. Therefore, all human beings should be respected. "So act as to treat humanity whether in thine own person or in that of any other, in every case as an end withal, never as means only."[14]

For example, Kant would argue that we have a duty to tell the truth, since persons ought to be respected and not used as a means to some other desired end. Thus, even if lying were to produce some desired outcome, it would be disrespectful of that person. It would be using a person as a means to that desired end and therefore should not be tolerated. However, Kant did not say that, as persons, we can never be used as means, for example, for some instrumental good. But, if we are used as an instrument toward some other good, we must also be regarded as ends in ourselves. Hence, for example, the notion of informed consent: Kant would probably agree that it was morally acceptable to use persons for research or organ donation, but only if our right to self-determination was respected.

Sometimes moral rules or principles are in conflict. When one is faced with a number of alternatives, the "right" alternative is the one consistent with all the rules. If a number of alternatives are consistent with the rules, then the choice is one of preference. When each choice is consistent with one rule but in conflict with another, then one attempts to appeal to the higher rule to resolve that conflict. For example, sanctity of life would have priority over the rule of veracity or truth telling.

To summarize, a rule, principle, or maxim is a fundamental, objective moral law grounded in pure practical reasoning, upon which all people would act if we were purely rational, moral agents.

Consequentialist Theory

Those who advocate *consequentialist theory* believe that the best alternative is the one with the best consequences, outcomes, or results. In consequentialist theories there are no absolute principles, moral codes, duties, or rules. There is the assumption that good can be quantified, and that we can calculate the relative good or harm that would result from our actions. One acts best by increasing the greatest good and the least amount of harm for the greatest number of people. Essentially, the consequences of an act consist of the sum total of differences that act will make in the world.

Consequentialist theories provide us with evaluative standards for assessing and ordering consequences. Consequentialists may choose to evaluate the moral value of an act based on outcomes that may be related to happiness, welfare, pleasure, pain, risk, or costs and benefits. The consequences of an act are measured in their totality. For example, in a situation where withdrawal of treatment is being considered, the consequences of this action would be evaluated not only in relation to the patient, but to the family, the health professionals involved, and society as a whole. Immediate and long-term consequences would be considered. The various consequentialist theories provide us with some evaluative standards for assessing consequences.

Utilitarianism

The best-known example of a consequentialist theory is *utilitarianism*, developed by John Stuart Mill (1806–1873) and based on the work of Jeremy Bentham (1748–1832).[15]

The theory articulated by Mill is founded on the principle of utility (the greatest happiness for the greatest number of people). Mill believed that most people desire unity and harmony with one other and essentially wish to benefit others. All rational beings strive to do their best. Mill argued that the principle of utility is grounded in the pursuit of pleasure and the avoidance of pain, which he believed are the main goals of life. He believed that actions are right when they promote happiness, wrong if they produce the reverse. In choosing between various alternatives, he believed an act to be right if and only if its utility is higher than the utility of any other act the person could have done instead.[16]

According to Mill, happiness is a realistic appraisal of the pleasurable moments afforded in life, whether experienced in tranquillity or passion. In order to evaluate happiness and to prioritize consequences, we should rely on our common sense, our habits, and our past experiences. Based on these factors we can then reasonably predict what would produce the most happiness and therefore the best consequences.[17]

Pluralistic utilitarian philosophers believe that no single goal or state constitutes "the good," and that many values besides happiness possess intrinsic worth, for example, friendship, knowledge, love, devotion, health, beauty, and such moral qualities as fairness. Utility, they say, is the total range of intrinsic values, the greatest aggregate good.

Act and Rule Utilitarianism

There are two approaches to utilitarian theory. In *act utilitarianism,* each act is judged on its consequences. In *rule utilitarianism,* one considers the utility of general patterns of behaviour rather than specific actions. A rule is correct provided that more utility would be produced by people following it, rather than by any other rule that would apply to the situation or act. Some argue that this is similar to Kant's notion of universality.

In practice, then, one would list the alternative actions available, consider the possible consequences or outcomes of each act, then quantify the consequences in relation to the "good," whether that be utility, pleasure, or happiness. The right alternative or rule would be the one that produced the most utility, the greatest good, or the least harm for the greatest number of people.

Ethical Principles

Ethical principles are derived from moral theory and serve as rules to guide moral conduct. As a framework for ethical decision making they are the most familiar to health professionals, as they are the foundation of many professional codes of ethics.

Biomedical ethical principles are well defined by Beauchamp and Childress (1983).[18] The important principles related to health care include autonomy, non-maleficence, beneficence, justice, and fidelity. Ethical principles are *prima facie,* that is, their application may be relative to another principle that may have more weight or priority in a given situation. However, some individuals may consider particular principles to be absolute. For example, some people advocate sanctity of life in all forms and at all costs, while others believe that quality of life may override sanctity of life in some circumstances.

Autonomy

The principle of *autonomy* (Greek: *autos,* "self"; *nomos,* "rule") recognizes that a capable and competent individual is free to determine, and to act in accordance with, a plan chosen by himself or herself.[19] This principle supports the Kantian view that individuals be respected as ends in and of themselves and never as means to some other end. As discussed earlier in this chapter, this view is based in Kant's belief that the existence of humanity has in itself absolute worth. Therefore, all human beings should be respected.[20]

This principle is consistent with Mill's utilitarian ethics. The utilitarian view states that autonomy maximizes the benefits of all concerned, and that social and political control over individual action is legitimate only if it is necessary to prevent harm to others.[21]

The legal doctrine of informed consent is based on respect for the principle of autonomy and an individual's right to the information required to make decisions about his or her own health care. Failure to provide a patient with adequate information limits that person's autonomy and interferes with that individual's rights. (The elements of informed consent will be discussed in Chapter 6.) The concept of the autonomous individual gives rise to the duty of respecting a person's values and choices. Autonomy assumes the person is competent, has the ability to decide rationally, rather than impulsively, and that he or she has the ability to act upon those decisions and choices.

As nurses know, illness puts limits on individual autonomy. The hospital environment further limits the patient's control. The views of the health care team may be readily apparent to the patient, leading to subtle forms of coercion in relation to the choices the patient must make. Patients may experience anxiety and stress, and may even be overwhelmed by uncertainty with regard to their future and the prognosis of their illness. It is the duty of the nurse to support the patient through this process, ensure the patient has the information he or she requires to make choices, and give the patient time to reflect on these choices to determine the best course of action for himself or herself. On occasion, autonomy conflicts with other principles such as beneficence, when a patient may refuse a treatment that the nurse and the health care team firmly believe is in the patient's best interest.

Non-Maleficence

The principle of *non-maleficence* is associated with the Latin maxim, *primum non nocere:* "above all (or first), do no harm." This is expressed in many professional codes of ethics and in the Hippocratic Oath: "I will use treatment to help the sick according to my ability and judgement, but I will never use it to injure or wrong them." This principle obliges us to act in such a way that we prevent or remove harm.[22] All members of society are obliged by law to respect this principle. In nursing, professional practice standards express the competencies that nurses must have to ensure the provision of safe patient care. Often, the actions of nurses may produce some temporary harm (e.g., the administration of medication by injection, restraining patients, painful procedures such as dressings or intravenous insertion). This temporary harm is justified if it is a means toward producing a good and if the principle of autonomy is respected.

Beneficence

The principle of *beneficence* sets a higher standard than non-maleficence in that one must make a positive move to produce some good or benefit for another. Beneficence asserts a duty or obligation to help others to further their important and legitimate interests.[23] Many thinkers argue that it is the ideal to be beneficent, but that we are not morally obliged to take positive action to benefit others. However, as professionals, nurses accept this duty to act in such a manner that not only protects patients from harm but produces some good or benefit. Failure to do this may violate professional duties and obligations.

At times, the principle of beneficence may conflict with that of autonomy. This is often a source of distress for health professionals when we know that a particular intervention is likely to benefit a patient yet the patient refuses consent. Health professionals have an obligation to ensure that the patient is provided with the information, support, and time to make the decision that is indeed (from the patient's perspective) in his or her best interests.

Traditionally, but less so in recent years, health professionals may have acted in a paternalistic ("father knows best") way toward patients, in an effort to protect them from the potentially harmful consequences of their choices. That is, out of a desire to be beneficent, physicians and nurses may have given that principle priority over others (autonomy, truth telling) in an effort to do what they think is best for the patient.

Fidelity

The principle of *fidelity* is the foundation of the nurse–patient relationship. This rule is about loyalty, keeping promises, truth telling, and being faithful to those entrusted in our care.[24] This principle is challenged when nurses are placed in situations where being loyal to a patient may compromise their own ethical principles, as when a terminally ill patient requests assistance to die when pain cannot be controlled and life has lost its dignity. Given the close nature of the nurse–patient relationship, the nurse would feel and understand the patient's physical and emotional pain, might even agree that this action would demonstrate care and compassion, but would be restricted by law (and perhaps by his or her own beliefs) from helping the patient in this circumstance.

Justice

The principle of *justice* obliges us to treat others fairly. It addresses questions of how to distribute resources equitably. This is a challenge when resources are scarce, as they increasingly are in health care. Nurses have to deal with such questions as how financial resources are distributed; which programs will be funded; how staff are allocated; how to organize patient assignments to ensure each patient access to the care required; how to decide who gets treatment first, who gets the scarce organ for transplantation, and many other issues.

In determining equitable distribution of resources, decisions may be based on one of several considerations, for example, giving each person an equal share, giving to the person with the most need, or to those who have tried the hardest, or who are the most deserving.[25] Even if we agree on an approach, we are challenged to define such terms as "deserving" or "need."

Feminist and Feminine Perspectives on Ethics

In recent years, feminine and feminist perspectives on ethics have emerged that offer alternatives to the traditional ethical theories that by and large have been developed or formulated by men. The deontological and utilitarian theories of morality place a strong emphasis on rationality and notions of justice, traditionally a male perspective. If, as some have argued, the moral development of women differs from that of men, then these approaches can be problematic for some women.[26] Further, given the patriarchal power structures within health care, and the fact that nursing continues to be dominated by women, nurses need to understand feminist perspectives.

Feminine and feminist perspectives are critical of the traditional ethical theories based on male perspectives, standards, biases, and experiences. Traditional ethics searches for a "systematic approach to evaluate the standards or justifications" of morality; the interest is in "determining which rules ideally should be followed."[27] Such rules may fail to fit the moral experience and intuitions of many women.[28] Just as men have historically been associated with reason, women have been associated with inclination, which Kant suggested has no moral value.[29] Feminine and feminist theorists resist the model of traditional rationalist ethics, believing instead that ethical analysis must make sense in the real world and not be primarily based on abstract notions.[30] That is, there is more to ethics than abstract reasoning: there is the context of the situation, and the relationships among all the individuals involved.

Feminist Theory[31]

There are many perspectives that fall under the broad category of feminist theory. Following is a brief sketch of three major lines of thought.

Liberal Feminism

This branch of feminism is concerned with the equality of women and the equitable distribution of wealth, position, and power. Though not critical of the "traditional" role of woman as wife and mother, there is concern about the social, political, and economic forces that channel women into these roles. The liberal feminist agenda, then, is to influence social and political forces that will overcome oppression and provide women with the same rights and opportunities as men. Some strategies include providing greater educational opportunities for women, ensuring that women have access to male-dominated professions (such as medicine), and implementing legislation that ensures equality for women.

Social Feminism

Social feminists analyze the cultural institutions that contribute to the oppression of women and the relationship between the private sphere of the home and the public domain of productive work. They argue that equity will never be attained until changes are made to structures such as the patriarchal family, motherhood, housework, and consumerism, since these influence the distribution of power, wealth, and privilege. The social and political structures must change so that responsibilities within the home and traditional female professions, such as nursing, are valued to the same extent as those of men.

Radical Feminism

This perspective challenges the patriarchal underpinnings of our society. Radical feminists seek to analyze and value women's experiences from the perspective of female rather than male standards and biases. The focus is on the development of women-defined thought, culture, and systems. In order for this to evolve, gender discrimination and sexual stereotyping need to be eliminated. Though the childbearing role of women and values such as nurturance are emphasized, they are also seen by radical feminists as the historical basis of oppression toward women.

Although these three perspectives embrace a broad range of feminist thought and practice, all share the following themes:

(1) recognition of the oppression of women,
(2) support for equal rights and opportunities for women, and
(3) an orientation to initiating change.[32]

Feminist theory is complex, as are the ethical perspectives it raises. Nurses as professionals can benefit through increased awareness of, and interest in, the ethical views that feminist theory offers.

Feminist Ethics

In feminist ethics, the oppression of women is felt to be an issue of utmost moral concern. It is derived from the "explicitly political perspective of feminism, wherein the oppression of women is seen to be morally and politically unacceptable."[33]

Feminists view individuals as unique yet part of a community. Their view of the individual is that of a complex product of a social structure defined within the context of relationships with others.[34]

Feminist ethics is committed to "eliminating the subordination of women."[35] In all contexts of ethical decision making, the question must be asked, "What does this mean for women?" The focus is on changing the status quo, empowering women, and escaping from oppression.[36] Unless this changes, feminists believe a truly ethical reality is not possible.

Feminine Ethics

Feminist thinker Carol Gilligan has suggested that women and men make ethical choices based on differing sets of values, perceptions, and concerns.[37] Feminine ethics considers the values, perceptions, and concerns that influence human interactions and relationships. Feminine views give significance to the nature of the relationships within a particular ethical context. When faced with a moral issue, women tend to seek out innovative solutions that will ensure that the needs of all parties are met, whereas men tend to seek the dominant rule, even when someone else's interests are sacrificed.[38]

Those with a feminine view on ethics argue that traditional theories are overly concerned with rational, logical, and objective thinking and acting. The feminine view focusses on values, feelings, and desires. There is emphasis on presence, listening, taking feelings seriously, searching for meaning, and seeing the person and the world from a more holistic perspective.[39] Ethical situations have more than one dimension, and encompass many principles and theories.

The view of feminine ethics expressed by Gilligan places greater importance on our emotive responses to ethical choices. Historically speaking, emotion has played a diminished role in ethical decision making. Given the caring nature of the nursing profession, and the intensity of the nurse–patient relationship, it is important that we consider this influence.

Tschudin and Marks-Maran, who draw on the work of Richard Niebuhr (1963), maintain that people function primarily through relationships as responsive, creative beings.[40] They start with the question, "What is happening?" and place emphasis on a person's response to a context or situation. Assuming that the wish to do the right thing is an inborn human urge, then a person's response—the feeling or the gut reaction—is the key indicator of morality.

Yarling, McElmurry, and Noddings focus on an "ethic of care."[41] Noddings in fact suggests that caring, which women take more into consideration because of their traditional role within the family, is the only moral consideration.[42] This view has been criticized since it seems to suggest the exclusion of women who do not share familial responsibilities for caring, and males, from the possibility of such caring and nurturing.[43]

A focus on caring requires us to examine all dynamics of a particular situation or context. An ethic of care requires our seeing as many aspects of a situation as possible. In this view, we enter another's world in order to see things as that person sees them. In that way, we can better understand the values and beliefs of others. The emphasis is on the process of self-understanding, whereby one offers explanations, rather than justifications, for choices. The sharing of unique perspectives facilitates a greater understanding of the dynamics of a situation and therefore provides greater insights to guide our choices.[44] This approach is not limited to the nurse's relationship with the patient. It is recommended as a means of understanding and respecting the various views and life experiences of all members of the health care team.[45]

Feminine ethical decision making is based on the desire to respond to each individual as an individual. The focus is on caring rather than on justice. Rather than treating all people alike in the name of fairness, some people need and want to be treated differently in the name of care and concern for each individual's personal context.

Some feminists have concerns about the feminine notion of caring, which they view as a gender trait and a survival skill of an oppressed group.[46] Too much emphasis on the welfare of others can drain the resources and energy of women. Feminists do not reject the relevance of caring, but instead attempt to identify criteria for determining when it should be offered and when not.

Feminists agree that feelings play a role in ethical decision making, but that these need to be balanced in relation to social justice.[47] When dealing with ethical issues, there is also the need to consider our experiences, the morally relevant features and responsibilities of the relationships involved, and the context of the situation.[48]

Professional Codes of Ethics

Professional groups have a duty to serve the public interest and the common good. As discussed in Chapter 3, members of professional groups have this obligation because their roles, missions, and ethical foundations focus not only on the individuals they serve, but on society as a whole.[49]

Codes of Ethics

Professional codes of ethics articulate the professional's ethical standards and obligations to clients and to society at large.[50] The public trusts that professionals will use their knowledge and skill in the best interests of the community and the individuals they serve. To maintain this trust, it is essential that professionals maintain scrupulous standards of conduct and be held accountable to the public and the individuals they serve.[51]

When nurses accept the professional role, they commit to these clearly articulated rules of practice and conduct. Professional codes of ethics express the moral and ethical standards we must uphold as members of our profession. They define acceptable and unacceptable behaviour and rules of conduct, and articulate general principles that guide our decisions and actions.

Many health care organizations have codes of ethics. These include institutions such as hospitals, community agencies, professional associations, and registration bodies.

The *Code of Ethics* of the CNA

The *Code of Ethics for Nursing* of the Canadian Nurses Association (see Appendix A, page 233) offers a framework and guide for ethical practice for Canadian nurses. First published in 1980 and revised in 1985 and 1991, the

Code affirms that each nurse must recognize his or her responsibility not only to individual patients but also to society, and must participate in activities that contribute to the community as a whole.

Nurses' commitment and allegiance to the individuals they serve may at times conflict with the interest of society and the common good, and this conflict may emerge in many everyday, practical decisions that nurses face. Such decisions may relate to standards of care, quality of life, and indeed to the very ethic of caring within the nursing profession and the health care system. Technology has altered the boundaries between living and dying. The irony is that major advances in health care delivery have brought caregivers not a sense of greater control, but rather, increased feelings of powerlessness. This has become a predominant theme in discussions among health care providers. For example, we can extend life, but at what cost? We can influence the creation of life, but should we?

The Canadian Nurses Association

The Canadian Nurses Association (CNA) is a national nursing organization with links to provincial professional associations such as the Registered Nurses Association of Ontario and the Manitoba Association of Registered Nurses. The CNA assists and supports the provinces in the development of standards of nursing practice, education, and ethical conduct. It initiates and influences legislation, government programs, and national and international health policy. It establishes and supports research priorities, facilitates information sharing, and represents the profession to health groups, government bodies, and the public.

Elements of the Code

The *Code of Ethics for Nursing* "seeks to clarify the obligations of nurses to use their knowledge and skills for the benefit of others, to minimize harm, to respect client autonomy and to provide fair and just care for their clients."[52] The Code identifies the basic moral commitments of nursing, serves as a source for education and reflection, provides a basis for self-evaluation and peer review, and establishes clear expectations for the ethical conduct of nurses.[53]

The Code is framed within twelve value statements that are clustered according to the sources of nursing obligations:

(1) Clients,
(2) Nursing Roles and Relationships,
(3) Nursing Ethics and Society, and
(4) The Nursing Profession.[54]

The values expressed in the Code provide a broad sense of the ideals of nursing. Specific direction is provided to the nurse through statements of moral obligations, which have their basis in nursing values. These standards provide direction for professional conduct and guidance for action within a specific context or circumstance. In some sections, limitations are described that identify "exceptional circumstances in which a value or obligation cannot be applied."[55]

The Code does not claim to provide rules of moral behaviour in all circumstances. It aims to provide guidance to the nurse in identifying areas of ethical violation, and in identifying and seeking some resolution to ethical dilemmas. In providing guidance for nurses in these areas, it is hoped that ethical distress can be minimized.[56] The rules of the Code are derived from the ethical principles described earlier in this chapter. A brief summary of the values and their application follows.

Value I: Respect for needs and values of clients

A nurse treats clients with respect for their individual needs and values.[57]

The Code emphasizes that it is the patient who decides what is in his or her best interest. This value demonstrates respect for the individual values, beliefs, and differences of the patients we care for. This is of particular significance given the multicultural and religious mosaic of Canadian society. The patient is recognized as part of a family unit (the definition of family in its broadest sense, to include same-sex spouses, significant others, friends, etc.) and that unit, with the patient's permission, may be involved in the delivery of care. Furthermore, this value makes explicit the requirement for informed consent, and respect for patient privacy.

Whether or not nurses behave in a manner consistent with this value may be apparent in our individual or organizational behaviours and policies. For example, the consistent application of rigid rules regarding visiting hours would not always demonstrate respect for the wishes and needs of the patient and family.

Value II: Respect for client choice

Based upon respect for clients and regard for their right to control their own care, nursing care reflects respect for the right of choice held by clients.[58]

Based on the principle of autonomy, this value stresses the significance of informed patient choice. Recognizing that consent may be given in writing or verbally, or simply implied (for example, holding out an arm to have blood drawn), a valid consent must be one that is based on the relevant information required to make that choice; it must be free from coercion; and it must be made by someone capable of that level of decision. For example, a patient may be able to make a decision about her activities of daily living, but may be incompetent to decide whether surgery is in her best interest. The challenge for health professionals is to determine competence and to ensure that choices are made in a non-coercive environment. Even if it is not the nurse's responsibility to obtain informed consent, it is the ethical duty of the nurse to ensure this standard is met.

Value III: Confidentiality

The nurse holds confidential all information about a client learned in the health care setting.[59]

Fundamental to the nurse–patient relationship is the nurse's professional obligation to respect patient confidentiality. Preservation of confidentiality ensures
that the nurse–patient relationship is maintained. The promise of confidentiality ensures full disclosure by the patient of information essential to achieving
the goals of care. A limitation to this rule arises if harm might result to the patient or others if confidentiality were maintained, or where statute law requires
disclosure (e.g., reporting child abuse).

Value IV: Dignity of clients

The nurse is guided by consideration for the dignity of clients.[60]

All patients deserve to be treated with respect, dignity, and compassion.
Disrespectful communication, disregard for patient privacy, and the failure to
involve patients in discussions that relate to them, violate our ethical responsibility to them. Patients require our care during very difficult and meaningful
periods in their lives, from birth to death.

The question of being treated with dignity arises especially in relation to the
dying patient. It is important that special attention be given to ensure that the
process of dying is dignified, and that the emotional, psychological, and physical needs of the patient, the family, and significant others are met. Nurses are
obligated to ensure optimal patient comfort and pain control, to deal compas-
sionately when in situations where treatment is being withdrawn, and to
provide the patient and family with the opportunity for home care if and when
this is possible. Based on this value, it would be the ethical obligation of the
nurse to ensure, for example, that everything possible be done so that a patient
does not die alone, unless he or she expresses this wish. The same priority
should be given to these situations as that provided to emergencies.
Assignments can be reorganized; help can be requested so that someone is there
with the patient.

Value V: Competent nursing care

The nurse provides competent care to clients.[61]

Nurses have a professional responsibility to ensure that they are competent to
practise. This requires continuing education to keep up with the many changes
and improvements in nursing care, and a regular review of skills. In non-emer-
gency situations requiring specialized skills that the nurse does not have, or
where the provision of care conflicts with the nurse's moral beliefs, the nurse is
required to refer that patient to another nurse. In situations of an emergency
nature, or where there is a lack of alternative resources, nurses may be called
on to provide care.

Value VI: Nursing practice, education, research, and administration

The nurse maintains trust in nurses and nursing.[62]

This value addresses the ethical responsibility of nursing leaders to ensure the
effective management and development of nursing staff, and to ensure that ad-

equate resources are available to secure the delivery of competent patient care. Furthermore, it deals with the ethical responsibilities related to nursing education, specifically with respect to the teacher–student relationship and the teacher–student relationship with the patient. As well, this value recognizes the importance of nursing research in developing the profession of nursing and in improving the quality of nursing care that patients receive.

Value VII: Co-operation in health care

The nurse recognizes the contribution and expertise of colleagues from nursing and other disciplines as essential to excellent health care.[63]

Collaboration among health care professionals ensures a higher level of patient care, improved continuity, and more effective management of health care resources. This value recognizes the role of the nurse as a member of the health care team. It makes explicit the nurse's responsibility to ensure licensure or registration and to affiliate with provincial and national associations and interest groups.

Value VIII: Protecting clients from incompetence

The nurse takes steps to ensure that the client receives competent and ethical care.[64]

The nurse has a duty to protect patients from harm. When the facts of a situation indicate incompetence on the part of another nurse or health professional, a nurse is required to take the most appropriate action, given the context of the situation, to ensure the safety of patients. When a nurse is aware of incompetence and neglects to take action, then he or she shares responsibility for the consequences of that incompetence. When delegating responsibility to others, the nurse must be assured that this delegation is appropriate and that those delegated to are competent to fulfil the delegated functions. Specific examples of these types of situations include delegation to students, the family, and other health care assistants.

Value IX: Conditions of employment

Conditions of employment should contribute in a positive way to client care and the professional satisfaction of the nurse.[65]

This value recognizes that the work environment and the existence of appropriate resources are critical to maintaining professional standards and ethical integrity. When supportive structures and mechanisms are not in place within the work environment, it is the shared responsibility of management and staff to ensure that improvements are made. For example, the nurse should not tolerate inadequate staffing patterns when patient care is being compromised. Though circumstances may require that nurses do their best in a unique situation when resources are not available (e.g., disasters, or when several staff call in ill), inadequate staffing patterns should not be tolerated on a regular basis. It is the ethical responsibility of nurses, management, and staff to take steps to rectify this situation.

Value X: Job action

Job action by nurses is directed toward securing conditions of employment that enable safe and appropriate care for clients and contribute to the professional satisfaction of nurses.[66]

The Code recognizes that some form of job action may be necessary to achieve outcomes that will ultimately improve or guarantee a high standard of care. In these circumstances, however, it would be the responsibility of nurses to ensure the safety of patients and to see that their care is not compromised. Situations where job action is initiated pose difficulties for nurses where personal and professional values may be in conflict.

Value XI: Advocacy of the interests of clients, the community, and society

The nurse advocates the interests of clients.[67]

This aspect of the Code focusses on the individual patient and society's right to health care. If the principles of the *Canada Health Act* are to be upheld, then issues related to fair distribution and equal access to health care have to be constantly addressed by nurses and other health care professionals. In order to gain access to the system and good health care, patients and society must be knowledgeable and informed about good health practices and the health care resources available to them.

Value XII: Representing nursing values and ethics

The nurse represents the values and ethics of nursing before colleagues and others.[68]

Essentially, the nurse must represent the profession when on committees that involve health care issues, and be involved in activities that fulfil nursing's obligation to society in general. For example, nurses should represent the profession on committees, groups, and organizations that shape public policy with respect to health care.

Value XIII: Responsibilities of professional nurses' associations

Professional nurses' organizations are responsible for clarifying, securing and sustaining ethical nursing conduct. The fulfilment of these tasks requires that professional nurses' organizations remain responsible to the rights, needs and legitimate interests of clients and nurses.[69]

This value outlines the ethical responsibilities of nursing organizations and associations. It makes explicit their responsibility to ensure co-operation, collaboration, and effective communication among one another and among other organizations that relate to nursing. The primary focus is on the patient, who is served through the influence the associations have on public policy, legislation, education, and the development of professional standards and codes.

An Ethical Decision-making Process

This chapter has attempted to introduce the theories, principles, rules, and codes that guide ethical decision making. The following framework is offered as a guide for ethical discussion within the context of health care practice. This framework provides the opportunity to incorporate one or more of the various theories, principles, and codes into the decision-making process. As well, it ensures the proper collection of the data relevant to that process, and that all aspects of the situation are considered. Decision-making frameworks provide a process or approach to guide ethical decision making. They serve as useful guides that assist individuals or groups to focus on the relevant questions and issues.

(1) Describe the Problem

Determine whether the situation constitutes an ethical dilemma, an ethical violation, or whether some significant gap in the care process, such as a breakdown in communication, has led to this problem.

(2) Gather the Facts

What is the patient's diagnosis? Prognosis? Age? What is the patient's cultural background and religion? Are there family or significant others? What is their relationship? Who is involved in the patient's care? Is the patient competent? Has a proxy decision maker been appointed? Is there a living will?

(3) Clarify Values

What are your beliefs about the situation? What are the values of other members of the team? Of the patient and family? Will the cultural and religious background influence what is happening and who should be involved in dealing with this problem?

(4) Note Reactions

How is everyone responding in this situation? What are their behaviours? Are there any emotive reactions? What is everybody feeling? Do they have a gut reaction to what is happening?

(5) Identify Ethical Principles

Which principles apply to this situation? Are any of these principles in conflict? Does one principle (or more) have priority over the others?

(6) Clarify Legal Rules

Are there any legal rules that govern this situation (as in release of confidential information)?

(7) Explore Options and Alternatives

How many options are available? Evaluate each in relation to ethical theories and principles. What are the potential consequences of each alternative? Are there rules that apply to these alternatives? Are they in conflict? How do they apply to the *Code of Ethics for Nursing*?

(8) Decide the Course of Action

Is one course of action more consistent with ethical theories, principles, and rules? Is there one consistent with your own values and beliefs? How do you feel about making this choice? Do you have a gut reaction to this decision? Can you live with the consequences of this decision?

(9) Develop an Action Plan

Once the choice has been made, how will it be carried out? How will the choice and the reasons behind it be communicated to others? Who will be involved? What are the responsibilities of the patient, the family, the nurse, and the health care team?

(10) Evaluate the Plan

Review the situation regularly. Modify the plan or strategy as required. In retrospect, is there anything you would have done differently? How might you improve this process next time? Is there anything in this process that should be incorporated into a guideline that could help others deal with a similar situation in the future?

Ethics Committees

Ideally, most ethical issues and dilemmas are resolved, and most decisions are made, by the patient, the family, and the health care providers most involved in that patient's care. However, these participants need education, guidelines, and supports to assist them. Sometimes the issues they face are complex and not easily resolved; or, they may have larger implications for the agency, the community, or society. Ethics committees exist to provide education, guidelines, advice, and support with respect to these issues.

The growth in number and complexity of ethical issues in health care has led to the growth in number of ethics committees in Canadian hospitals. Surveys of Canadian hospitals completed in 1984, 1989, and 1991 provide evidence of this growth.[70,71] A poll of 215 Canadian hospitals with more than 300 beds conducted in 1984 found that 36 (26 English, 10 French) of the 196 who responded had ethics committees.[72] A similar study of 142 English-language hospitals having more than 300 beds indicated that 70 of the 120 (84.5%) who responded had an ethics committee.[73] In 1991 in Quebec, 60 institutions surveyed had some form of a clinical ethics committee, while 144 did not. The busier hospitals seemed more likely to have a committee, and 77% of those who did had more than 400 beds. The majority of these ethics committees were instituted between 1985 and 1990.[74]

Clinical Ethics Committees

A *clinical ethics committee* is defined as "any committee that is recognized as being primarily involved in ethical issues regarding patient care."[75] Unlike *research ethics committees,* who have the function of reviewing the ethical aspects of research proposals, clinical ethics committees deal primarily with the ethical perspectives of patient care. The roles of clinical ethics committees vary and may include one or more of the following functions.

Consultation

Rarely are ethics committees in Canada involved in decisions regarding patient care. Rather, they offer advice about how a situation may be approached, or they assist those seeking help in working through the decision process. Essentially, it is the patient, the family, and the caregivers who must make and act on decisions, but they can obtain support and assistance from ethics committees. Referrals to ethics committees are made by patients, families, physicians, nurses, other caregivers, and administrators.

Education

Most clinical ethics committees play a role in the education of staff. In fact, this is their most important function, given the increased need for staff to be knowledgeable about these issues. Education is provided through interest sessions or in-services, workshops, case presentations, and internal publications.

Policy

Ethics committees may have the responsibility of establishing policies or guidelines to assist staff in dealing with complex issues, or to help clarify the ethical values and duties within an organization or agency. These may include policies on confidentiality, and guidelines respecting resuscitation, withdrawal of treatment, the use of reproductive technologies, and consent. Guidelines developed by ethics committees can also serve as educational tools for staff if the ethical rules and principles involved in developing the guidelines are made explicit.

Research

Ethics committees may also conduct research on ethical issues. For example, a committee may survey provider attitudes on withdrawal of treatment or organ donation in order to develop guidelines in these areas, or they may be interested in determining the extent of ethical problems that caregivers face and the decision processes they use.

Composition of Ethics Committees

Most ethics committees have representation from physicians, nurses, chaplains, lawyers, administrators, social workers, and other care providers. Some also have ethicists, board members, and community representatives on the committee. Ethics committees tend to report to either the board of directors of the hospital or the medical advisory committee.

Implications for Nurses

Surprisingly, it was demonstrated in a pilot study by Storch et al. (1990) that nurses in general had limited awareness of, and experience with, ethics committees. This phenomenon has been linked to the power structures within hospitals and the narrow focus of nurses at the bedside.[76]

Nurses, more than any other health professionals, have prolonged exposure to the patient. Consequently, nurses are likely to understand more than other members of the health care team how the patient feels. Their knowledge of the patient is critical when making ethical decisions. Further, nurses are involved in the outcomes of these decisions. For example, when treatment is withdrawn, or when "no CPR" orders are written, nurses implement these decisions and participate in their consequences.

Nurses are aware of the extent of ethical problems and violations because they face them daily. Therefore, nurses must be involved in ethics committees. They must pursue their issues or concerns. Though due process should be followed, nurses need to be aware that when satisfaction is not achieved they have access to ethics committees. Furthermore, as professionals who are held accountable for their practice, nurses have the right (and often the responsibility) to go directly to ethics committees for advice and consultation. These committees can also support nurses in determining the most appropriate process to follow, and can provide the information or knowledge required. Representatives from ethics committees may also be invited to participate in discussions with other care providers, patients, and families in direct care environments.

Summary

The key points introduced in this chapter include:
- the complexity of ethical choices nurses make
- the influence of values on ethical decision making
- the relevance of a solid understanding of ethical theory
- a basic introduction to ethical theory and principles
- the *Code of Ethics* of the Canadian Nurses Association as a guide to ethical practice
- the tools and process to assist in identifying, understanding, and working through ethical challenges
- when and how to utilize hospital ethics committees.

References

1. The Code is reproduced in Appendix A, page 233.
2. Gilligan, C. (1988). *In a different voice* (pp. 5–23). Cambridge: Harvard University Press.
3. Beauchamp, T.L., & Childress, J.F. (1983). *Principles of biomedical ethics* (p. 19). New York: Oxford University Press.
4. Albert, E., Denise, T., & Peterfreund, S. (1975). *Great traditions in ethics* (pp. 210–212). New York: Van Nostrand.
5. Ibid., pp. 204–207.
6. Ibid.
7. Ibid., p. 205.
8. Ibid., p. 207.
9. Ibid., pp. 207–208.
10. Ibid., pp. 210–212.
11. Ibid., pp. 215–216.
12. Ibid., p. 216.
13. Ibid., p. 215.
14. Ibid., p. 223.
15. Mill, J.S. (1987). *Utilitarianism. On liberty and considerations on representative government.* London: Everyman Classics.
16. Mill, J.S. (1993). *On liberty and utilitarianism* (pp. 145–148). New York: Bantam.
17. Ibid.
18. Beauchamp & Childress, supra footnote 3.
19. Ibid., p. 59.
20. Ibid.
21. Ibid., pp. 59–61.
22. Ibid., pp. 106–107.
23. Ibid., p. 148.
24. Ibid., p. 237.
25. Ibid., p. 187.
26. Gilligan, supra footnote 2.
27. Sherwin, S. (1992). *No longer patient* (p. 35). Philadelphia: Temple University Press.
28. Ibid., p. 42.
29. Ibid., p. 43.
30. Ibid., p. 55.
31. For the following précis of feminist theories, the authors are indebted to P.E. Valentine, "A Female Profession: A Feminist Management Perspective," Chapter 20 in J.M. Hibberd & M.E. Kyle, *Nursing Management in Canada* (Toronto: W.B. Saunders, 1994).
32. Adamson, N., Briskin, L., & McPhail, M. (1988). *Feminists organizing for change: The contemporary women's movement in Canada* (p. 9). Toronto: Oxford University Press.
33. Sherwin, supra footnote 27, p. 49.
34. Ibid., p. 53.
35. Ibid., p. 54.
36. Ibid.
37. Gilligan, supra footnote 2.
38. Sherwin, supra footnote 27, p. 46.
39. Lind, A., Wilburn, S., & Pate, E. (1986, Spring). Power from within: Feminism and the ethical decision-making process in nursing. *Nursing Administration Quarterly, 10*(3), 50–57.
40. Tschudin, V., & Marks-Maran, D. (1993). *Ethics: A primer for nurses.* London: Balliere Tindal. See also Niebuhr, R. (1963), *The responsible self.* New York: Harper & Row.
41. Crowley, M.A. (1989, April). Feminist pedagogy: Nurturing the ethical ideal. *Advances in Nursing Science, 11*(3), 53–61.
42. Sherwin, supra footnote 27, p. 46.
43. Condon, E.H. (1992). Nursing and the caring metaphor: Gender and political influences on

an ethics of care." *Nursing Outlook, 40*(1), 14–19.

44. Crowley, supra footnote 33.

45. Baker, C., Diekelmann, N. (1994). Connecting conversations of caring: Recalling the narrative to clinical practice. *Nursing Outlook, 42,* 65–70.

46. Sherwin, supra footnote 27, p. 50.

47. Ibid., p. 52.

48. Ibid.

49. Jennings, B., Callaghan, D., & Wolfe, S. (1987, February). The professions: Public interest and common good. *Hastings Centre Report* (Special Supplement).

50. Ibid.

51. Ibid.

52. Canadian Nurses Association. (1991). *Code of ethics for nursing.* Preamble (p. ii).

53. Ibid.

54. Ibid., p. vii.

55. Ibid., pp. iv–v.

56. Ibid., pp. ii–iii.

57. Ibid., pp. 1–2.

58. Ibid., pp. 3–4.

59. Ibid., pp. 5–6.

60. Ibid., p. 7.

61. Ibid., pp. 9–10.

62. Ibid., pp. 11–12.

63. Ibid., p. 13.

64. Ibid., pp. 15–16.

65. Ibid., p. 17.

66. Ibid., pp. 19–20.

67. Ibid., p. 21.

68. Ibid., p. 23.

69. Ibid., pp. 25–26.

70. Jean, A., Pare, S., & Parizeau, M. (1991). Hospital ethics committees in Quebec: An overview. HEC *Forum, 3*(6), 339–346.

71. Storch, J.L., Griener, G.G., Marshall, A., & Olineck, B.A. (1990, Winter). Ethics committees in Canadian hospitals: Report of the 1989 survey. *Healthcare Management Forum, 3*(4), 3–8.

72. Ibid.

73. Ibid.

74. Jean et al., supra footnote 66.

75. Storch et al., supra footnote 67.

76. Storch, J.L., & Griener, G.G. (1992, Spring). Ethics committees in Canadian hospitals: Report of the 1990 pilot study. *Healthcare Management Forum, 5*(1).

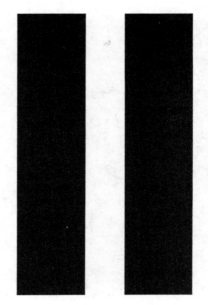

Selected Ethical and Legal Issues in Nursing

Professional Competence, Misconduct, and Malpractice

CHAPTER OBJECTIVES

The purpose of this chapter is to enable the reader to:
- appreciate the professional responsibilities and accountabilities of the nurse
- understand the ethical and legal aspects of professional competence, misconduct, and malpractice
- clarify the nurse's ethical and legal responsibilities to the patient and to other health care practitioners
- appreciate the implications of "whistle-blowing"
- apply legal rules and ethical theory to hypothetical case studies and actual situations
- explain the legal concepts of negligence, duty of care, vicarious liability, standard of care, and causation
- appreciate the significance of documentation
- clarify the criminal law with respect to standard of care and negligence
- know the role of the coroner's office and the implications of a coroner's inquest.

The ethical and legal aspects of professional competence, misconduct, and malpractice are interrelated. Two means by which the skill and conduct of nurses are gauged are the civil law (as in the civil lawsuit) and the complaints procedures related to the disciplinary powers of the nursing regulatory bodies (as discussed in Chapter 3). By these regulatory and self-governing mechanisms, nurses are made accountable to their patients and to the public in general.

The following case study sets out a situation in which an individual nurse and her colleagues are called upon to make ethical judgements and decisions that may have unforeseen legal consequences.

CASE STUDY

"Whistle-blowing" and duty of care

Several nurses in a nursing team work and rotate together through the same schedule in a busy Intensive Care Unit (ICU) of a major hospital. Recently, one of the nurses, Kathy, has been under extreme personal stress owing to the break-up of a relationship and the death of a close family member.

Over the last four to five weeks, her colleagues have noticed occasions on which Kathy has arrived for night shift smelling of alcohol. When the other nurses raise this with her, Kathy explains that she has had a glass or two of wine over dinner with some friends. As the weeks go by, such incidents increase in frequency. At times, Kathy's speech seems slurred. The other nurses on the team hesitate to report these experiences to the nurse manager, as they do not wish to add to Kathy's stress. They hope that as she deals with her personal problems, this issue will resolve itself. To protect Kathy and to minimize the risks to her patients, she is given easy assignments and is sent on a break whenever the night supervisor visits the unit.

In this particular ICU, the nurses are expected to perform specialized skills and are assigned certain delegated medical acts. As well, under the nursing standards policy of the hospital, each nurse is subject to annual review of knowledge and skills. Kathy is three months overdue for this review. The unit teacher has scheduled her for a review three times, but on each occasion, Kathy has cancelled, citing illness or heavy workload.

One night, Kathy arrives, once again smelling of alcohol. She is assigned a patient who is experiencing cardiac arrhythmias. During her shift, Kathy notes an arrhythmia on the patient's monitor, which she identifies as runs of ventricular tachycardia. In this unit, the nurses have been delegated the act of administering lidocaine in response to such an arrhythmia. Kathy prepares and administers the intravenous bolus of lidocaine. A few minutes later, the patient has a respiratory and cardiac arrest. Fortunately, he is easily resuscitated.

Upon review of the patient's status, it is noted that he had in fact experienced supraventricular tachycardia, for which lidocaine is not indicated. Furthermore, one of the other nurses noticed that the empty drug ampoule contained pavulon, not lidocaine. These drugs are contained in similar-sized ampoules, and the labelling is the same colour. Pavulon causes paralysis and is used during general anaesthesia or with some patients who are being mechanically ventilated in an ICU. Clearly, the drug led to the patient's arrest.

ISSUES

Some of the legal and ethical issues that arise out of this complex scenario include:

1. Have the nurses in the unit an obligation to report Kathy's alcohol use? To evaluate Kathy's risk to her patients?

2. What are Kathy's responsibilities for reviewing her knowledge and skills? The hospital's responsibilities?
3. What is the teacher's responsibility to ensure that Kathy's review takes place?
4. What responsibility, if any, has the second nurse to report that the incorrect drug was given?
5. What is the specific duty of the charge nurse (as distinct from Kathy's colleagues)?
6. What responsibility has the hospital to report the occurrence to the family (and the patient, if living?)
7. What is the legal, civil, and criminal liability of Kathy, the hospital, and the other nurses to the patient and his family?
8. What disciplinary action will Kathy or the other nurses face?

DISCUSSION

Negligence and the Duty of Care

This case study highlights a number of major ethical and legal challenges for nurses. What is the nurse's ethical and legal responsibility when a colleague demonstrates incompetence? What is the individual professional's responsibility to maintain competence, and what is the organization's responsibility to ensure the overall competence of staff? Furthermore, what are nurses' responsibilities to colleagues who are in need of help?

Chapter 4 discussed the elements of the *Code of Ethics* of the Canadian Nurses Association. Value v, Competent Nursing Care, states that nurses have a professional responsibility to ensure that they are competent to practise and must take the required education and skill review to ensure that competence is maintained. Value VIII, Protecting Clients from Incompetence, clearly states that nurses have an obligation to protect patients from harm.

When aware of incompetence on the part of another nurse or other health professional, nurses are required to take action to ensure the safety of the patient. When a nurse fails to take such action, then he or she shares responsibility for any subsequent consequences of that incompetence. Further, when health professionals delegate added responsibilities, that delegation should be appropriate and there should be assurance that those to whom the act is delegated are competent to carry out that act. In this case study, then, Kathy, her colleagues, and the teacher reviewing her skills had a shared professional responsibility to ensure that she was competent to care for her patients.

Individual nurses have a responsibility to maintain their professional competence, and must also maintain the minimum standards of their regulatory body. When other health care organizations, such as hospitals or community agencies, impose a higher standard, then that also must be met. In this case study, both Kathy and the hospital bear responsibility for review of her skills.

The leadership within any organization must take steps to ensure compliance with this expectation. If the employee does not respond to the requirement for reassessment or recertification, then reminders, counselling, and if required, disciplinary action must take place.

What was happening to Kathy in this case study? Did her colleagues understand the significance of her behaviour? Were they aware of the warning signs that Kathy was in crisis and needed help? Here, Kathy's colleagues, concerned about her personal situation, decided to protect her. Hoping that Kathy's crisis would resolve, they made efforts to shield her from further harm. Though one might sympathize with their concern, their strategy was counter-productive to Kathy's needs, placed the lives of patients in jeopardy, and compromised their own professional integrity.

Nurses function within a high-stress work environment. When personal stresses add to this, some nurses (as others in society) may become vulnerable to the misuse of substances such as alcohol or drugs to provide short-term relief of their symptoms. Some may become vulnerable to controlled substances such as narcotics, since nurses have ready access to such drugs. Nurses such as Kathy require early intervention. Rather than be concerned that she might be subject to discipline, Kathy's colleagues should be aware that support groups, counselling, and therapy are available for nurses in crisis.

Kathy's colleagues, if unsuccessful in dealing directly with her, have a responsibility both to Kathy and to her patients to take their concerns forward to the manager, a staff counsellor, or other professional or union representative. For example, a concerned and astute manager would recognize Kathy's need for help. It is better to provide counselling and therapy early on than to wait until patient care is compromised and Kathy's future career is in jeopardy.

General Principles

Recall the discussion of the general principles of negligence in Chapter 2 (pages 22–26). Basically, three elements are required to prove that a person is negligent and liable to another for damages. First, the person who is aggrieved (the plaintiff) must demonstrate that the person whom he or she is suing (the defendant) owed him or her a duty of care. Secondly, it must be established that the defendant breached that duty of care by engaging in conduct that did not meet a reasonable standard. Thirdly, the plaintiff must demonstrate that he or she has suffered physical harm or damage to either person or property, as a result of the defendant's breach of duty of care. If all three of these requirements are met, the plaintiff will have a case of negligence against the defendant.

Statutory Duty of Care

Most provincial nursing statutes explicitly or implicitly impose certain duties that nurses owe to patients in their care. Among these is the duty to report a fellow nurse whose conduct displays a lack of proper skill, judgement, knowledge, or training.[1] This also includes, in many provinces, a duty to report a nurse who is under the influence of alcohol or drugs.

In Ontario, for example, regulations under the *Nursing Act, 1991*[2] define certain acts of professional misconduct: "contravening a standard of practice of the profession or failing to meet the standard of practice of the profession" is one such act;[3] failing to report an incident of unsafe practice or unethical conduct of a health care provider to that provider's employer or to the College of Nurses is another.[4]

Thus, in our case study, Kathy's colleagues clearly have engaged in professional misconduct by failing to report incidents of her being intoxicated. In covering up a potentially harmful situation, they are ethically and legally culpable for any harm that may arise. Kathy has also breached her duty not to practise her profession while her ability to do so was impaired by alcohol.

Common Law Duty of Care

The common law also imposes a duty of care. In any negligence lawsuit involving a nurse or other health care professional, the trial will essentially amount to an evaluation of the nurse's conduct and the degree to which the nurse has met an accepted standard of care. The nurse, as a professional, is legally required to operate and act at a level that meets or exceeds that of a reasonably prudent caregiver or health practitioner. This, of course, implies that the nurse has a duty to maintain a level of expertise through continuing education to ensure that he or she practises in accordance with the latest standards. It would not do, for example, for a nurse trained in the 1960s to continue to operate and practise according to the standards of that decade in the 1990s. These standards would be such as those laid out by the provincial regulatory body (e.g., the Registered Nurses Association of British Columbia, the College of Nurses of Ontario) and the agency or hospital in which the nurse is employed.

As the nurse in our case study is representing herself as a qualified health practitioner, she owes a duty of proper care to all her patients. This duty has been described in case law as "the duty to exercise a reasonable degree of skill, knowledge and care in the treatment of a patient."[5] Quite apart from the issue of Kathy's practising her profession while under the influence of alcohol is the issue of her having mistakenly identified the arrythmia on the patient's monitor as ventricular tachycardia, when in fact the patient was experiencing supraventricular tachycardia. Kathy has not fulfilled her duty to read and interpret the monitor signs correctly. Has she lived up to the standard of care required of her?

An interesting illustration of the court's role in determining the standard of care and in assessing nursing conduct is found in the Nova Scotia Supreme Court decision of *Thompson Estate v. Byrne.*[6] In that case, the plaintiff, a middle-aged woman, had undergone quadruple heart by-pass surgery and was sent to the Cardiovascular Intensive Care Unit (CVICU) of the hospital following a successful operation. The patient was then placed in the care of the defendant, a nurse in the CVICU.

The defendant worked with several other nurses in this ward and, while every nurse had specific patients to care for, each would help the others as needed. While in the CVICU and while still anaesthetized, the plaintiff dislodged her endotracheal tube, which had been inserted to assist her breathing following the surgery. Upon seeing this, the nurse immediately announced to her colleagues that the patient had extubated herself, and went to the plaintiff to attend to her. As in any hospital, nurses were not permitted to perform an intubation upon a patient, as such a procedure could be performed only by a physician. However, the patient was being "bagged" pending the re-establishment of the endotracheal tube.

The extubation occurred at approximately 16:30 hours. A second nurse on duty, upon hearing the nurse's remark, called for assistance. A resident soon arrived and attempted to re-intubate the patient. With the first try, he had difficulty in locating the patient's vocal chords so that he could position the tube. He remarked that this would be a difficult intubation and requested that an anaesthetist be called to assist. The second nurse, who made the call, had difficulty locating the anaesthetist on duty. Thus, she went to the nearby Operating Room to get the anaesthetist. (This was a common means of seeking help, as the anaesthetists were usually there and the Operating Room was near the ICU.)

Meanwhile, the resident made a second, apparently successful attempt to re-intubate the patient. However, the tube was lodged in the patient's oesophagus, a fact that became apparent only some time later, when a respiratory technician who was "bagging" the patient noticed resistance in the flow of air and that the patient's abdomen was beginning to swell. At this point, the patient was observed to be turning cyanotic from lack of oxygen. Her heart rate had dropped, and she was given cardiac massage by the anaesthetist, who had arrived by then. It was now approximately 16:45 hours, that is, fifteen minutes since the patient had extubated herself.

The anaesthetist made a third, very difficult but ultimately successful attempt to re-intubate the patient, and an airway was re-established by 17:00 hours. The patient's colour returned to normal. Unfortunately, it was soon discovered that she had suffered severe brain damage as a result of hypoxia. She remained in a coma until she died two years later.

Her estate brought a negligence action against the resident, the anaesthetist, the hospital, and two of the nurses in the ICU ward in whose care she had been placed following the heart surgery. The claim alleged that the second nurse, who had gone to get the help of the anaesthetist on the resident's instructions, had been negligent in not making sufficient efforts to obtain help promptly, and that the injury to the patient would not have occurred but for the delay in the arrival of the anaesthetist. The claims against the nurses alleged that they had failed in their duty (1) to prevent the patient from extubating herself, (2) to attend the patient properly and particularly at all times, knowing that she had attempted to remove the tube on prior occasions, and (3) to live up to standards in cardiovascular intensive care units.[7]

The claims against the doctors were dismissed for lack of evidence of negligence. However, the claims against the nurses and the hospital remained. The testimony of several doctors and one nurse educator (herself an RN) was received by the court in order to assist it in assessing the conduct of the nurses and to determine the appropriate nursing standards against which to measure that conduct.

The doctors and nursing expert were unanimous in stating that the nurses had functioned in an entirely appropriate and professional manner throughout, under very difficult circumstances. There was no duty upon the nurse, as it was judged that to find such duty would, in such circumstances, place an inordinate burden upon nurses. Of course, such a finding would depend on the size, organization, and staffing of the unit, factors that vary from institution to institution, depending upon financial and human resources. In this case, the CVICU had seven patients in seven patient beds. There was a total of five nurses on duty in the unit.

The nursing expert stated that the nursing care was comprehensive, the nursing assessments were thorough, the problems had been identified by the nurses, and the physicians were kept informed at all times. Under these circumstances, the expert felt that the nurses had not breached any standards of nursing practice in an ICU ward.[8] With respect to the nurse, the court found that she did not have a duty to do any more than she had done to obtain the help of staff physicians. Had she done more, she would have been in breach of her primary duty to stay with her patient and assist the doctor who was attempting the re-intubation.[9] The court accepted the expert's opinion, and thus found no negligence on the nurses' part.

In discussing the duty of care owed by nurses, the court stressed that health care professionals are not insurers or guarantors of the success of the treatment that they undertake to provide. Thus, the standard of care to which they are held is not a standard of perfection. The court reiterated the distinction in law between carelessness in one's conduct and a genuine error in judgement. The law does not hold a professional responsible for the latter but will hold him or her responsible for the former if, in acting carelessly, harm ensues. Carelessness would be behaviour that did not accord with or conform to the approved and customary practices of similar institutions or professionals in the community (in this case, Canada).[10] In *Thompson Estate v. Byrne,* the nurses' conduct did not depart from such customary practices, as evidenced by the facts and analyzed by the expert testimony.

Application to Case Study

Similar analytical process will apply in examining Kathy's conduct. Her actions would be re-examined with the aid of expert testimony to determine whether and how she had breached her duty of care to her patient. As the hospital is likewise under a duty to provide proper and competent medical and nursing staff to patients in its care,[11] it also would likely be named as a defendant in any subsequent lawsuit, assuming the patient had suffered harm.

Kathy and the hospital may be sued by the patient, his family, or his estate, if he subsequently died. The plaintiff might allege that the hospital had breached its duty toward him to provide proper care and to ensure competent nursing and other health care staff. Thus, the hospital could be held directly liable for any damage or injury caused by Kathy as a result of her negligence.

For example, it may be held negligent in failing to ensure adequate and safe emergency procedures and, in this case study, in failing to ensure that drugs were safely and properly stored (e.g., pavulon may have been placed in the container labelled lidocaine). The finding of liability is also possible as the hospital, through Kathy's supervisor, failed to review Kathy's skills to ensure that she was competent and able to carry out her duties properly and effectively. She was an employee of the hospital, and her actions were under its control. This is known as the doctrine of **vicarious liability**.

Similarly, Kathy is under a duty to ensure that she arrives at work in a fit and proper condition. She clearly breached her duty in arriving at the hospital in an impaired state, and her condition may have placed the patient in jeopardy and contributed to the risks of harm.

Another aspect of vicarious liability as it relates to hospitals is that physicians who provide instructions to nursing staff in the care of their patients are entitled to rely on the assumption that the hospital has hired duly qualified, competent, and properly trained nursing staff. The doctors are not responsible for ensuring that the nurses carry out those instructions properly unless they have actual knowledge that the nursing staff are not competent to carry out those instructions. Thus, in cases where instructions are not properly followed, the doctor may argue as a defence that the nurse was negligent, if any claim of negligence is brought against the physician. In such a case, the instructions provided by the physician must not be negligent in and of themselves.

The Standard of Care and Causation

The nurse's conduct must be examined and compared to normal, competent, and reasonable standards of nursing practice to determine whether his or her conduct was or was not in conformity with that expected of a reasonably competent and skilled nurse. Of course, standards of practice change over time as new knowledge and technology are introduced and become widely available. Standards also differ from one institution to another, and from one treatment setting to another. For example, the standards of practice and expectations of a nurse in a critical care setting, such as a Cardiovascular Intensive Care Unit, will differ from those in a rehabilitation setting. Patients have a right to expect that a nurse employed in an ICU will have the knowledge and skill required to provide the necessary care in such a specialized area of practice.

In many cases, hospitals and other health care institutions that employ nurses have policies and procedures in place for the annual review of the nurses' skills. This practice would be recognized as a standard of care in any negligence suit brought against such an institution. Thus, to ensure that the hospital's duty is fulfilled, it is vital that the institution enforce nursing staff reviews. The hospital is responsible for ensuring that these reviews take place, and nurses cannot refuse to participate in them.

For example, in our case study, the nurses in the CVICU were expected to perform certain delegated medical acts, including the interpretation of arrhythmias and, when required, the administration of lidocaine. Kathy's skills should have been reviewed to ensure that she was competent and knowledgeable in the proper interpretation of arrhythmias. This inability led Kathy to conclude that lidocaine was needed when it was not. The fact that she administered the wrong drug (and, even if it had been the drug she intended, one that was not indicated for this patient's condition) shows that she did not meet the basic standard of care with respect to the administration of medication (i.e., checking the label carefully prior to administering the drug).

Employers also have a common law duty to take active steps to ensure that nurses falling short of the standard come to meet the expected standard. Such steps may include counselling, additional education, and, in some cases, disciplinary measures. The duty also includes ensuring that the nurse's skills are reviewed on a regular basis (although the nurse also has such a duty). In Kathy's case, counselling would be in order, but the hospital may have to resort to disciplinary measures if Kathy persistently fails to meet the standards of practice expected of her. (These standards include the separate issue of her arriving at work in an impaired condition.)

In some institutions, the review of skills is completely the responsibility of the nurse. If this is the case, this stipulation should be made explicit at the outset of the nurse's employment with the institution or agency. Appropriate action must be taken if these expectations are not met. Standards of care provide a baseline for assessment, planning, decision making, and action. They help to ensure the provision of safe and efficient nursing care within the institution or health care agency.

One of the errors committed in the case study is that Kathy failed to ensure that she was giving the correct medication to the patient. Furthermore, she failed to assess the patient's condition correctly prior to administering medication that, even if it had been correct, was not indicated for this type of cardiac problem. This case illustrates two crucial duties that the nurse must discharge properly: (1) to assess a patient's condition and problems correctly and accurately, and (2) to ensure that the correct medication is administered when required. In failing to do these things, Kathy has not met the standard of care required of her and has breached her common law duty to provide reasonably competent, knowledgeable, and skilled nursing services to her patient. She is thus negligent.

Duty to Make Correct Assessment and Accurately Recorded Observations

The former of these two duties was one of several aspects of nursing conduct to be examined in a case decided by the British Columbia Supreme Court in 1981. In *Meyer v. Gordon*,[12] the parents of a newborn infant who suffered severe brain damage and ensuing cerebral palsy as a result of a negligent delivery brought an action for negligence against two of the participating nurses, the hospital, and the attending physician. In all, three nurses were involved in some way in the delivery. The plaintiff had previously had a very fast labour, her first child having been born within four hours of the onset of labour. The plaintiff's doctor knew this, but had not advised the nursing or hospital staff that this might be a fast delivery when he had his patient admitted to the hospital on the morning when her labour began. Ascertaining the patient's birth history would be a normal and standard part of any labour assessment to be performed by a nurse. The plaintiff was admitted at approximately 11:30 hours.

The first nurse who examined the plaintiff, Nurse W., did not ascertain whether this was her first or second birth, and in fact failed to obtain any obstetrical history. It was clear at the trial that, had she done so, the history would have indicated that this patient should be closely watched. As well, there was evidence that the charting done by the two nurses who attended the plaintiff was inaccurate and incomplete. As a result, the nurses' notes were rejected by the trial judge as unreliable. Nurse W.'s failure to ascertain the obstetrical history of the mother in this case shows a marked departure from acceptable standards of practice in Canada.

At approximately 11:30 hours, Nurse W. performed the first examination of the plaintiff and ascertained that she was in the early stages of labour. She did not record this, however, and was imprecise as to the position of the foetus at that time, noting the position only as "mid." Neither did the nurse record the duration of the contractions during her first, and only, vaginal examination. At this point, she ascertained that dilation was three centimetres, but the character of the cervix (an important indication of the progress of labour) was not recorded accurately.

A second nurse, Nurse M., assisted Nurse W. in these examinations. Neither nurse appears to have recognized the danger of leaving the mother lying on her back, in which position she remained until delivery. The court found, among other things, that permitting the plaintiff to remain in this position contributed greatly to foetal distress and constituted a marked departure from the standard of care at that hospital, which was known for excellence in obstetrics. The mother should clearly have been repositioned on her side.

The foetal heart rate was checked at 11:50 hours and again at 12:00 hours. However, this information does not appear to have been recorded until much later. The court noted that both nurses had gone back and altered the chart some hours after the delivery to make the record appear more complete than it actually was. These facts meant that the court was unable to rely upon the nurses' notes as an accurate account of what had happened. (The problems connected with accuracy of documentation will be discussed more fully in Chapter 9.)

At noon, the patient's doctor prescribed an injection of Demerol and Gravol to ease her pain and nausea. Although this was not explicitly stated by the court or in the evidence as reported, the giving of Demerol would no doubt have had a sedative effect not only on the mother, but also on the foetus. This could have contributed to the onset of foetal distress. He did not instruct Nurse M. to conduct a vaginal examination prior to administering the Demerol and, in fact, none was conducted before the drug was given at 12:05 hours. This was also against generally accepted practice.

From the time the Demerol was given until the child was born at 12:32 hours, the plaintiff was left lying on her back, alone and completely unattended despite her excruciating and rapid labour pains and despite Nurse W.'s opinion that the foetal heart rate ought to have been checked every fifteen minutes at that point. The court noted that, although the obstetrical ward appeared to have been extremely busy that day, the plaintiff did not appear to have been anyone's patient in particular from that point on.

At 12:15 hours, the plaintiff's husband, noticing his wife's extreme pain, sought out Nurse W.. He told her that he believed his wife was about to give birth and needed assistance. The evidence at trial indicates that Nurse W. may have brushed off his concern, dismissing him as a nervous husband. The court found it deplorable that there was no nursing care available to the plaintiff when her husband sought it.[13]

At approximately 12:30 hours, the plaintiff's husband again sought out a nurse, saying that his wife was giving birth. A third nurse (Nurse T.) responded and went to the plaintiff. She found the baby's head already born with a very large amount of meconium about the baby's head. She completed the delivery; however, as Nurse M. (who assisted her) had failed to include a suction bulb in the emergency bundle, Nurse T. was unable to suction the meconium from the baby's nose and mouth. This was also deemed a serious oversight by the expert physicians who testified at trial.

It is clear that the baby was not breathing when she was born. Nurse T. described the baby as "very flaccid and limp." Further time was lost in bringing the baby to the caseroom for resuscitation. Another doctor was involved in resuscitation using initial suctioning, positive pressure ventilation, and oxygen with endotracheal suctioning. As the court noted later, all of these factors contributed to the risk of brain damage as a result of foetal distress. The resuscitation efforts continued for some time with the assistance of two other physicians and were ultimately successful. The child was moved to the Intensive Care Nursery of the hospital. It was soon discovered, however, that she had suffered brain damage as a result of foetal distress and resulting asphyxia in conjunction with meconium aspiration.[14]

The plaintiffs sued the mother's doctor, the doctors involved in the resuscitation efforts and, more importantly, the nurses and hospital that had provided the nursing care. The court dismissed the suit against the doctors (except the plaintiffs' own doctor, whom it found 25% liable on the basis that he had failed to instruct Nurse M. to conduct a vaginal examination of the plaintiff prior to administering the Demerol). The hospital was found 75% responsible for the baby's brain damage, as a result of its negligence in failing to provide adequate and proper nursing care. Among its findings, the court listed the particulars of the nurses' negligence:

(1) The nurses' observations were insufficient;

(2) the mother was left lying on her side unattended until the time of birth;

(3) no nursing care, apart from the injection of Demerol, was made available to the mother in the last thirty minutes prior to birth;

(4) the Demerol was given to the plaintiff without a vaginal examination and without changing her supine position;

(5) the child was covered in meconium, and there was no suctioning device available in the emergency bundle in order to suction it from the child's nose and mouth as she was being born; and

(6) there was some time lost before suctioning procedures were started by the second doctor.[15]

The court concluded that:

> ... the foetal distress which caused the brain damage was a direct result of the inadequate observations that were made initially, coupled with leaving [the plaintiff] in a supine position, unattended. That lack of care, followed by the failure of the nursing staff to be in attendance at the time of the birth of the head to assist the child by suctioning the meconium from the nose and mouth, all contributed to causing the foetal distress which caused the brain damage.[16]

Of course, as discussed in Chapter 2, one of the elements of any negligence action is that the defendant's breach must be the cause of the plaintiff's injury and that injury must be a reasonably foreseeable consequence of that breach. In the *Meyer* case, the court relied on the rule that a person who, in acting negligently, increases materially the risks of injury to another will be liable to that other for negligence even though there may have been other factors that contributed to those injuries and for which the defendant was not responsible.[17] In the *Meyer* case, the court found that the failure of the nursing staff to examine the mother properly and care for her, as well as their leaving her unattended in a supine position, materially increased the risk of injury to the child and the risk of foetal distress and resulting hypoxia. Since the nursing staff clearly created these risks, the hospital was thus liable for the consequences.[18]

The court in this case made use of procedural manuals prepared by the hospital for guidance of nursing and medical staff in various treatment situations. In particular, one manual itemized the problems associated with leaving a woman in labour in the supine position. Such manuals, if authoritative and directory, are often referred to by courts in assessing the conduct of a health practitioner accused of negligence. It is therefore wise for any nurse to study all available procedural guides and manuals (including hospital policy statements and regulations covering various treatment situations) and to follow them as closely as possible. Indeed, if they are authoritative, such manuals will set out the standard of care expected of nursing staff, and the hospital will be under a duty to enforce these standards. It follows that any deviation from such standards to a lower standard of practice could also constitute a breach on the part of the hospital, thereby leaving it open to a negligence action. Following the manuals will also demonstrate that the nurse has adhered to standard and widely accepted procedures in a particular emergency or treatment situation.

Duty to Check and Ensure Proper Medication

The second duty, to ensure that the proper medication is given, was discussed in *Bugden v. Harbour View Hospital.*[19] Although the case was decided in 1947, it illustrates the duty of care required of nurses when preparing or dealing in medication. It also illustrates the fact that the physician was once entitled to rely upon a nurse's competence in the dispensing and administration of medication. This standard has now changed, since physicians are now equally under a duty to ensure that the correct medication is given. The current practice is for the nurse to show the physician the medication (or, during surgery, the surgical instrument) that he or she has requested. When dispensing medication, a nurse today would normally check the bottle or ampoule up to three times to ensure accuracy. In this way, there are more opportunities to catch a mistake.

The *Bugden* case originated in Nova Scotia. The patient, a miner, dislocated his thumb and went to the defendant hospital to have it treated. The doctor on duty examined the thumb and decided he would reset it using a local anaesthetic. He was assisted by an experienced graduate nurse (Nurse A.), whom he asked to give the patient morphine and atropine. This she did. He then decided to have X-rays taken of the thumb prior to beginning the re-setting, and asked the nurse to get Novocain (a local anaesthetic).

Nurse A. immediately went to another part of the hospital and asked a second nurse (Nurse B.) for Novocain. Nurse B. gave Nurse A. a labelled bottle, but neither she nor Nurse A. examined the label. Nurse A. took the bottle back to the doctor who, without checking it, filled his syringe with the solution it contained and injected it into the patient's thumb. Upon seeing that the thumb was not yet properly anaesthetized, he injected more of the solution. A total of 4 mL of this solution was injected into the patient. The doctor then proceeded to set the thumb.

A short while later, Nurse A. noticed that the patient looked ill and called the doctor, who attempted an unspecified treatment that failed. Thirty minutes later, the patient died. It was subsequently discovered that the bottle from which the doctor had filled his syringe and which was thought to contain Novocain in fact had contained epinephrine hydrochloride, a heart stimulant (also known as adrenaline). A 4-mL dose of this drug was fatal: the patient had died of heart failure as a result of having been given adrenaline by mistake.

The patient's wife sued in negligence for damages, naming the doctor, the hospital, and the two nurses as defendants. The Supreme Court of Nova Scotia stated that where it was the duty of several persons to guard against danger, any one of them who failed to take precautions could not escape by saying that another person should have caught his error.[20] The court elucidated upon the duty of care of each nurse involved in this case and stated:

> Persons who are in charge of dangerous things under which category, I think, drugs are included are under a duty to handle them with such care that harm will not arise to those who depend upon their skill. At the least they must exercise reasonable care to avoid such harm.... The liability in any particular case arises from the foreseeability of damage, and the duty to take care.[21]

In this case, the court noted that it was impossible for a competent nurse not to realize that if adrenaline were used instead of Novocain, the danger of death would be great. There was, therefore, a duty upon each nurse to avoid what in fact had happened. The failure of Nurse B. to verify that she was giving the correct drug did not absolve Nurse A. from a similar duty. Although Nurse B.

was not directly involved in treating the patient, she was the nurse in charge of drugs at the hospital and owed a duty to all potential patients to ensure that they were given the proper medication. Since drugs are articles dangerous in and of themselves, there is a duty upon anyone handling them to take precautions so that others coming into proximity with them are not hurt.[22]

Both nurses, as well as the hospital, were found negligent. The doctor escaped liability in that expert evidence from other doctors indicated it was reasonable for him to rely on Nurse A. to give him the proper medication. It would have been unreasonable to impose upon the doctor a duty to supervise nurses who were hospital employees (not his own) while treating patients. As we have said, the standard of care today in such a situation has been increased to require the nurse to show the bottle or container of medication to the physician or other person administering it. Further, there would probably be an obligation today on the physician to check the medication as well.

In another Ontario case, *Fiege v. Cornwall General Hospital et al.,*[23] a nurse was found negligent when she improperly administered an injection of Talwin into the left buttock of a patient. The nurse, contrary to standard procedure, administered the injection directly into the site of the patient's sciatic nerve, causing the patient an injury. The trial judge concluded that it was improper for an injection to be made over the sciatic nerve and that if the plaintiff's injury could be attributed to this injection, the nurse was negligent in administering it.[24]

Application to Case Study

Applying the principles of general negligence to our case study, it is fairly certain that, if any damage or injury resulted from the administration of pavulon to the heart patient, Kathy would be responsible. She did not take proper precautions in administering the correct drug. Furthermore, she failed to make a proper assessment of the patient's condition, for which lidocaine was not indicated. In failing to do these things, Kathy breached the standard of competent nursing care. Finally, she breached her professional obligation not to work while impaired.

Most provincial nursing statutes frown heavily upon a nurse's working while impaired. For example, in Ontario, Prince Edward Island, and Saskatchewan, practising nursing while one's ability to do so is impaired by any substance constitutes professional misconduct.[25] It would also likely constitute misconduct under the legislation of the remaining provinces and territories (even though these statutes do not expressly refer to impairment of the nurse while on duty), as it would adversely influence the nurse's ability to practise safely and properly. It may also constitute a threat to the safety of patients.

Furthermore, Kathy's fellow nurses may also be negligent. Since they know of Kathy's possible impairment when caring for the cardiac patient, they may, in permitting her to continue to provide care, be contributing to the risk of injury to that patient. It is clearly their professional and ethical duty to alert Kathy's manager of the fact that Kathy may have a drinking problem and, more importantly, that she may be under the influence of alcohol as she provides care to patients. In some cases, the failure to report improper, negligent, or unethical conduct could in and of itself constitute professional misconduct. The matter, in most cases, will then be taken up according to the disciplinary procedures and mechanisms of the provincial regulatory body (as discussed in greater detail in Chapter 3).

Criminal Law Sources of Liability

The criminal law also holds significant consequences for nurses and other health practitioners who act carelessly or with recklessness. In Chapter 2, we mentioned the *Criminal Code* provisions concerning the omission to do that which a health practitioner has undertaken to do. Section 216 of the *Criminal Code* provides:

> 216. Every one who undertakes to administer surgical or medical treatment to another person or to do any other lawful act that may endanger the life of another person is, except in cases of necessity, under a legal duty to have and to use reasonable knowledge, skill and care in so doing.

In specific relation to the practice of nursing, this places an obligation upon people who represent themselves as qualified and competent nurses to ensure that their skills and education are adequate to perform properly the medical treatment that they are called upon to administer. The section excludes cases of necessity, which imply emergency or life-threatening situations. Here, however, a nurse would not normally act to administer such treatment if there were a more qualified practitioner, such as a physician, available to administer (for example) emergency surgery. Otherwise a nurse, acting in good faith, could proceed if he or she performed to the best of his or her ability. The legal policy here is to encourage people to render emergency treatment to those in urgent need of it. In some extreme cases, such treatment could include surgery under circumstances where the aid of a qualified surgeon was unavailable.

Criminal Law Standard of Care

A person who represents herself or himself as a duly qualified health practitioner will, if serious injury or bodily harm ensues, be held to the standard of the reasonably qualified practitioner. The decision of the British Columbia County Court in the case of *R v. Sullivan and Lemay*[26] illustrates this point. Although that case involved two midwives, the point is equally applicable to nurses. In that case, the midwives were assisting in a home birth. The child died as a result of their negligent delivery, and they were each charged with criminal negligence causing death (with respect to the infant) and with criminal negligence causing bodily harm (to the mother, as a result of their negligent delivery procedures).

In addressing the standard of expertise to which the defendants would be held, the court said that the midwives' conduct constituted a lawful act that might endanger the life of another person within the meaning of this section.

Therefore, they were under a legal duty to have and use reasonable skill, care, and knowledge in performing the delivery, and their conduct would be held to the standard of a competent childbirth attendant, even though they had no formal training as midwives.

Criminal Negligence

Section 219 of the Code defines **criminal negligence** thus:

> 219(1). Every one is criminally negligent who (a) in doing anything, or (b) in omitting to do anything that it is his duty to do, shows wanton or reckless disregard for the lives or safety of other persons.

The "duty" of which this section speaks is a duty imposed by law, either statute law or common law.[27] This section must be read in conjunction with section 217 of the Code, which states:

> 217. Every one who undertakes to do an act is under a legal duty to do it if an omission to do the act is or may be dangerous to life.

Thus, if a nurse fails to perform some act that is part of his or her nursing procedures and duties, and as a result someone dies or suffers serious bodily harm, the nurse's omission may be characterized as criminally negligent and would constitute a criminal offence of either criminal negligence causing death or criminal negligence causing bodily harm, depending on the impact on the patient. Before the conduct could be characterized as negligent, however, it would have to demonstrate a marked or substantial departure from conduct that one would expect from a reasonable and competent nurse. There would have to be extreme carelessness, or recklessness (i.e., a complete disregard for consequences of one's actions), or such grave and serious omission as to show that the nurse failed to recognize obvious risks or, if aware of those risks, that he or she chose to take them anyway, "reckless" and oblivious to the consequences. Such a formulation in the law shows how extreme and outrageous the carelessness must be in order to be judged criminally negligent. In Kathy's case, being intoxicated and failing to see she was administering the wrong drug might be classified as reckless behaviour.

Necessity for Causation

By definition, criminal negligence must cause death[28] or bodily harm[29] to another. If we assume that the patient in our case study died as a result of being administered the wrong drug, it is possible that Kathy might be charged with criminal negligence causing death. The fact that she was working while impaired would be taken into consideration in assessing whether her conduct showed a reckless disregard for the lives or safety of others within the meaning of the Code.

In many cases, impairment has been a factor in finding drunk drivers criminally negligent when they have operated motor vehicles while under the influence of alcohol and have either hurt or killed others in accidents. In such cases, the fact that the accused was intoxicated of his or her own volition is evidence that may lead a court to decide that he or she acted with wanton or reckless disregard for the lives or safety of others.[30] Intoxication is therefore a relevant factor in determining whether a person acted wantonly or recklessly.

In Kathy's case, the fact that she was impaired would be relevant in a charge of criminal negligence causing death. The fact that her intoxication rendered her incapable of appreciating the probable consequences of her actions would not be a defence. Whether a conviction could be successfully obtained, however, would depend on whether the mistake in administering the wrong drug demonstrated a wanton or reckless disregard for the life or safety of the patient. Even if Kathy's conduct was negligent according to civil law, if it was not negligent according to this criminal law standard, she would not be convicted of criminal negligence. And even if Kathy's conduct was found to be grossly negligent in a civil law context, that conduct may not be sufficient so as to show the degree of wanton or reckless disregard required to convict her of criminal negligence. The patient would also have to suffer some harm, or die.

There is a substantial difference between being negligent in a civil lawsuit and being criminally negligent. The latter type of negligence requires conduct that exceeds what one would normally expect of a reasonable person (in this case, a reasonable nurse). The intent of the accused is irrelevant. It is sufficient that the accused acted in such a manner as to demonstrate that he or she either recognized the obvious risk of danger to another and took that risk anyway, or that he or she ought reasonably to have foreseen such a risk and failed to do so.[31] In other words, the accused was completely indifferent to the risks that his or her actions posed to the life or safety of others who might reasonably be expected to be so affected.

The Provincial Coroner's and Medical Examiner's Systems

In every province, the consequences of an unexplained death must be investigated with a view to determining its causes and identifying ways to prevent similar occurrences in the future. The coroner's and medical examiner's systems of the various provinces merit discussion, as these are concurrently integral components of both the criminal justice system and provincial constitutional responsibility for administering justice within the province. Thus, if there is any evidence of serious negligence on the part of nursing or medical staff that is attributed to the death of a person, an inquest may be ordered by a coroner, or a court, to determine all possible causes and circumstances of the death. It is therefore important for nurses to have a basic understanding of both the coroner's and medical examiner's systems in use across Canada, since nurses may be called upon to testify at such inquests.

The **coroner's inquest** is primarily a fact-finding and investigatory endeavour. In earlier times, a coroner's court could also find criminal or civil responsibility; however, the modern coroner's inquest is not a criminal trial. There is no accused person. In some provinces, the coroner has the authority, upon conclusion of an inquest, to order the arrest of anyone who has been found by the coroner to be responsible for the death of any person whose death forms the subject of the inquest.

Ontario, Quebec, New Brunswick, Prince Edward Island, Saskatchewan, British Columbia, the Yukon Territory, and the Northwest Territories use the traditional coroner's system adopted from English common law. The remaining provinces have moved away from this system to a more modernized medical examiner's system. Both systems, however, are broadly similar in their workings as a means to investigate suspicious deaths. In the medical examiner's system, the function of holding an inquiry is usually left to a judge, or, in the case of Alberta, the Fatality Review Board.[32]

A detailed review of each province's system is beyond the scope of this book. However, as an example, Ontario's system will be briefly described. Under Ontario's *Coroner's Act*,[33] a Chief Coroner for Ontario is appointed to supervise a number of coroners throughout the province. Each such coroner will be appointed for a particular region and each is a legally qualified medical practitioner. A coroner appointed for a specific region is required to live in that region.

Under the Act, everyone who has reason to believe that a person has died:

(1) as a result of violence, misadventure (e.g., an accident), negligence, misconduct or malpractice,
(2) by unfair means,
(3) during pregnancy or following pregnancy in such circumstances to which the death could be attributed,
(4) suddenly and unexpectedly,
(5) from disease or sickness for which the person was not treated by a legally qualified medical practitioner,
(6) from any cause other than disease, or
(7) under circumstances that require investigation

must report the death either to a coroner or to the police.[34] Similarly, if a person dies while in a home for the aged, a children's residence, a home for retarded persons, a mental institution, a nursing home, or a public or private hospital to which the person was transferred from one of those previously mentioned institutions, the person in charge of such institution must notify the coroner in writing of the death.[35] Pending an order from the coroner, no person may in any way alter the condition of, or interfere with the body of, the deceased.

Once notified, the local coroner will issue a warrant to take possession of the body as part of his or her investigation. The investigation and fact finding into the circumstances of the death begin at this point. The coroner has the power to enter into any place where the death occurred, inspect and extract information from any records or writings relating to the deceased, and seize anything that he or she believes is material to the purposes of the investigation.

In cases where someone has died in a health care institution or agency, it is likely that the coroner would seize the deceased's medical records immediately upon being notified of the death. This is a precaution to preserve the character of the evidence and to avoid the possibility of additions being made to such records that might obscure the medical circumstances and condition of the deceased at the moment of death.

It is important, therefore, to ensure that records are made as contemporaneously as possible with the act being recorded. The nurse involved in the care of the deceased is at the very least a potential witness to the circumstances surrounding the treatment, care, and condition of that person immediately prior to the death. At most, such a nurse may be called upon to testify at the coroner's inquest and will have to rely upon the records to refresh his or her memory as to the events leading up to the death. Questions asked of witnesses in such cases may be quite detailed and require precise interpretation of the nursing notes and other records. Therefore (and as we will discuss further in Chapter 9), the necessity of making clear and accurate records as close as possible to the time when the nursing act was performed cannot be overstressed.

If the coroner deems it advisable, he or she can order an inquest to be held into the circumstances of the deceased's death. Otherwise, the matter will proceed no further.

If an inquest is held, the coroner will hold a hearing, in some provinces, with the aid of a jury (usually smaller than a criminal trial jury of twelve). The jury's function is to aid in making recommendations as to any improvements to procedures, policies, and standards that may help to prevent similar occurrences.

The inquest will usually proceed along the same lines as a trial. However, the inquest is not a criminal trial; there is no prosecution and no accused. The Crown attorney may be a participant, and any other parties who are material witnesses or participants in the events leading up to the person's death may be called to testify at the inquest.

A person cannot be compelled to testify at an inquest once he or she has been charged with a criminal offence. If a person is called to testify, he or she will have the right to the aid of a lawyer. However, the lawyer's involvement may be limited to advising on answers to questions and the rights of the witness. In most provinces, the witness has the right not to have any evidence that he or she gives at an inquest used against him or her in any ensuing criminal proceedings. This is to ensure that the witness' rights (under the *Charter of Rights and Freedoms*) against self-incrimination are maintained. This does not mean, however, that the witness has the right to refuse any proper questions put to him or her. A refusal to answer may place that witness in danger of being found in contempt of court, a judgement that carries with it fines and a possible jail term.

The inquest is more relaxed in terms of following the strict rules of evidence normally applied in a court. However, coroners tend to follow such rules, especially in recent years.

In provinces with a medical examiner's system, the medical examiner takes the place of the coroner. Such a person is appointed by the provincial government and is usually a trained physician, given the medical complexities and technicalities that tend to be the focus of such inquests. Historically, however, coroners were laymen, untrained in medical matters. In the past few decades there has been a trend away from lay coroners, and now most are doctors. The procedures across the country are fairly similar, except that in some provinces (such as Nova Scotia or Manitoba) the inquest may be held by a provincial court judge. The investigative and inquiry functions are thus kept separate.

Once the inquest is concluded, the coroner, or judicial officer conducting the hearing, may give a decision (taking into consideration any recommendations made by the jury) on the causes of the deceased's death, and anything that could have been done to prevent it. For example, if the inquest is into the death of a patient at a hospital, the coroner's jury might recommend changes to certain policies or procedures that it feels may have contributed to the death. Further, if anyone is suspected, as a result of the coroner's decision, of criminal responsibility, it is possible that criminal charges may be laid in the wake of the coroner's decision. The criminal justice process would then take over to determine the guilt or innocence of any accused person.

Summary

The key points introduced in this chapter include:
- the professional responsibilities and accountabilities of the nurse
- the ethical and legal aspects of professional competence, misconduct, and malpractice
- the nurse's ethical and legal responsibilities to the patient and to other health practitioners
- the implications of "whistle-blowing"
- legal rules and ethical theory as they apply to hypothetical case studies and actual situations
- the legal concepts of negligence, duty of care, vicarious liability, standard of care, and causation
- the significance of documentation
- the criminal law with respect to standard of care and negligence
- the role of the coroner's office and the implications of a coroner's inquest.

References

1. See, e.g., Alberta: *Nursing Profession Act*, SA 1983, c. N-14.5, section 103(1); Ontario: O. Reg. 799/93, section 1, paragraph 25; Saskatchewan: *Registered Nurses Act, 1988*, SS 1988, c. R-12.2, section 26(2)(k); Manitoba: *Registered Nurses Act*, RSM 1987, c. R40, CCSM, c. R40, section 46(1).
2. See O. Reg. 799/93, section 1.
3. Ibid., section 1, paragraph 6.
4. Ibid., paragraph 25.

5. *Thompson Estate v. Byrne et al.* (1993), 114 NSR (2d) 395, at 423 (SCTD).

6. Ibid.

7. Ibid., p. 397.

8. Ibid., p. 421.

9. Ibid., p. 424.

10. Ibid., citing McCormick v. Marcotte, [1972] SCR 18, at p. 21, per Abbott J.

11. *Kolesar v. Jeffries* (1974), 59 DLR (3d) 367, at p. 376.

12. (1981), 17 CCLT 1 (BC SC).

13. Ibid., p. 15.

14. Ibid., p. 9.

15. Ibid., p. 37.

16. Ibid.

17. Ibid., p. 42, citing *McGhee v. Nat. Coal Bd.*, [1972] 3 All ER 1008 (HL).

18. Ibid., pp. 42–43.

19. [1947] 2 DLR 338 (NS SC).

20. Ibid., per Doull J., at p. 30.

21. Ibid., pp. 340–341.

22. Ibid., citing *Dominion Natural Gas Co. v. Collins,* [1909] AC 640 (JCPC), at p. 646-647.

23. (1980) 30 or (2d) 691 (HCJ).

24. Ibid., per Carruthers J., at p. 692.

25. Ontario: supra footnote 1, section 1, paragraph 6; Saskatchewan: supra footnote 1, section 26(2)(n); and Prince Edward Island: Reg. No. EC504/89, section 2(a)(ii).

26. (1986), 31 CCC (3d) 62; 55 CR (3d) 48 (B.C. Co. Ct.), appeal dismissed on other grounds (1988), 43 CCC (3d) 65; 65 CR (3d) 256; 31 BCLR (2d) 145 (CA).

27. *R v. Coyne* (1958), 124 CCC 176; 31 CR 335 (NB SCAD).

28. *Criminal Code of Canada,* RSC 1985, c. C-46, as amended, section 220.

29. Ibid., section 221.

30. See *R v. Anderson* (1985), 35 MVR 128, at p. 133 (Man. CA).

31. *R v. Sharpe* (1984), 12 CCC (3d) 428; 39 CR (3d) 367; 26 MVR 279 (Ont. CA).

32. Alberta: *Fatality Inquiries Act,* RSA 1989, c. F-6, as amended.

33. RSO 1990, c. C.37.

34. Ibid., section 10(1).

35. Ibid., section 10(2).

Six

Consent to Treatment

CHAPTER OBJECTIVES

The purpose of this chapter is to enable the reader to:
- understand the foundation of consent in law and ethics
- explain the principle of autonomy and its role in consent
- appreciate the concept of competence or capacity
- understand the tort of battery
- explain the concept of informed consent
- clarify the various types of, and approaches to, consent
- understand the rights of patients to refuse consent to medical or health care
- describe the nurse's role in ensuring that informed consent takes place
- apply the legal rules and ethical theory to hypothetical case studies and real case law
- understand the consent challenges with respect to the incompetent adult and to children
- clarify professional responsibilities in emergency situations
- understand the concept of proxy or substitute consent
- clarify existing new and impending consent legislation in the various provinces.

Basis in Ethics and Law

Rights

As we saw in Chapters 2 and 4, in Canada the rights of patients extend to personal autonomy, and the right to be informed of all risks material to a particular medical procedure, including the risks, both real and probable, in forgoing such treatment. (A *material risk* is one which a reasonable person would wish to know in deciding whether to consent to or forgo a given medical procedure.) These rights include the right of a patient not to be subjected to any treatment to which he or she has not given a free and informed consent if mentally capable, and the moral right to be treated with respect, dignity, and courtesy by all health care professionals. Legal rights are enforceable by the courts via the lawsuit. Moral rights are guaranteed by professionals who deem these part of their ethical and professional duty.

Autonomy

The principle of autonomy supports the capable and competent patient's right to determine and act on a self-chosen plan. Informed consent represents autonomy and ensures the individual's right to the information required to make personal decisions about health care. Nurses are obliged to respect the choices of their patients. However, there are situations when nurses may face a conflict between respect for the individual's wishes and their obligation to help their patients and protect them from harm.

Patients have the right to refuse consent to treatment, regardless of whether that treatment is in their best interests. It is the duty of the nurse to support the patient through such decisions. It is also the nurse's duty to ensure that the patient has the information required to make such choices, as well as sufficient time to reflect on the alternatives available. Whether or not the nurse is part of an informed consent process, he or she is obligated to advocate for the patient where the patient has not been duly informed, or where the patient's wishes have not been respected.

Patient autonomy is the hallmark of free and informed consent to treatment. It is recognized in both civil law and common law throughout Canada. In Quebec, for example, the new *Civil Code* proclaims this principle. Article 3 declares that every person possesses personality rights, which include the right to life, the right to personal integrity and inviolability, and respect of name, reputation, and privacy. This last-mentioned right of privacy is interesting in that it implies that individuals have the right to make decisions about their life and affairs free of governmental scrutiny and interference (except as permitted by law). This right to privacy is likewise implied in the United States Constitution, and has been used to strike down laws restricting abortion rights in that country.

If a patient is mentally competent, the law requires health practitioners, including nurses, to respect any decision he or she makes, no matter how potentially harmful that decision may be to the patient. Yet, autonomy can be meaningful only when patients are given full and complete information as to their medical condition, the risks which that condition poses to their life, and the benefits and drawbacks of any proposed treatment that health care professionals may offer. The risks, material facts, and alternatives, including the consequences of non-treatment, must be explained to the patient.

For example, if a patient refuses to ambulate, or to practise deep breathing and coughing exercises prior to surgery, the nurse must explain the benefits and risks of such procedures and the consequences of not doing them. The explanation must be respectful and courteous, and the nurse must give the patient an opportunity to change his or her mind. Such interventions as injections, medications, and so forth cannot be forced on a competent patient.

Suppose a patient is in the final phases of metastatic cancer: the cancer has spread to her bones, and she is in severe pain. The care plan is to turn her every two hours to prevent pressure sores and to minimize the likelihood of pneumonia. Turning causes her great pain such that she requires additional sedation, which causes extended drowsiness. Should the nurses give this patient the choice of being turned or not? Are there alternatives? As long as the patient understands and is willing to accept the consequences of not being turned, her decision is valid. She may choose to refuse turning in order to avoid the pain and the need for increased sedation.

If the patient is ill informed, or is misled by the information provided, any consent given is, in law, no consent at all. He or she may have decided differently if informed fully and properly. Hence, that patient's right to autonomy will have been infringed, as he or she has not been able to make a free and informed decision as to whether to undergo or forgo treatment.

Respect for the patient's autonomy is likewise compromised when, in the absence of consent, the health care professional presumes to decide whether treatment should proceed. This includes decisions as to what is and is not a material risk, all of which should be disclosed to the patient. (There are exceptions to the need for such consent in emergencies, as we will see later in this chapter.)

Battery

As discussed in Chapter 2, **battery** is a category of intentional **tort**, and is legally defined as the touching of another, however slight, without that person's consent. Thus, it is an unwanted intrusion on the physical person of another. In a medical context, the administration of any medical treatment, diagnostic test, nursing care, surgical procedure, or other such medical intervention, no matter how necessary or beneficial to the patient's health and well-being in the health practitioner's opinion, is forbidden unless the professional who is administering the treatment has obtained the patient's prior consent, or unless the patient has suffered a serious injury that renders him or her unable to give consent, and a lack of prompt medical attention would result in serious bodily harm or death.

It is a fundamental principle of ethics and the law that people who are mentally competent have the right to their bodily integrity and personal autonomy respecting medical treatment. This right applies even to mentally incompetent persons to the extent that their wishes, when they were competent, are known. If the patient is not competent, his or her prior wishes, as expressed to others or in an advance directive must be respected to the greatest extent possible. The final decision as to whether any nursing care, medical treatment, or plan of care should or should not proceed rests with the patient. The nurse or other health practitioner who proceeds without the patient's consent runs the risk of being found liable in a civil lawsuit for battery or, if he or she has carelessly informed the patient and harm results, for negligence.

To summarize, a truly **informed consent** requires the following conditions to be met:

(1) The consent must be given voluntarily. There must be no coercion or undue pressure from another person to obtain that consent.

(2) The patient must be told of all material and possible risks inherent in a proposed procedure, together with its benefits and drawbacks, as well as the risks of forgoing the treatment.

(3) The consent given must be specific to the proposed treatment or procedure. For example, a consent to an appendectomy does not authorize the removal of other infected or diseased tissues unrelated to that condition.

(4) The consent must specify who will perform the procedure or treatment. If a patient has consented to its performance by a particular specialist, this would not authorize the substitution of another, less qualified, or different type of health practitioner.

(5) The patient must be legally capable. A minor under a certain age may not be legally qualified to consent, depending on the province.

(6) Similarly, in most provinces, mental incompetency renders persons legally incapable of consenting unless they are capable of understanding the nature and consequences of the procedure, notwithstanding their mental condition.

Types of Consent

There are two basic types of consent: expressed and implied. *Expressed consent* is a clear statement of consent from the patient. No specific wording is required; an expression such as, "Okay, nurse, go ahead" is sufficient. Many provinces require that a written consent also be obtained as evidence that the patient has consented to a medical procedure or treatment. It is important to remember that the patient has the right to withdraw consent or revoke (cancel) a previously given consent at any time, even orally, provided he or she is mentally competent to do so.

Implied consent is inferred from a patient's conduct. For example, a nurse advises a patient whose hand has just been punctured by a rusty nail that she will be administering a tetanus vaccine as a precaution to prevent "lockjaw." The patient then holds out his arm to receive the injection. Clearly, through this action, he has consented to the treatment without written or verbal means.

Record and Timing of Consent

Many nurses may be concerned when no expressed written consent is found in the patient's chart and the patient is ready for surgery and perhaps already sedated. Must a written consent be obtained in this instance? The written consent form itself does not stand alone; it is merely documentary evidence. What matters is the fact that an informed consent has been given. If the physician has documented somewhere in the patient's chart the fact of the patient's consent and the disclosure relating to the risks, consequences, and benefits of the procedure, this will usually be sufficient. Moreover, the written consent can be revoked at any time by the patient provided he or she is mentally competent to do so.

Written Consent Forms

The blanket consent form used in some hospitals should not be solely relied upon, since it may not be specific to the particular procedure or treatment. The physician should document the fact that the procedure was explained to the patient along with its risks and consequences, and that the patient verbally consented. In many cases, the gravity of the situation or the risks in delaying treatment may preclude the obtaining of a signed consent; thus, documenting the fact of an informed consent is very important. Any such note should be signed and dated by the physician. It can also be signed by the nurse who is present at the time when such disclosure is made to the patient.

CASE STUDY

Consent to treatment

Doris, a widow seventy-five years of age, lives alone in a suburban bungalow that she and her late husband owned for thirty years. Her few close friends have died in the past few years. She has two grown children, a son and a daughter, who both live in another city. Over the past six or seven months, her general health has declined. She has lost weight, has grown weak, and finds it difficult to leave home to go about her daily activities.

One week, Sam, her postman, notices that Doris's mail has not been taken in for two days. Sam is concerned; he knows Doris's daily routine, and she always informs him when she plans to go out of town. He knocks on Doris's door but receives no answer. Alarmed, Sam calls the police, who, upon arrival at Doris's home, discover her lying semi-conscious on the kitchen floor.

Doris is rushed to a nearby hospital. A preliminary diagnosis of gastrointestinal bleeding is made by the attending physician and, since it is an emergency, she is given a blood transfusion as part of the initial treatment to stabilize her. A few days later, when Doris is awake and alert, the physician in charge of her case advises her that he wishes further investigations to determine what is wrong. Though she is apparently alert and competent, the nurses caring for Doris have noted some occasions when she seems confused as to her surroundings, doesn't seem to realize where she is, and does not know what day it is.

When the physician tells Doris that her condition urgently warrants further tests, she becomes agitated and upset. She fears that the doctors will find that she has cancer and that she will soon die. Consequently, she refuses to authorize any further tests. The members of the team know that any number of easily treated factors could be causing the bleeding, and they are concerned that Doris's refusal of further investigation and treatment is not in her best interests. Some nurses question whether Doris, in her present state of mind, is capable of making such a decision. The team wishes to involve her son and daughter, but Doris refuses to give them any information that would enable them to contact her children. She does not want her family involved, as she feels she has always been able to take care of herself and does not wish to worry her children.

Over the next few days, the team members find further evidence that Doris's bleeding is recurring. Something must be done soon or she may die.

ISSUES

1. Does Doris have the mental (and hence legal) capacity to make the decision to accept or refuse treatment?
2. Has Doris been given adequate opportunity to make an informed decision with respect to consent to treatment?
3. May the nurses or other team members legally and ethically disclose information pertaining to Doris's condition to her children, assuming they are able to contact them through their own efforts?
4. What are the competing ethical interests in this situation and how can they be resolved?
5. May the team proceed with the investigation of Doris's condition on their own, on their assumption that she is not capable of giving or withholding consent?
6. What legal procedures must be followed to obtain permission to proceed with further investigation of Doris's condition, assuming she is not mentally competent?

DISCUSSION

In this case study, it is clear that the health care team cannot proceed legally without Doris's consent. If they do so, they may be liable for battery, as there is absolutely no consent here, let alone an informed one. Although the nurses and physicians are genuinely motivated by good faith and have Doris's best interests at heart, they are not free to substitute their own judgement and proceed on their own authority. Even if Doris is not mentally competent to consent (which is unclear, based on the details given), this would still not authorize the medical team to proceed of its own accord. If Doris is indeed mentally incapable of giving consent, and failing an advance directive signed by her, the consent of a substitute decision maker would have to be obtained.

The law and practice in this area require that, as a first step, a nurse or physician must explain the procedures and their importance, as well as the risks of forgoing them, to Doris. Also, as suggested earlier, Doris needs to be given enough time to make her decision. The team needs to respond to her questions and clarify any misconceptions. Nurses can play a role in exploring with patients the factors that might motivate their decisions (e.g., fear, past experiences, misconceptions, etc.). If Doris does consent, any subsequent withdrawal of that consent must be respected by the team members. A resumption of treatment would require disclosure of any material change in the risks.

Informed Consent

The most celebrated case dealing with the requirement of informed consent to medical treatment is *Reibl v. Hughes*.[1] In the Reibl decision, the plaintiff suffered from a blocked left carotid artery. Accordingly, he was booked for an elective internal carotid endarterectomy, which was performed by the defendant, a neurosurgeon. During the surgery, or immediately thereafter, the plaintiff suffered a stroke which resulted in unilateral paralysis, impotence, and permanent disability. The plaintiff sued the neurosurgeon for negligently performing the operation and for the surgeon's failure to inform him adequately of the risks of the surgery.

The case ultimately reached the Supreme Court of Canada, where the court held that the surgeon was liable in that he had indeed failed to inform the plaintiff of all material risks atttending the surgery. In this case, although there was a real risk of stroke, paralysis, and possibly death, the surgeon had told the patient only that it would be better for him to have the surgery. He did not inform him of the risks. Furthermore, as the plaintiff had difficulty with the English language, it was incumbent upon the surgeon to ensure that the information conveyed was fully understood.

If such disclosure is not made, the health practitioner in a case such as this risks being found liable for negligence. The complete failure to obtain any consent at all, or the obtaining of consent through fraud, would leave the practitioner open to a civil suit for battery.

Refusal of Consent on Religious or Other Grounds

Along with the issue of informed consent is that of an instruction or limitation by which the patient refuses consent to certain procedures or treatment on moral or religious grounds. The Ontario Court of Appeal dealt with such a case in its decision in *Malette v. Shulman*.[2] In that case, the plaintiff had been seriously injured in a motor vehicle accident and rushed to a nearby hospital. She had sustained serious injuries to her head and face and was bleeding profusely. The physician on duty in the Emergency Department, who attended her upon her arrival, determined that she would need blood transfusions to maintain her blood volume and blood pressure lest she succumb to irreversible shock. The surgeon who examined her prior to X-rays being taken also determined that she would require a blood transfusion. She was barely conscious at the time.

Meanwhile, shortly after the patient's arrival at the hospital, a nurse discovered a card in the patient's purse printed in French, signed by the patient and identifying her as a Jehovah's Witness. The card read:[3]

NO BLOOD TRANSFUSION!

As one of Jehovah's Witnesses with firm religious convictions, I request that no blood or blood products be administered to me under any circumstances. I fully realize the implications of this position, but I have resolutely decided to obey the Bible command: "Keep abstaining … from blood." (Acts 15:28, 29) However, I have no religious objections to use the non-blood alternatives, such as Dextran, Haemaccel [sic], PVP, Ringer's Lactate, or saline solution.

The card was brought by the nurse to the attention of the physician who had first seen the patient.

Before X-rays could be completed, the patient's blood pressure dropped markedly, her respiration became increasingly distressed, and her level of consciousness dropped. She continued to bleed profusely. At that moment, the physician determined that blood transfusions were necessary to preserve her life. He decided to administer the transfusions to her personally and on his own responsibility, notwithstanding the card that had been brought to his attention.

Usually, nurses would administer a blood transfusion pursuant to an order drawn up by a physician. The question then becomes: What is the legal obligation of a nurse to follow a physician's order when he or she knows that order to be contrary to the patient's wishes and that the patient has not consented to such treatment? In such a case, the law would apply equally to the nurse as well as to the physician. Both must respect the patient's wishes, and may not proceed to administer treatment to which consent has been withheld, no matter how necessary that treatment, or how irrational the patient's decision may seem.

Returning to the *Malette* case, shortly after the physician administered the transfusion, the patient's daughter arrived at the hospital and became furious when told that blood transfusions had been administered to her mother. She affirmed her mother's instructions that no blood be given to her, and signed a document specifically prohibiting the giving of further blood to the patient, saying that her mother's faith forbade blood transfusions and that she would not wish them.

Despite these objections, the physician refused to follow the daughter's instructions. In his professional opinion, the transfusions were absolutely necessary to save the patient's life, and it was his professional duty to ensure that she receive them. He did not believe that the card signed by the patient expressed her current wishes. He could not be sure that she had not changed her religious beliefs, or that she had been fully informed of all the risks of forgoing a blood transfusion. (Again, if a nurse were carrying out an order for a blood transfusion under similar circumstances, despite the fact that he or she may have similar misgivings about the instructions, that nurse would be bound by the patient's limitations on consent to treatment.)

The plaintiff recovered fully from her injuries. Despite this, she brought a lawsuit for battery, negligence, and religious discrimination against the physician and the hospital. Her action was allowed, and she was awarded damages on the grounds that the administration of the blood transfusions had been done against her specific wishes and that this constituted a battery upon her. The physician appealed this judgement in the Ontario Court of Appeal.

The Court of Appeal reviewed the law dealing with informed consent. It found that the common law recognized the right of a patient to refuse consent to medical treatment, and that this right was paramount to the health practitioner's professional opinion about what might be best for that patient. The Court stated that, while it is true that informed consent is not required in emergencies where the patient is unable to give consent (and the physician has no reason to believe that the patient would refuse consent if conscious or able to do so), in the presence of clear instructions such as those contained in the Jehovah's Witness card in this case, the physician was not free to disregard the patient's instructions. There is no corresponding doctrine of "informed refusal" requiring or authorizing a health practitioner to proceed with emergency treatment where the practitioner has not been able to inform the patient of all the consequences and risks of refusing treatment.[4]

The Court upheld the trial judge's finding that there was no rational basis or evidence upon which the physician could found a belief that the card was not valid or that the patient's religious views had changed. Hence, there was no justification for the doctor's refusal to adhere to the patient's advance instructions. The treatment having thus been administered without the patient's consent, the Court of Appeal upheld the finding of liability for battery against the physician.[5]

Of course, the Court made clear the fact that, in this case, it was not deciding the enforceability of advance directives regarding euthanasia or withdrawal of treatment. The patient here asked only that her spiritual beliefs be respected, and she was willing to risk death for them. She did not wish to die, as she consented to the use of non-blood alternatives. This case thus imposes a limit on the doctrine of emergency treatment wherein the requirement for consent is waived. It further reinforces the principle that a patient's wishes are the final say on whether or not treatment shall be administered, no matter how necessary to life that treatment may be.

Withdrawal of Consent

Recently, the Supreme Court of Canada reviewed the law of informed consent in a situation where the patient withdrew consent during a medical procedure to which she had previously consented. Although this case involved an action for battery and negligence against the attending physicians, the principles contained in this decision and developed by the Supreme Court are equally applicable to nursing professionals.

In *Ciarlariello v. Schacter*,[6] the court was asked to consider whether a doctor still owed a duty of disclosure to a patient of all material risks inherent in a medical procedure where the patient withdraws a previously given informed consent during that procedure.[7] The plaintiff was asked to attend at a hospital for the purpose of undergoing the first of two angiograms meant to determine the exact location of a suspected aneurysm. On the patient's arrival at the hospital, the physician who was to administer the test explained the risks inherent in the procedure, including possible blindness, paralysis, and death. Although the plaintiff's first language was Italian and her English was poor, she claimed at that time to have understood the doctor's explanation. The plaintiff's daughter acted as interpreter during these explanations. The patient thereupon signed a consent to the tests. Despite this, the doctor had misgivings as to the free and informed nature of the consent.

The doctor therefore destroyed the patient's consent and asked her to go back to her family to consult with them. This she did, and later returned with a consent signed by her daughter. The patient took the test; it failed to reveal the aneurysm conclusively but indicated a possible site. The doctors in charge of her case decided that a second angiogram would likely pinpoint the site of the aneurysm.

In the meantime, the plaintiff suffered a second severe headache indicating a "re-bleed" of the aneurysm, and it was decided that a second angiogram was needed. The patient consented to this second test. Beforehand, a second radiologist (who had worked with the radiologist who administered the first test), carefully explained the test to her, including all possible material risks (skin rash, and on rare occasions, death, blindness, stroke, and/or paralysis). He stated that the patient appeared to understand, and proceeded with the angiogram.

During the procedure, the plaintiff began moaning and yelling. She began to hyperventilate and flex her legs. She calmed down sufficiently to tell the doctor, "Enough, no more, stop the test." The test was stopped, and both radiologists proceeded to examine her complaint that her right hand was numb. She was unable to move it or grasp with it. Her left hand was also slightly weak. Gradually, the strength returned to her left hand and both arms, though her left hand remained weak. Her sensory perception was normal. Both radiologists concluded that the residual weakness in her left hand was due to her hyperventilating. Both expected the weakness to be temporary. The rest of her motor function appeared to return to normal.

At this point, the plaintiff became quiet and co-operative. The first radiologist took over the test and explained to her that one more area needed investigation and that this procedure would take five more minutes. She asked the plaintiff if she wished to continue the test, to which the plaintiff replied: "Please go ahead." The final injection of dye was administered, during which the plaintiff suffered an immediate reaction, rendering her a quadriplegic. She sued all the doctors involved in treating her for damages for negligence and battery. She died soon after her lawsuit came to trial, and her family and estate continued the suit.

This case is of some relevance to nursing in that it illustrates that a patient has the right at any time to withdraw consent to treatment. Such withdrawal may occur in difficult circumstances, as in the *Ciarlariello* case, and it is important for the health practitioner to ascertain whether or not the consent has been withdrawn. This may not always be clear. A professional who continues to administer treatment, regardless of a patient's instructions to stop, risks being found liable to the patient for battery. In the *Ciarlariello* case, the patient clearly withdrew her consent. She had given an informed consent within the requirements laid down in *Reibl v. Hughes*.[8] Thus, the doctors had not been negligent in explaining the risks of the procedure to her.

A further issue with respect to resumption of treatment after consent to it has been withdrawn is also crucial. The criteria laid down by the court governing the health professional's actions in such a case include a consideration of whether or not the risks have changed materially during the procedure, and whether a reasonable patient would wish to know of such changes.[9] In the *Ciarlariello* case, there was no evidence that the patient's condition had deteriorated such that she could not properly consent to the resumption of the treatment. Thus, her consent to resume the tests was valid.

As discussed in Chapter 2, one of the elements that must be proven in a negligence action is that the plaintiff's injury must have resulted from the defendant's breach of duty toward the plaintiff. In an action for negligence such as that in *Reibl v. Hughes* or the *Ciarlariello* case, the question becomes whether or not a reasonable person in the plaintiff's position would still have consented to the procedure if he or she had known the information and risks that the health practitioner failed to disclose.

In *Ciarlariello v. Schacter,* the court found that the plaintiff's consent was an informed one and that there was no negligence on the doctors' part. It also found that, as the risk of quadriplegia resulting from an angiogram was far less than the risks of not locating the aneurysm, a reasonable patient in the plaintiff's position would still have consented to the procedure.

Competency to Consent

Incompetent Adults

To return to our case study, before her children can be consulted, Doris's attending physicians must determine whether she is mentally competent to make an informed decision respecting the diagnostic tests. If Doris is competent, her wishes that her children not be contacted must be respected.

In cases involving elderly patients, the initial and seemingly irrational refusal to consent may not necessarily be evidence of an incompetent mind. The nurse or other practitioner must remain patient (if the situation is not urgent or life-threatening). Elderly patients are often fearful of impending illness. Many may have friends or relatives, even a spouse, who have recently succumbed to a serious illness. For example, a patient whose brother has died of cancer may fear that he himself will be stricken with the disease. This fear may paralyze some people's thinking. They may be in a state of denial and may rationalize their refusal to consent on the basis that "if cancer is not detected, then that means I don't have it." This may be all that is going on in a patient's mind when he or she says: "No! I don't want to go through those tests; leave me alone, I'm all right!"

The law allows any mentally competent adult to refuse consent to medical treatment. How, then, can the mental capacity of a patient be determined? Some have suggested the following test: "... can the patient appreciate the nature and consequences of the proposed treatment so as to be capable of rendering an informed judgement?"[10] A method of testing for this appreciation is to explain to the patient, carefully and in detail, the risks and nature of the proposed procedure and then to ask the patient to repeat his or her understanding of the risks and treatment, while carefully noting the responses and words used.[11] On this basis, the health practitioner is then able to form an opinion of the patient's ability to appreciate the nature, risks, and consequences of the proposed procedure.

Of course, patients may be capable of making decisions concerning some matters yet not others, and their mental capacity may fluctuate over time. Even when the patient has stated an intention that the procedure should commence but has displayed an irrational or confused understanding of that procedure, the health practitioner should be reluctant to proceed. If the patient's responses demonstrate a mental incapacity to comprehend the nature of the risks of the procedure, however beneficial it may be to the patient, the practitioner should not proceed without the consent of an authorized substitute decision maker.

In some provinces, any health care professional faced with a question of administering treatment to a mentally incompetent patient must obtain the consent of the patient's spouse, parent, a person in lawful custody of that patient, or the patient's next of kin.[12] If no such persons are available, and the situation is not an emergency, a physician may have to obtain the consent of the patient's committee, appointed under statute (e.g., Ontario's *Mental Incompetency Act*[13]; this law will soon change in Ontario with the passage of the *Substitute Decisions Act, 1992*). Under such a law, a court may be asked by any interested party, usually a spouse or relative, to appoint a *committee of the person* (one or more persons, often relatives of the patient) to act in that person's best interests, including the giving or withholding of consent to medical treatment. This committee then has the authority to consent to any medical treatment on behalf of the patient, who will legally have been found incompetent by the court. In such a case, the physician may obtain the necessary consent from the committee.

For example, the Quebec *Civil Code* provides that where a person is incapable of giving consent, such consent may be given by a curator (or tutor, in the case of a child). A curator in Quebec is similar to a committee of the person in Ontario and other common law provinces with similar provisions. He or she (or they) are appointed by the court to act in the incapable person's best interests and to ensure proper care for that person. In the absence of a curator, the person's spouse or, if there is no spouse or the spouse cannot consent, a close relative or adult showing a special interest in the patient may give consent.[14] If such a person (including the patient) either cannot consent or refuses consent, a health care professional in Quebec cannot proceed with such treatment until and unless he or she obtains an order from the court authorizing such procedure.[15]

For example, suppose a patient in the later stages of Alzheimer's disease is rushed to the emergency department suffering from sharp abdominal pain. The patient's son is with him and has been appointed committee over the person of his father. The father exhibits classic symptoms of Alzheimer's: he is confused and incoherent, and at times does not recognize his son. The emergency team will have to obtain the son's consent to tests and treatment for the father. In such consultation, the son should be encouraged to make any decisions as his father would have made them when he was competent.

Children

There are likewise competency issues with respect to children. In some provinces, a child who is old enough and mature enough to understand the nature and risks inherent in a medical procedure is given the right to consent to such treatment of his or her own accord.

For example, in Ontario, regulations made under the *Public Hospitals Act*[16] require health care personnel to obtain a written and signed consent from a patient before administering any treatment to that person. Under those regulations, any mentally competent person sixteen years of age or older may consent in writing to medical treatment.[17] (However, the recent *Consent to Treatment Act, 1992,* proposes that capacity to consent, rather than age, be the relevant consideration.) In Quebec, any child over the age of fourteen may give consent freely without need for recourse to his or her parents or guardians.[18] However, if such a child refuses consent, a court order is necessary before treatment may proceed, even if the health care professional has obtained the consent of that child's parent or guardian.[19]

In Ontario, persons under sixteen may consent on their own if they are married. Since the vast majority of children under sixteen are unmarried, the law in Ontario requires the consent of a parent or other adult with lawful custody of the child or, in the absence of such a person, the child's next of kin.[20] Where such persons are unavailable or refuse to consent to treatment that, in the physician's or nurse's opinion, is necessary for the child's health, the doctor or nurse may have to apply for a court's consent under the children's welfare statutes of the province. In Ontario, this might be done under the *Child and Family Services Act.*[21]

A Children's Aid Society (CAS) may apply to a court to have a child in need of protection made its ward so that it can make treatment decisions on that child's behalf. This has been done in cases involving parents who had refused medical treatment for their children on religious grounds. If the refusal places the child's life at risk by denying life-saving treatment, the court can deem such a child a "child in need of protection" and can authorize the CAS or other such body (in some provinces, the director of child welfare) to give the required consent where it is in the child's best interests.

Emergency Treatment

In all cases, the law in all the common law provinces and Quebec allows physicians and other health care professionals to administer treatment in an emergency where the patient's consent cannot be obtained. Such a situation might arise because of the nature of the injuries or illness, or because no time can be spared in administering such emergency treatment. Health professionals acting in extreme emergencies will be absolved of any liability for administering treatment, provided there is no gross negligence on their part.

Proxy Consent

The common law traditionally did not allow **proxy consent** to treatment—that is, a consent granted by a third party designated by the incapable person (when capable) to make decisions on his or her behalf. The only situations in which third-party consent was recognized was in the case of parents consenting on behalf of minors and committees appointed over mentally incompetent persons. However, situations may arise where the patient is unable to consent, not because of some current or progressive mental infirmity, but owing to a physical condition, for example, when a patient is comatose.

A proxy decision maker is clearly desirable in such situations. In our case study, the medical team would have to resort to a proxy if Doris were not competent to give or withhold consent.

We will discuss Ontario's recent legislation in this respect, as it is presently the most detailed such legislation in the country.

Ontario

The main components of the Ontario legislation affecting consent to treatment are contained in the *Consent to Treatment Act, 1992,*[22] the *Substitute Decisions Act, 1992,*[23] and the *Advocacy Act, 1992.*[24] Only parts of these Acts were in force at the time of preparing this text; however, they were expected to come fully into force by April 1995.

The *Consent to Treatment Act* enshrines into statute law the common law requirements for an informed consent to treatment, as discussed above. It preserves the right and duty of health care providers to restrain or confine persons when necessary to prevent serious bodily harm either to themselves or to others.[25] The Act requires all health practitioners (including nurses) to ensure, firstly, that the patient to be treated is capable of consenting, and secondly, that the patient in fact consents. If the patient is not capable, the health practitioner must obtain the consent from another person authorized to give consent under the Act.[26]

Ontario's statute defines informed consent in much the same way as discussed earlier in this chapter, that is, it allows the consent to be expressed or implied, provided that an informed consent has been given, that it relates to the treatment proposed, and that it has not been obtained through fraud or misrepresentation.[27]

The legislation also defines when a person is capable of giving consent. A person is capable if he or she understands the information given that is relevant to making a decision concerning the treatment, and can appreciate the reasonably foreseeable consequences of a decision or lack thereof.[28] The statute provides that persons can be capable with respect to certain treatments and incapable for others, and capable and incapable at different times.[29] This provision addresses concerns that arise when a capable person has not yet given consent and then later may no longer be capable, for example, while under heavy sedation. It also addresses such situations as Alzheimer's patients who have periods of lucidity, only to relapse into a confused state moments later.

The health practitioner in charge of the patient's care is responsible for determining whether the patient is capable or incapable of consenting to a proposed treatment. If the patient's capacity to consent returns after another person has made a decision with respect to the patient's treatment, the patient's own decision to give or refuse consent will govern.[30] This rule would not apply, however, to a **guardian of the person** appointed by court order, or an attorney acting under a validated **power of attorney for personal care**.[31] The health practitioner's determination of incapacity must be made in accordance with government-prescribed criteria and procedures. (These criteria and procedures had not yet been passed at the time this text was prepared.)

If the physician examining the patient determines that he or she is not capable of consenting to treatment, the patient must be informed of that fact.[32] At this point, the procedures for obtaining consent vary depending on the nature of the treatment proposed. If the health practitioner (including a nurse) finds the patient is incapable with respect to a treatment that is a "controlled act" under section 27(2) of the *Regulated Health Professions Act*[33] (see the discussion in Chapter 3 of controlled acts under the RHPA, pages 74–77) but is not a "prescribed act" (a specific medical act designated by the government by regulation), the patient must be given written notice advising that he or she has the right to meet with a government-appointed *rights adviser* and to make an application to the Consent and Capacity Review Board for a review of the health practitioner's finding that the person is incapable.[34]

The health practitioner must also notify a rights adviser of the finding of incapacity in respect of a particular treatment under the Act. The rights adviser may be another health care professional prescribed by regulation as a rights adviser, or an advocate appointed under the *Advocacy Act, 1992*.

The rights adviser must then meet with the patient and advise him or her of the consequences of the finding of incapacity and of the patient's right to challenge the finding before the Consent and Capacity Review Board. (This does not apply to an unconscious patient.) The patient need not understand the rights adviser's explanation, but the adviser must explain to the best of his or her ability and in a manner that addresses the patient's needs.

The health practitioner may proceed with treatment only if no application has been made to the Board for a review of the finding of incapacity and forty-eight hours have elapsed, or after the Board has made a decision in the matter.

If the proposed treatment is not one requiring notification of a rights adviser, the patient may still make an application to the Board, and the practitioner must ensure that no treatment be administered until the same conditions are met as those where a rights adviser must be notified.

These provisions have been the subject of much criticism by the College of Physicians and Surgeons and the Registered Nurses Association of Ontario. With respect to treatment administered by nurses, it was felt that if the nurse judged the client incapable, the nurse would have no practical way of knowing whether there was a guardian or other substitute decision maker available to give or withhold consent on the patient's behalf. Without any consent whatsoever, not even the simplest treatment or basic comfort measures (a drink of water, a cold cloth for the patient's head) could be administered. Despite these objections and a request that the definition of "treatment" in the proposed legislation be amended to distinguish between invasive, high-risk procedures and basic assessment and care measures, no such amendment was made.

There was great concern that the time involved in securing a rights adviser would delay the commencement of basic care measures and compromise the patient's health, especially in serious cases, which may quickly develop into emergencies.[35] This is no less true of the delays caused by the review application to the Consent and Capacity Review Board. A patient's medical condition can rapidly worsen in the forty-eight-hour period required by the statute.

Further, the scheme places a burden on already overworked health practitioners with respect to notification requirements. In most cases, it is felt that adequate treatment decisions could be made by a relative or spouse of the patient without resorting to a cumbersome bureaucratic maze. Indeed, the proposed scheme could do more harm than good to people who cannot give consent yet urgently require treatment. In such situations, nurses would be more than competent to assume the role of advocate on the patient's behalf.

These special provisions do not apply where an incapable person has appointed an attorney who is acting under a validated power of attorney for personal care, or to a court-appointed guardian of the person. Such persons are free to give the required consent but only in accordance with the instructions, limitations, and authority contained in such power of attorney or court order.[36] The legislation provides, however, that no one may give consent to electroshock therapy on behalf of an incapable person.

Where a substitute decision maker gives consent, the known wishes of the patient must be taken into account and must govern the substitute's decision to give or refuse consent to treatment. The wishes may be contained in the power of attorney itself or any other document, or may be known orally. Such documents are commonly known as **living wills** because they provide directions on behalf of the maker after that person has lost the ability to make those decisions on his or her own behalf. The substitute decision maker must make the decision in the patient's best interests and in accordance with the patient's values and beliefs. As well, the substitute must consider whether:

(1) the proposed treatment will likely improve the patient's condition or well-being;

(2) the patient's well-being or condition would likely improve without the treatment;

(3) the benefits of treatment outweigh the risks; and

(4) a less intrusive treatment would be as beneficial as the one proposed.[37]

Once the procedures respecting notification of the rights adviser have been met and time for an application for review to the Consent and Capacity Review Board has elapsed, the practitioner will have to consider from which person to obtain the necessary consent. This will be fairly straightforward when the person has an attorney with a validated power of attorney for personal care or a court-appointed guardian. The Act establishes a hierarchy of alternative substitute decision makers:[38]

(1) a guardian appointed by the court under the *Substitute Decisions Act, 1992;*

(2) an attorney for personal care acting under a validated power of attorney for personal care that confers that authority;

(3) an attorney for personal care acting under a power of attorney for personal care that confers the authority but is not validated;

(4) the incapable person's representative, appointed by the Board pursuant to an application by the incapable person;

(5) the incapable person's spouse or partner[39];

(6) the incapable person's child;

(7) the person's parent, or another who is lawfully entitled to give or refuse consent if the person is under sixteen;

(8) the person's brother or sister;

(9) any other relative of the incapable person.

Other requirements are that the substitute decision maker be at least sixteen years of age[40] and, if there is a conflict between two or more persons mentioned in any of these categories, each claiming to have the authority to give consent, the person who ranks highest on the above list prevails.[41] However, if the higher-ranking person refuses to assume responsibility for giving or refusing consent or is himself or herself incapable, the lower-ranking person may give the consent. If no such persons are available, the Public Guardian and Trustee may give or refuse consent.

With respect to minors, any person over fourteen may give or refuse consent on his or her own behalf if that person is capable. This means that parental wishes will not necessarily govern situations where a minor fourteen or older refuses treatment, even if the treatment is necessary.

Emergency treatment poses a special challenge for the health practitioner, and the Act provides special rules for such situations. If a patient is found incapable, in the health practitioner's opinion, with respect to proposed treatment necessary to alleviate severe suffering, or the patient is at risk of serious bodily harm if the treatment is not administered promptly, and it is not possible to find a substitute decision maker without delaying such treatment, then the practitioner may administer the treatment. He or she may do so even when an application has been made to the Consent and Capacity Review Board for the appointment of a representative to give such consent on the patient's behalf.

The authority to proceed extends to any examination of the patient or diagnostic procedures (if these are reasonably necessary) to determine whether the patient is at risk of serious bodily harm or is experiencing severe suffering. The emergency treatment can continue for as long as is reasonably required to find someone who can give the necessary consent from among the list of persons authorized to do so. The Act obliges the health practitioner to ensure that a continuing search is made for any substitute decision makers willing to assume responsibility to give or refuse consent. In the event that the patient becomes capable once again, his or her wishes govern.

The notice requirements described above do not apply to emergency treatment. The health practitioner, when acting in accordance with these rules, is required to note in the patient's chart that the treatment was necessary to avoid the risk of serious bodily harm or to alleviate severe suffering, and that the person was incapable of giving consent.[42] If the health practitioner is informed by a person falling in categories 1, 2, or 3 of the list of authorized people, or has reason to know of the incapable patient's wishes (expressed at any time after the person reached the age of sixteen) with respect to administering emergency treatment, the practitioner may proceed only in accordance with those wishes. Thus, for example, if the patient is unconscious, and an attorney for personal care advises the practitioner that this patient once expressed the desire that no blood transfusions be administered in an emergency, the practitioner may not administer such treatment.[43] Notwithstanding a refusal of consent by someone in the above list, the practitioner may proceed if he or she continues to believe that the treatment is necessary to alleviate suffering or avoid serious bodily harm, and that the person refusing the consent has done so against the patient's previous wishes, values, or beliefs.

Attorneys for Personal Care

With respect to substitute decision makers, Ontario's *Substitute Decisions Act, 1992* provides that a person over the age of sixteen may exercise power of decision on behalf of an incapacitated person who is also at least sixteen years old.[44] In most cases, the parents of an incapacitated adolescent would presumably continue to make treatment decisions and give the necessary consents, as is currently the case. The test under this statute for incapacity (thus the need for a substitute decision maker) is similar to that under the *Consent to Treatment Act,* but in this case, the patient must be unable to understand information regarding his or her health care, nutrition, shelter, clothing, hygiene, or safety, or be unable to appreciate the reasonably foreseeable consequences of a decision (or lack of decision) respecting these matters.[45]

Under this statute, there are two methods of providing a substitute decision maker for an incapable person. The first is an appointment of a person or persons in a written document (power of attorney for personal care) in advance of the subject's becoming incapable. Those named in the power of attorney are authorized by the person making it (the grantor) to make decisions concerning the grantor's personal care on his or her behalf.[46] The person named in the power of attorney (the attorney[47]) for personal care may only be the grantor's spouse, partner[48], or a relative. It cannot be any other person if that other provides health care to the grantor for compensation or provides residential, social, training, advocacy or support services to the grantor for compensation.[49] This provision is important, since in some situations the grantor may be tempted to name his or her physician, or a respected and trusted nurse, as an attorney. The legislation prevents any such conflict of interest arising. However, critics point out that a nurse may be one of the more knowledgeable persons relative to care and treatment issues concerning the incapable patient, and thus a practical and beneficial choice of attorneys. This provision may therefore be viewed as a questionable limitation on the incapable patient's rights to choose and appoint an attorney.

The attorney may act only in accordance with this statute and the limitations stipulated by the grantor in the power of attorney. In the case of a person who has neither a trusted friend, partner, spouse nor relatives to name as attorney, he or she can name the Public Guardian and Trustee of Ontario (with that person's permission).[50] This is a government official charged with ensuring that mentally incompetent persons, orphaned children having no legal guardians, and their property are cared for and their legal rights protected when there is no one else available to act in their interest.

Before a power of attorney for personal care can be acted upon, it must be validated according to the procedures set out in the statute. However, if the attorney has reason to believe that the grantor is incapable of making a decision respecting his or her personal care, the attorney explains to the grantor:

(1) the need for a decision;
(2) the decision the attorney intends to make; and
(3) the right of the grantor to object to the decision.

If the grantor does not object to the decision, the power of attorney need not be validated.

Lack of formal validation under the Act has consequences. If the grantor at any time objects to the attorney's decision, and the decision is unaffected by the health practitioner's assessment of incapacity, the power of attorney can be contested. For instance, if the incapacitated person objects to an attorney's decision regarding nutrition (which is not a "medical treatment" decision), that person's wishes prevail over the attorney's decision, unless the power of attorney has been formally validated under the *Substitute Decisions Act*.[51] Again, this allows the incapable patient maximum autonomy and control.

Of course, the grantor making the power of attorney must be mentally capable of giving it. The test for determining this capacity is: Does the grantor understand whether the proposed attorney has a genuine concern for his or her welfare, and does the grantor appreciate that he or she may need to rely on the attorney to make decisions?[52] The power of attorney for personal care can be revoked at any time, provided the grantor is mentally capable when he or she does so. The grantor must also have had the capacity to make decisions with respect to any instructions contained in the power of attorney for personal care.

The formalities for making a legally valid power of attorney for personal care in Ontario are not complicated, but should be carefully observed. Otherwise, there is a risk that the power of attorney might be declared invalid by a court. The power of attorney for personal care must be signed by the grantor in the presence of two witnesses. The witnesses cannot be any of the following: the proposed attorney or that person's spouse or partner; the grantor's spouse or partner; a child of the grantor or a person that the grantor has treated as if that person were his or her child; someone whose own property is under a guardianship (this prevents a potentially incompetent person from being a witness); or a person under eighteen years of age.[53] A witness may sign the document only if he or she has no reason to believe that the grantor is incapable of making the power of attorney or is incapable of giving the instructions provided in that document.

In an application to validate a power of attorney for personal care, the Public Guardian and Trustee may require that an advocate explain to the grantor:

(1) that the power of attorney is to be validated, and that assessors have made statements in support respecting the grantor's mental capacity;
(2) the powers that the attorney will have if the power of attorney is validated; and
(3) the grantor's right to oppose the validation of the power of attorney.

The *advocate* is a person appointed by the Advocacy Commission of Ontario (under the *Advocacy Act, 1992*[54]) to provide advocacy services to persons who are vulnerable because of a physical or mental disability that prevents them from expressing their wishes and ascertaining their rights. If the advocate advises the Public Guardian and Trustee that the incapable person does not object, the power of attorney may be validated.

The Public Guardian and Trustee validates the document by issuing a certificate outlining those matters of personal care in which the grantor has been found incapable. The validation then applies only to decisions concerning those matters and functions. For example, if the power of attorney authorizes the attorney to make decisions respecting medical treatment and nutrition, and the grantor is found incapable only with respect to medical care, the attorney may make decisions only respecting the grantor's medical care. In this way, the grantor's autonomy is respected and preserved, and the attorneyship is as unobtrusive as possible in the grantor's life.

The legislation allows maximum protection for the grantor. For example, the grantor has the right to request an assessment by an assessor who may be a physician, a psychologist, or a psychiatrist, as designated by government regulation to make such an assessment. The assessor is responsible for determining whether or not the grantor is in fact incapable with respect to some, if not all, treatment decisions. The grantor is free to nominate a preferred assessor in the power of attorney for personal care. The assessment may also determine whether the grantor continues to be incapable. An attorney must have the grantor assessed at the grantor's request. A grantor can also be assessed if the attorney believes that the grantor is once again capable of personal care.[55]

Once an assessor makes a finding that the grantor is again capable, the power of attorney for personal care ceases to have effect. Such power of attorney may again become valid if the grantor again becomes incapable of personal care. When the court appoints a guardian of the person, any power of attorney, even if validated, ceases to be valid. Similarly, the grantor may revoke the power of attorney if he or she is mentally capable of doing so, that is, the grantor must not be incapacitated in order for the revocation to be valid.

Court-appointed Guardians of the Person

The second method of providing a substitute decision maker under the *Substitute Decisions Act* in Ontario is through an application to the Ontario Court (General Division) for the appointment of a guardian of the person.[56] This route is more difficult. In such an application, the court must consider whether there is an alternative course of action for making decisions that does not require the court to declare the applicant incapable of his or her personal care. Such an alternative may be less restrictive of the patient's decision-making rights than appointing a guardian.[57] Thus, the legislation is aimed at encouraging alternatives to court proceedings in these matters.

Any person may bring the application for the appointment of a guardian, which conceivably might include the applicant's physician, a close friend, relative, spouse, partner, or any person who has an interest in the applicant's care. In any event, the appointed guardian cannot be someone who provides health care for compensation,[58] but may include the applicant's attorney for personal care. Such an appointment could expand the attorney's decision-making power over and above the authorization contained in the power of attorney for personal care. If it is made in a court order for full guardianship, it might include the power to determine the person's living arrangements, shelter, and safety; take charge of any lawsuits by or against the applicant; gain access to personal information about the applicant; make decisions about the applicant's health care, nutrition, and hygiene; give or refuse consent to medical treatment on the person's behalf; make decisions about the applicant's employment, education, training, clothing, and recreation, and any other duties and powers specified in the order. In short, a full guardianship may (depending on the exact provisions of the court order) grant power to the guardian over all facets of the incapable person's life.

Before appointing a guardian, the court must find that the subject is in fact incapable according to the definition outlined above. The appointment of the guardian may be for a limited time, or may have such conditions attached to it as the court considers appropriate. In deciding the application, the court must consider whether the proposed guardian is the attorney under a power of attorney; the incapable person's wishes, to the extent that these can be ascertained; and the closeness of the relationship between the person applying for the guardianship and the incapable person.

A partial guardianship order may also be made where the court considers that the patient is incapable with respect to some but not all aspects of personal care and health. In such a case, the guardianship order will specify those matters in which the guardian has the power to make decisions, leaving other matters to the patient's own discretion. In this way, any court order can be tailored to be as unobtrusive as possible to the incapable patient's life, while still affording the protection of a competent guardian to make crucial decisions on his or her behalf.

Duties of Guardians and Attorneys for Personal Care[59]

The philosophy behind the law is to involve the incapable person in the process to the greatest extent possible in the circumstances. Thus, both guardians and attorneys are required to exercise their powers diligently and in good faith. They are required to explain their powers and duties to the incapable person. His or her wishes, made while capable, must guide the guardian or attorney when faced with decisions relevant to these wishes. The guardian or attorney must make diligent efforts to ascertain the existence of prior wishes and what those wishes or instructions might be. The most recent wish made while the person was capable must prevail over an earlier such wish. In determining those prior wishes, the incapable person's values and beliefs must be taken into account.

If it is not possible to make a decision in accordance with such a wish, or if such wishes or instructions cannot be determined, the guardian or attorney must make the decision in the incapable person's best interests. The least restrictive and least intrusive course of action under the circumstances must be chosen and, in making any decision, the guardian should foster the incapable person's independence as far as possible. The guardian should involve the incapable person in making this determination to the greatest extent possible, and should likewise consult with the person's family, friends, and health care providers. Here, nurses caring for such patients have an opportunity to make their perspectives and views known and to contribute to the quality of care.

Manitoba and British Columbia

Manitoba's substitute decision-maker legislation, the *Health Care Directives Act*[60] (in force as of July 23, 1993), is similar to that of Ontario. In Manitoba, the document signed by the grantor is called a *directive,* and the grantor is referred to as the *maker* of the directive. The person who is appointed to be the substitute decision maker is the *proxy.* A significant difference between the Ontario and Manitoba legislation is the fact that in Manitoba there is no provision for formal validation of the directive.

Validation is a legal process that will be initiated in Ontario when the *Substitute Decisions Act, 1992* comes into force. It is akin to the process of obtaining probate for a will after the death of the maker of the will. In the

validation process, a court has the opportunity to review the circumstances behind the making of the proxy, the mental condition of the maker, the details of
the care required by that maker, and the adequacy of the document. If all is in
order, the court validates the document and the proxy decision maker thereby
acquires full authority to make treatment decisions on behalf of the incapacitated person within the limits outlined in the document.

The Manitoba Act is silent on court-appointed guardians; however, this area
is covered through other legislation. There is no advocacy legislation of the
kind passed in Ontario, and the Manitoba Act makes no provision for the participation of advocates, as in Ontario. Finally, the directive need not be
witnessed so long as the maker has signed it. However, the Manitoba Act does
permit another person to sign for the maker in the maker's presence and in the
presence of a witness. Neither the person who signs for the maker nor the witness may be nominated as proxies in the directive. This is intended to cover
directives made by blind persons or others who, though mentally competent,
are physically unable to sign the document. No such provisions are contained
in the Ontario law per se, though regulations might possibly provide for this
once they are passed.

British Columbia recently passed an *Adult Guardianship Act*[61] and a
Representation Agreement Act,[62] which establish procedures respecting substitute
decision making, similar to those of the Ontario and Manitoba statutes. The
Adult Guardianship Act provides for the appointment of a guardian or substitute
decision maker on behalf of the incapable person. Under the *Representation
Agreement Act,* a competent adult also has the right to appoint a substitute decision maker (called a *representative*) to make treatment and care decisions on
his or her behalf. The document making the appointment is called a *representation agreement,* which must be signed by the patient's representative (unlike
Ontario's or Manitoba's legislation). The signatures of each party to the agreement must be witnessed by two persons. The representative of the incapable
person is also supervised by a *monitor* whose duty it is to ensure that the representative carries out all his or her duties under the agreement and in
accordance with the wishes of the incapable person (as expressed when he or
she was capable). British Columbia's legislation is similar to Ontario's, but was
not yet proclaimed at the time this book was written.

British Columbia has also recently passed the *Health Care (Consent) and
Care Facility (Admission) Act,*[63] which codifies much of the law on informed consent and is broadly similar to Ontario's *Consent to Treatment Act, 1992.* As in
Ontario, the British Columbia legislation provides for the participation of an
"advocacy organization" on behalf of an incapable person, but at a later stage.
In British Columbia, an advocate becomes involved only if major treatment
(e.g., surgery, major diagnostic testing or investigation) is contemplated, and
then only if other substitute decision makers (such as the person's spouse, including same-sex spouses, or a child, parent, or other relative) dispute among
themselves what treatment should be administered.

British Columbia's legislation also provides for consent to admission to a
health care facility only upon acceptance of a proposal from the institution out-

lining the activities and programs that are offered and its treatment policies. A substitute decision maker may accept such a proposal on behalf of an incapable person. No person may be admitted to a facility in British Columbia without acceptance of such a proposal.

Summary

The key points introduced in this chapter include:
- the foundation of consent in law and ethics
- the principle of autonomy and its role in consent
- the concept of competence or capacity
- the tort of battery
- the concept of informed consent
- the various types of, and approaches to, consent
- the rights of patients to refuse consent to medical or health care
- the nurse's role in ensuring that informed consent takes place
- how the legal rules and ethical theory apply to hypothetical case studies and real case law
- consent challenges with respect to the incompetent adult and to children
- professional responsibilities in emergency situations
- the concept of proxy or substitute consent
- existing new and impending consent legislation in the various provinces.

References

1. [1980] 2 scr 880; (1980) 14 cclt 1; 114 dlr (3d) 1; 33 nr 361.
2. (1990), 72 or (2d) 417 (ca), aff'g. 63 or (3d) 243; 47 dlr (4th) 18; 43 cclt 62 (hcj).
3. Ibid., p. 419.
4. Ibid., p. 432.
5. Ibid., p. 434.
6. [1993] 2 scr 119, aff'g. (1991), 44 oac 385; 76 dlr (4th) 449; 5 cclt (2d) 221 (ca), aff'g. (1987), 7 acws (3d) 51 (Ont. hcj).
7. Ibid., per Cory J., p. 123 (scr).
8. Supra footnote 1.
9. Supra footnote 6, p. 139.
10. This is a formulation suggested by Sharpe, G. (1987), *Canadian medical law*, p. 77.
11. Ibid.
12. Infra footnote 13.
13. rso 1990, c. M.9. This statute is repealed effective April 1995, at which time new procedures and provisions under the *Consent to Treatment Act, 1992*, so 1992, c. 31, and the *Substitute Decisions Act, 1992*, so 1992, c. 30, are expected to come into force.
14. *Quebec Civil Code*, article 15.
15. Ibid., article 16, paragraph 1.
16. rso 1990, c. P.40, section 32(1)(g).
17. rro 1990, Reg. 965, section 26(1)(a).

18. *Quebec Civil Code,* article 14, paragraph 2.
19. *Ibid.,* article 16, paragraph 2.
20. Supra n. 17, section 26(1)(b).
21. RSO 1990, c. C.11, as amended.
22. Supra footnote 13.
23. Supra footnote 13.
24. SO 1992, c. 26.
25. *Consent to Treatment Act,* supra footnote 13, section 3.
26. Ibid., section 4.
27. Ibid., sections 5(1) and (2).
28. Ibid., section 6(1).
29. Ibid., sections 6(2) and (3).
30. Ibid., section 7(1).
31. Ibid., section 7(2).
32. Ibid., section 9(1).
33. SO 1991, c. 18, section 27(2).
34. *Consent to Treatment Act,* supra footnote 13, sections 9(3) and 28(1).
35. See: Standing Committee on Administration of Justice, *Advocacy Act, 1991,* and *Companion Legislation,* Legislative Assembly of Ontario, Transcript March 10, 1992, pp. 945-1 to 1010-2.
36. *Consent to Treatment Act,* supra footnote 13, section 11.
37. Ibid., section 13(2).
38. Ibid., section 17(1).
39. A *partner* is defined as one with whom the incapable person has lived for at least one year and with whom he or she has a close personal relationship of primary importance to both their lives. This is would apply to homosexual couples.
40. *Consent to Treatment Act,* supra footnote 13, section 17(2).
41. Ibid., section 17(5).
42. Ibid., section 23.
43. Ibid., section 24.
44. *Substitute Decisions Act,* supra footnote 13, sections 43 and 44.
45. Ibid., section 45.
46. Ibid., section 46(1).
47. The term "attorney" is not used in this legislation in the sense commonly understood to mean "a lawyer." The person appointed as attorney need not be a lawyer, and his or her office, as such, should not be confused with that of a lawyer who is a practising member of the provincial bar. In Ontario, as in many other provinces, a lawyer is never referred to as an "attorney" (except in Quebec). The term "attorney" is customarily used in the United States to mean and refer to a licensed lawyer.
48. Supra footnote 39.
49. Supra footnote 20, section 46(3).
50. Ibid., section 46(2).
51. Ibid., section 46(11).
52. Ibid., section 47(1).
53. Ibid., sections 10(2) and 48(2).
54. Supra footnote 24, section 7(4).
55. *Substitute Decisions Act,* supra footnote 13, section 51(1).
56. Ibid., section 55(1).
57. Ibid., section 55(2).
58. Ibid., section 57(1).
59. Ibid., sections 66 to 68.
60. *Health Care Directives Act,* SM 1992, c. 33, CCSM, c. H27.
61. SBC 1993, c. 35.
62. SBC 1993, c. 67, not yet proclaimed into law.
63. SBC 1993, c. 48.

CHAPTER Seven

Death and Dying

CHAPTER OBJECTIVES

The purpose of this chapter is to enable the reader to:
- appreciate some of the legal and ethical issues surrounding death and the process of dying
- distinguish among the legal definitions of death, euthanasia, and assisted suicide
- articulate the legal and ethical issues surrounding tissue donation and organ transplantation
- understand the legal and ethical implications of withdrawal of treatment
- appreciate the use and legality of advance directives (living wills)
- consider some possible redefinitions of death.

Some of the most challenging ethical and legal decisions in health care relate to death and dying. Recent, extraordinary advances in medical technology have made it possible to extend life in cases where death would once have been certain. Yet, there is a heavy cost when extending a person's life also diminishes the quality and dignity that give life its meaning.

Today, even the process of dying has become more complex. In many hospitals, patients don't "die" anymore; they "have cardiac arrests." Advanced technology allows parts of us to continue after death through organ donation. This is possible because we can now keep bodies alive, even though what makes us persons—the capacity to interact with the world—is gone. Recently, various special interest groups have begun to demand that patients be given back their right to die, or at least, the right to decide how that dying process will unfold. Consequently, health care professionals have been obliged to explore and redefine the very meaning and definition of life and death.

In this chapter, we will examine the complex ethical and legal challenges that relate to death and dying and to organ donation.

Withdrawal of Treatment and Euthanasia

Sometimes, patients, families, and caregivers are asked to choose between extending a painful, undignified life, or death. When death is preferred, the means toward achieving that choice may place caregivers and family under great moral stress—for example, in the case of withholding food and fluids at a patient's own request. These decisions become even more problematic when the patient is incompetent and has left no advance directive. Hence, it is not surprising that questions regarding advance directives, withdrawal of treatment, euthanasia, and assisted suicide have surfaced in recent years.

Many ethical principles ground decisions about these issues. Often, these principles conflict. On the one hand, we have the principle of autonomy, or respect for the rights of individuals to make decisions that affect their lives. But the law places limits on that autonomy and draws the line when it comes to individuals' determining how and when their lives will end. In such cases, the principle of autonomy conflicts with the principle of the sanctity of life, which for many is an absolute principle, that is, it cannot be overridden in any circumstances.

Nurses placed in such situations undergo extreme emotional and moral distress. Conflict occurs when the patient's wishes, the nurse's loyalty to the patient, and the principle of beneficence (e.g., concern over providing a good and avoiding harm when pain control and symptom relief fail) clash with the principle of sanctity of life and the law. These situations, more than any others that nurses face in their practice, represent true dilemmas and provide a poignant reminder that what is legal may not, for some, be what is right.

The issue of withdrawal of treatment first gained prominence in the mid-1970s with the case of Karen Ann Quinlan in the United States.[1] More recently, the deaths of Sue Rodriguez[2] in British Columbia and "Nancy B."[3] in Quebec have renewed and re-energized the controversy over the ethical and legal justifications for and against euthanasia, withdrawal of treatment, and "physician-assisted suicide." In the United States, pathologist Dr. Jack Kevorkian publicly admitted assisting the deaths of a number of patients using the "suicide machine" that he designed and built; while in Canada, the federal government promised a full legislative debate and public hearings on the issue.

There is an important distinction between euthanasia or assisted suicide, and withdrawal of treatment. In euthanasia, active steps are taken to help end the life of a patient who requests this. Such a request might arise in the case of irreversible injury or terminal illness, when the patient has deemed his or her quality of life unacceptable. This may be due to complete loss of mobility and the ability to perform even the most basic tasks of everyday life (as in the case of patients with ALS), or extreme confusion and forgetfulness limiting the capacity to communicate (as is the case with Alzheimer's patients), or severe and unendurable pain that requires heavy medication, rendering the patient too sedated and disoriented to take an active part in life.

In assisted suicide, the patient is mentally competent to decide to end his or her life because of its deteriorating quality, yet is too debilitated by illness to act on this decision without the assistance of a third party (e.g., a physician, nurse, relative, or friend).

In withdrawal of treatment, nothing active is done to end the patient's life; rather, all treatment necessary to sustain life is withdrawn, and nature is permitted to take its course. Indeed, it is this approach, previously labelled "passive euthanasia," which the Quebec Superior Court adopted in the *Nancy B.* decision, as discussed in Chapter 2.

The following case study explores the issues surrounding euthanasia, assisted suicide, and withdrawal of treatment.

CASE STUDY

Assisted suicide

Joan, a forty-year-old mother of two teenage children was diagnosed two years ago with cancer of the ovaries. She has always been independent and active, a devoted mother who ran a corporate law practice and participated in civic organizations.

Early in her illness, Joan was treated with chemotherapy, radiotherapy, and surgery, and for a time, the cancer seemed to be in remission. After a year, however, she suffered a relapse. The cancer had metastasized to her liver and lower intestines.

Since then, Joan has been in and out of hospital receiving one form of treatment or another, to no avail. Over the last two months, Joan's health has deteriorated such that she is in constant and intense pain, especially in her bones. During her last admission to hospital, the team decided that nothing they could do would slow the growth of the tumour. After discussions with the team and her family, Joan decided to enter a home palliative care program. This provides her with home care services, a pain control protocol, and the services of a home care nurse. As well, Joan's husband Bob has taken leave of absence from work to remain at home with his wife.

For the past few weeks Joan's condition has remained unchanged, although the pain is becoming difficult to control and she suffers frequent bouts of nausea and constipation (which are side effects of the medication). She has become despondent and distressed with respect to her loss of dignity and the effect her illness is having on her family.

One day Joan exclaims to the home care nurse: "I've had enough! I can't stand the pain, I have become a burden on my husband and children. Please help me end it!"

ISSUES

1. What can the home care nurse do legally, and what should she do ethically, in this situation?
2. What are the alternatives available to the nurse?

DISCUSSION

This case study is a moving example of a situation that challenges the ethical and professional integrity of the nurse and the nature of the nurse–patient relationship. Nurses are encouraged to empathize, that is, to enter into the patient's way of seeing and being, so that the nurse can feel what the patient feels and can understand from the patient's perspective. A nurse working closely with a patient such as this might then understand the patient's pain and be sensitive to her request. Regardless of their ethical values and beliefs, most nurses would feel frustrated by their limited ability to reduce the patient's physical and emotional pain, and to respect and support her wishes.

Nurses have a duty to care for the physical, emotional, and psychological needs of the patients and families entrusted to them. The *Code of Ethics* of the CNA states:

> As ways of dealing with death and the dying process change, nursing is challenged to find new ways to preserve human values, autonomy and dignity. In assisting the dying client, measures must be taken to afford the client as much comfort, dignity and freedom from anxiety and pain as possible. Special consideration must be given to the need of the client's family or significant others to cope with their loss.[4]

The nurse in this case study cannot immediately assume that Joan has thought through all the issues and the choices available to her and has made a reasoned decision to end her life. The nurse caring for Joan has a responsibility to explore with her the reasons behind this request. Has it arisen out of fear and uncertainty about the future and how her death will occur? Has her pain become unbearable? Does she believe she is a burden to her husband and family? Is she angry about her illness and its inevitable outcome? Is she frustrated with the growing lack of control she has over her life? Finally, does she believe she has little or no dignity left?

Based on the reasons behind Joan's request, the nurse may be able to intervene to assist in making her dying more tolerable. Joan is already receiving palliative care, but perhaps her symptoms can be managed more effectively; for example, she may require better pain control.

Patients dying with cancer can tolerate extremely high levels of pain medication. Nurses should ensure that such patients receive the level of analgesia they require while attempting to minimize the related complications of drowsiness, confusion, constipation, and diarrhoea. Patients should be given choices regarding the level of pain control they receive. Some may elect to experience some pain in order to remain lucid and to continue communicating with others. For other patients, the pain may be so severe that they want it controlled even if that means falling into a semi- or unconscious state. Nurses may be concerned that high levels of pain medication may bring about or hasten the patient's death. From an ethical perspective, the nurse's primary obligation is to respect the patient's wishes and to provide a good by minimizing the pain, even if this hastens death. The obligation to provide palliative care and to provide adequate pain control is also supported in law.[5]

Joan's nurse should assist her in taking control over the time she has left. There are ways that her family and caregivers can give her back some control. Perhaps she needs more opportunity to talk about her feelings and the meaning this experience has for her. Joan's husband and family may have similar needs; the nurse could help them talk about these matters with Joan.

There may be many other nursing interventions that might help Joan. Occasionally, there is nothing else we can do to relieve someone's physical and emotional suffering. It is in these situations that we face one of the most challenging ethical and legal dilemmas in health care today.

From an ethical perspective, there is little consensus on the morality of euthanasia and assisted suicide.

Euthanasia

Euthanasia, or "painless death," is defined as an act that brings about the immediate death of a terminally ill patient. Commonly referred to as "mercy killing," it is seen as a means to end the suffering and pain of patients who otherwise would experience a difficult, undignified death. It is viewed as an act of compassion, as the intention is to do a good by relieving pain and suffering.

Today's heightened awareness of euthanasia arises partly out of advances in health care technology, and partly out of the growing number of patients with terminal conditions (such as cancer and AIDS), where the quality and dignity of the dying process are a concern. The recent court case involving Saskatchewan farmer Robert Latimer's conviction for the first-degree murder of his severely disabled daughter is a case in point.[6] The attention given to patient rights and respect for patient autonomy has provoked questions regarding the right to die and the right of patients to choose the time and means of their death.

Some who argue against euthanasia base their reasoning on the principle of sanctity of life and the traditional rules and laws prohibiting the taking of life except in situations of self-defence or war. (Strong advocates of this principle would argue that even in these circumstances, it is unacceptable to kill.) Others are concerned about the potential for abuse if euthanasia were permitted. It would be difficult to limit the act to situations where patients were terminally ill and actively dying; conceivably, it might extend to the chronically ill, the infirm, the elderly, and the demented. (This is the "slippery slope" argument.)

Those who support euthanasia believe that not all life is worth living. They believe that when someone is dying and it is no longer possible to eliminate their physical, emotional, and psychological pain, then euthanasia should be permitted at the request and with the consent of the competent patient. Supporters believe that sanctity of life is not an absolute principle and can be overridden out of respect both for patient autonomy and for the dignity of human life. They believe that, since death will occur anyway, euthanasia only makes that process more compassionate and dignified. If rules were in place to control euthanasia, such as in the Netherlands, they argue, then the potential for abuse would be lessened.

Assisted Suicide

Suicide is defined as the act of taking one's own life. In *assisted suicide,* the person lacks the means of completing the act and requires the assistance of someone else. For example, an accomplice might provide the patient with a lethal dose of medication, or help the patient to ingest it. This issue has arisen in cases where patients with a chronic disease have desired the means to control the time of their own death prior to falling into a state where such action is no longer possible. An example is the patient with amyotrophic lateral sclerosis (ALS) who wishes to live as long as possible, yet not end up in a state of total paralysis, dependent on artificial ventilation. Such persons would require assistance to commit suicide, since generalized weakness would limit their ability to do this on their own.

The arguments for and against assisted suicide are similar to those of euthanasia. However, those who support assisted suicide also argue that by not providing assistance we set limits on these persons' autonomy by denying them the opportunity to perform an act that able-bodied persons are capable of doing.

Public Opinion on Euthanasia and Assisted Suicide

A number of polls have been conducted to determine the public's attitudes with respect to euthanasia and assisted suicide. These polls indicate that the level of support for physician assistance in relation to euthanasia or assisted suicide for terminally ill patients ranges from 54% to 75%.[7] A poll published in the *Journal of the Canadian Medical Association* (March, 1994) found that 65% of respondents supported active euthanasia for patients experiencing severe pain and terminal illness. However, these same respondents (63%) expressed concern that the legalization of euthanasia might lead to its use in other situations. Only 34% were against euthanasia in all situations.[8]

Since nurses are representative of society at large, it is unlikely that their views differ statistically from the opinions expressed in this survey. Some nurses hold strong views on one side of the debate; others are confused by the shades of grey and the arguments on both sides. Regardless of their perspective, all nurses experience moral distress in these situations, which are likely to increase over the next few years.

The Current Law in Canada

The case of *Rodriguez v. British Columbia (Attorney General)*[9] has received tremendous public attention. Mrs. Rodriguez was diagnosed with amyotrophic lateral sclerosis (ALS), a progressive disease of the nervous system that eventually results in complete paralysis and the loss of the ability to speak, swallow, or breathe without a respirator. The patient afflicted with ALS gradually loses control of all bodily functions. Finally, even the heart muscle succumbs to paralysis, and the person dies. Throughout the course of the disease, the patient's mind remains clear. The ability to reason is unaffected by the deterioration of the nervous system, although the disease can take a heavy emotional toll on the patient, family, and friends. The disease is accompanied by painful muscle spasms, though these can be controlled to a degree with appropriate medication.

Mrs. Rodriguez was married and the mother of a young son. At the time of her Supreme Court hearing, she had been given a life expectancy of between two and fourteen months (without the assistance of a respirator).[10] Her concern throughout was that, while she wished to live as long as possible, she did not wish to live through the last and most debilitating stages of ALS and die as a result of asphyxiation. Such a death would have been very painful and unbearable. Fearing the complete loss of control over her bodily functions, and hence the ability to end her own life when she wished to do so, she brought an application before the Supreme Court of British Columbia for an order declaring section 241(b) of the *Criminal Code* unconstitutional.

Section 241(b) makes it an offence, punishable by up to fourteen years' imprisonment on conviction, for anyone to counsel, aid, or abet another person to commit suicide, whether or not the suicide is successful. Mrs. Rodriguez sought that declaration on the grounds that the effect of that section was to deprive her of several of her rights under the *Canadian Charter of Rights and Freedoms,* namely, her right to life, liberty, security of person,[11] equality before the law,[12] and freedom from any cruel or unusual treatment.[13] She argued that the effect of the law was to deprive her of control over her body and her life. Further, she argued that section 241(b) prevented her from obtaining the assistance of another person in ending her life when she could no longer do so on her own, and that this subjected her to cruel and unusual treatment at the hands of the state. Finally, she argued that since suicide was no longer a criminal offence in Canada,[14] she was being discriminated against and treated unequally by the law solely by reason of her physical disability, because she was effectively being prevented from doing that which able-bodied people could do legally.

Mrs. Rodriguez's application was dismissed by the Supreme Court of British Columbia and again by the B.C. Court of Appeal. A final appeal to the Supreme Court of Canada was heard on May 20, 1993, and the Court rendered its decision in September of that year.

The Court delivered a five-to-four decision against Mrs. Rodriguez's application. The closeness of the vote illustrates the difficulty of the issues and the lack of consensus in the courts. The majority of the judges felt that while the effect of section 241(b) was to impinge on Mrs. Rodriguez's right to life, liberty, and security of person, such intrusion was not contrary to the principles of fundamental justice. The majority also felt that her right to equal treatment was violated, but that this was permitted as being a "reasonable limit which [was] demonstrably justified in a free and democratic society."[15] The minority judges opined that both her right to life, liberty, and security of person, as well as her right to equality before the law, had been infringed, and that the infringement by the state through section 241(b) could not be justified in any way under the *Charter*. Thus, they felt that the section could not stand as valid under the Constitution and that therefore, Mrs. Rodriguez should be free to seek assistance in committing suicide when she wished it.

Mr. Justice Sopinka, writing the decision for the majority, undertook a historical review of the ethical and legal principles behind the legislative prohibitions against both suicide and assisted suicide. The chief ethical principle that he identified was the state's and society's concern for the sanctity and value of human life and human dignity,[16] as well as society's role in protecting those who are vulnerable and who could be coerced or encouraged, in a moment of weakness, to commit suicide. The purpose of section 241(b) was to protect such members of society. In recent times, the concept of protecting human life at all costs has become tempered with limitations premised on personal independence and dignity and with quality-of-life considerations.[17] Further, the common law has recognized the right of an individual to withdraw or withhold consent to medical treatment, even where such lack of treatment would likely result in death. Mr. Justice Sopinka's decision relied on the decision of the Supreme Court of Canada in *Ciarlariello v. Schacter*,[18] the *Nancy B. v. Hôtel-Dieu de Québec*[19] decision of the Quebec Superior Court, and the decision of the Ontario Court of Appeal in *Malette v. Shulman*.[20]

The majority judgement suggests that the law recognizes a form of "passive euthanasia," for example, inadvertently hastening a terminally ill patient's death by administering larger and larger doses of pain medication where the intent was to control pain. Another example might be withdrawing (with the patient's consent) all treatment and artificial means to prolong life where such treatment has become therapeutically useless. The distinction between passive and active euthanasia is thus seen as a basis for upholding the law's continued prohibition against assisted suicide.

In response, the majority judgement of the Supreme Court notes that the law has always had a great aversion to the participation of one person in the death of another, but passive euthanasia is considered acceptable because *artificial* means to prolong life are withdrawn on the patient's request and death ensues as a *natural* consequence. While some have criticized the distinction between passive and active euthanasia as artificial (since both take place with the full knowledge that death will ensue),[21] in the case of passive euthanasia the exact time of death cannot be known, and death does not result directly from the actions of another. Critics of the active/passive distinction and proponents of euthanasia also note that the outcome in either situation is ethically the same, but that in a case where treatment is merely withdrawn, death can come more slowly and may be more painful.

Another legal concern that justifies maintaining the blanket prohibition on assisted suicide, in the majority's opinion, is that of preventing abuse, together with the difficulties in formulating guidelines and conditions under which assisted suicide would be legally permissible. Mr. Justice Sopinka cites a working paper of the Law Reform Commission of Canada[22] which points out examples of mass suicides, or of one person taking advantage of the depressed state of another to encourage him to commit suicide for the other's financial gain, as reasons justifying the continued prohibition. Further, he reviews the record in the Netherlands, which has the most liberal guidelines on euthanasia and physician-assisted suicide, and notes evidence (he does not state his source) of a disturbing rise in cases of involuntary active euthanasia (which is not permitted by those guidelines).[23] Thus, the "slippery slope" argument, in the opinion of the majority, justifies a complete prohibition on physician-assisted suicide. To Mr. Justice Sopinka, to hold otherwise would "send a signal that there are circumstances in which the state approves of suicide."[24]

The minority Justices wrote equally compelling dissenting opinions. The Chief Justice, Mr. Justice Lamer, opined that section 241(b) of the *Criminal Code* infringed on the rights of disabled persons such as Sue Rodriguez because it effectively deprives them of choosing suicide, an option available to able-bodied persons.[25] As such, they were not being treated equally before the law as guaranteed under the *Charter*. Lamer also relied on the fact that it is a fundamental aspect of personal autonomy in the common law that citizens have the right to make free and informed decisions about their bodies and to consent or withhold consent to specific medical treatment, even when to do so would likely result in death.

The next consideration was whether such violation was "a reasonable limit ... demonstrably justified in a free and democratic society" within the meaning of section 1 of the *Charter*. Here Mr. Justice Lamer undertakes an interesting review of the values and objectives of the prohibition against assisted suicide. He points out that the repeal of the attempted-suicide prohibition by Parliament in 1972[26] reflected its belief that self-determination was now a paramount factor in the regulation of suicide. Thus, if no outside interference with an individual's decision could be shown, then that person's attempting suicide would no longer be a criminal offence.[27]

With respect to the "slippery slope" argument, His Lordship felt that despite the concern that decriminalizing assisted suicide would leave the physically disabled vulnerable and open to manipulation by others, this still would not justify depriving a disadvantaged group (i.e., the disabled) of equality before the law, specifically, the right to determine the circumstances in which they end their life. In Mrs. Rodriguez's case, there was no evidence of such vulnerability and plenty of evidence of her free consent.[28] He thus concluded that the limit placed by section 241(b) of the *Criminal Code* upon Sue Rodriguez's right to equality was not reasonable and could not be justified under the *Charter*.

Hence, the section was constitutionally invalid. However, he was inclined to suspend the declaration of unconstitutionality for one year, until such time as Parliament could address the issue and either enact legislation that would deal with assisted suicide in cases such as Sue Rodriguez's, or simply enact no constitutional legislation to replace section 241(b). This effectively meant that, while the law was unconstitutional, it would nevertheless remain in effect for one year so that the "floodgates" would not be opened, thus negating the objective of protecting the vulnerable from the influence and coercion of others in consenting to assisted suicide.

In the meantime, he would have granted Mrs. Rodriguez an exemption to compliance with section 241(b), provided that:

(1) she had applied to a superior court for authorization;
(2) she had been certified by her attending physician and a psychiatrist to be competent and had made her decision freely and voluntarily, and that at least one physician be with her when she commits assisted suicide;
(3) the physicians also certify that (a) she is or will become physically incapable of committing suicide unaided and (b) they have informed her of her continuing right to change her mind about terminating her life;
(4) notice and access be given to the Regional Coroner at the time;
(5) she be examined daily by the physicians;
(6) the exemption would expire thirty-one days after the date of the physicians' certificate in (1) above; and
(7) the act actually causing her death must be her act alone, unaided by anyone else.[29] The conditions were described as having been designed with Mrs. Rodriguez's circumstances in mind. However, Mr. Justice Lamer advanced them as guidelines to future applicants in similar circumstances.

The approach taken by two of the dissenting Justices (Madam Justice McLachlin, who wrote the dissent, and Madam Justice L'Heureux-Dubé, who concurred in that dissent) is also interesting. Madam Justice McLachlin felt that security of person entails personal autonomy, which protects the dignity and privacy of individuals with respect to decisions surrounding their own bodies.[30] Part of that autonomy involves the right of the person to decide what is best for him or her. There was thus no rational basis upon which to deny Mrs. Rodriguez a right that was freely available to others who were more able-bodied than she was.

CASE STUDY

Withdrawal of treatment

A patient in the Critical Care Unit, Mr. C. is seventy years old and has end-stage cardiac disease. He is intubated and dependent on medication to sustain an adequate blood pressure. Though his case is seemingly futile, the medical team plans to continue aggressive therapy. One of the patient's sons would like treatment to be withdrawn. The patient's wife and daughter disagree. Mr. C. is unable to speak for himself and has made no decisions respecting care in advance, while competent. The treatment plan and the rules of the unit mean visiting is kept to a minimum of ten minutes per hour.

ISSUES

1. In the absence of direction from the patient, how should the medical team make their decision?
2. Who has the right to make the decision in this situation?
3. Would an advance directive have helped? How?
4. What are the responsibilities of Mr. C.'s nurse?

DISCUSSION

Situations like the one described in this case study often give rise to conflict among family members, and this is stressful for all involved. The health care team may feel torn between their primary focus—the best interests of the patient—and the competing interests of the family. Decisions regarding withdrawal of treatment are more difficult when the patient is incompetent and unable to participate. Unfortunately, this is often the case in Intensive Care Units. The nurse may experience moral distress when the wishes of the most appropriate next of kin or substitute decision maker conflict with what the nurse believes is in the patient's best interest. This distress is alleviated if the nurse is confident that decisions regarding care are based on the previously expressed wishes or values of the patient.

In this case study, the fact that the treatment being administered is futile and that the patient seems near death raise an interesting legal point with respect to withdrawal of treatment. The Quebec Superior Court's decision in *Nancy B. v. Hôtel-Dieu de Québec* dealt with the legality of a lucid patient's request not to be subjected to further medical treatment when that person deems such treatment no longer appropriate. (The details of this case are reviewed in Chapter 2.) This ruling was made in the context of Quebec's *Civil Code,* which places ultimate responsibility for treatment decisions with the patient. Thus, consent-to-treatment issues (as discussed in Chapter 6) may be inseparable from the issue of withdrawal of treatment.

In point of fact, withdrawal of treatment in these circumstances is supported by the common law. For example, in the United States, the Superior Court of New Jersey ultimately supported the concept of withdrawal of treatment in the case of Karen Quinlan. The problem is that the common law has historically been hesitant to recognize the right of a spouse or next of kin to make treatment decisions on behalf of an incapable person. In Manitoba, this situation has been remedied in the *Health Care Directives Act*[31]; in Nova Scotia (to an extent), in the *Medical Consent Act*[32]; in British Columbia, in the recently enacted *Adult Guardianship Act*[33]; and in Ontario, in the *Substitute Decisions Act, 1992*,[34] which will enable another person to make decisions on behalf of those who cannot make them for themselves. It is too early to tell yet how the recent Ontario legislation will affect this issue.

At present, the practice is to accept treatment decisions made by an incapable person's spouse or, if there is no spouse, that person's closest living relative. For example, the patient's closest living relative may make the decision on the basis of what the patient would have wished. This means that the **proxy** (the person making the decision for the incapable patient) must make every effort to determine what the patient's wishes would have been.[35]

In the case study, the conflict between the son on the one hand, and the wife and daughter on the other, suggests that the matter may have to be resolved in court through committeeship proceedings (as discussed in Chapter 6). The committee would be authorized to make treatment decisions respecting the patient. This is a sad, costly, and needless development. Otherwise, it is fairly certain that the law would not interfere with the decision to withdraw treatment in such a case, especially where such treatment is demonstrably futile. However, it draws the line at positive acts in the nature of assisted suicide.

In the majority of cases, the resolution should not end up in court. It is the health care team's responsibility to meet with the family to weigh the alternatives and to explore their feelings and views. It is important that the family be fully informed of all the medical facts relevant to the patient's situation. It is also helpful to share with them a framework that might assist them to reach consensus on the best course of action.

Through discussion, the family might remember occasions when Mr. C. expressed thoughts on what he would want in such a situation as this—for example, a comment made about a similar case on television or in the newspapers. Or, they might talk about Mr. C.'s lifelong values in order to get some sense of his likely decision, were he capable. With the support of the health care team, clear communication, and time, most situations like this can be resolved.

Advance directives are always helpful in cases of incompetence. In future, it is likely that these will play a greater role in treatment decisions, especially when legislative reform encourages them.

Advance Directives (Living Wills)

An **advance directive** is a person's instruction regarding decisions about care if he or she is ever rendered incompetent. Advance directives can take the form of verbal discussion with someone whom the person has identified as a substitute decision maker.

Currently, this practice does not have legal sanction in most provinces. However, it will soon be legally recognized in Ontario with the passing of the *Substitute Decisions Act, 1992.*[36] It is currently recognized in Manitoba under the *Health Care Directives Act,*[37] and in Nova Scotia under the *Medical Consent Act.*[38] Substitute-decision legislation has been passed in British Columbia (the *Adult Guardianship Act*[39]). That statute contemplates an application to a court for the appointment of a guardian or substitute decision maker. Despite this, a living will is still a very useful document, even for a person living in a province or territory that as yet has no such legislation.

A written advance directive may be obtained in the form of a **living will,** a document that enables a patient to specify his or her informed choices well in advance of requiring such care. The living will takes effect only when the patient is incapable of making decisions. People with living wills usually update and revise them on a regular basis. Regardless of whether they are sanctioned by law, living wills are a useful resource for health care professionals.

The University of Toronto Centre for Bioethics has published and distributed a succinct living will (reproduced in full in Appendix B, pages 249–259). This tool defines the salient points of a living will and frames a process whereby an individual can make informed choices with respect to possible health care situations in the future.

There are two components to this living will. An *instruction directive* allows the person to specify which life-sustaining treatments he or she would not wish in various situations. The *proxy directive* allows individuals to identify a substitute decision maker, should they ever be rendered incompetent.

Individuals who complete the living will are advised to ensure that several appropriate people know the will exists and that copies are distributed, particularly to their doctor, lawyer, and family members. The will should be reviewed and updated on a regular basis to ensure that it continues to reflect the person's current wishes.

The University of Toronto Centre for Bioethics's living will, unlike most published to date, specifies many health situations that individuals could face. These include permanent coma, terminal illness, stroke, and dementia. Within each problem a mild, moderate, and severe state is defined. The life-sustaining options with respect to these conditions are outlined and explained with the lay person in mind, for example, cardiopulmonary resuscitation, respirators, dialysis, surgery, blood transfusions, antibiotics, and tube feeding. Space is included for the individual to provide further instructions with respect to other health care situations that might arise.

Ideally, individuals who complete a living will consult with physicians, nurses, and perhaps their lawyer or other persons, so that they fully anticipate the situations that might arise, and comprehend the treatments available to them. This helps them to make choices that are right for them, and ensures that these choices are clearly expressed in the living will.

CASE STUDY

Organ donation

Mr. R., a patient who has ingested a large quantity of barbiturates, is admitted to an Intensive Care Unit (ICU). The drugs have damaged his brain to such a degree that he has been declared brain-dead. He remains on a ventilator and is presently haemodynamically stable. In the same hospital, another patient, Mr. S., is dying as a result of a rejection episode following a heart transplant. Mr. S. has less than twenty-four hours to live unless another suitable heart is found for re-transplantation. Mr. R. is judged by the ICU team to be a suitable donor for the urgently required heart. Further, a signed organ donor card was found in his wallet. As is the practice in most hospitals, and despite the existence of this card, the ICU team approaches Mr. R.'s parents and requests them to consent to donating their son's organs. The parents categorically refuse consent. They are not informed about Mr. S., for fear that this would constitute coercion. Mr. S. dies the next day.

ISSUES

1. What is the legal status of a signed organ donor card?
2. Is the consent of the donor's family required?
3. Could health care professionals be more aggressive in encouraging the donor's family to give consent? Should family be told about the recipient in need?
4. Might further legislation in the area of consent help? How?

DISCUSSION

The field of transplantation has grown tremendously in recent years. The long-term survival rates for lung, heart, kidney, and liver transplants have improved remarkably. Patients who would have died otherwise may live more than five years longer with good quality of life. Transplantation in general has become a proven, cost-effective alternative to other treatments, especially in the case of renal transplantation.

In Canada, organ donation is generally viewed as morally justified when treatment alternatives to transplantation are not readily available, and respect for the autonomy of the donor and his or her family is maintained through appropriate legislation and guidelines.

The ethical issues associated with organ donation include the determination of brain death, consent, and donor management. The organ donation process, if not managed properly, can be highly stressful for the nurses involved.

Ironically, recent successes of transplant programs have contributed to the problem of limited availability of organs. The supply of donor organs has not kept pace with the growing need. Furthermore, advances in the field of neurosciences, compliance with seat-belt legislation, and a reduction in drinking and driving have reduced the numbers of deaths where there is a potential for organ donation. This situation has led to efforts to maximize all potential donors. Strategies explored have included changes to the legislation regarding the consent process, donor incentives, education, and a further redefinition of death.

The nurses caring for a donor patient may experience moral conflict during the donation process. It is important that nurses understand all aspects of this process and the relevant ethical issues so that they can deal more effectively with the difficult transition from trying to save the life of a patient to managing that patient's organs for the benefit of others. Greater understanding, together with ethical management of the process by all members of the team, can make this an enriching experience for all involved.

Legal Definition of Death

Removal of organ tissues from deceased donors is bound up with the legal and medical determination of death. Few jurisdictions in Canada or the United States provide a legislative definition of the moment of death. Historically, physicians have concurred that a person is dead when all vital signs (heartbeat, pulse, respiration) have ceased. In religious terms, death was seen as the moment when the soul leaves the body, generally at the time when the person's heart ceases to beat. Until well into the twentieth century, the courts recognized that a person was legally dead when the "vital functions had ceased to operate. The heart [had] always been regarded as a vital organ" in this determination.[40]

In the last half century, sophisticated medical technology has allowed physicians to sustain the lives of seriously ill patients in situations where previously such persons would have died. A patient who can no longer breathe on his or her own or whose heart function has ceased can now be kept alive with the aid of respirators and other devices to sustain blood circulation. As well, advances in medical transplant technology have made possible the transplantation of viable organs from deceased donors into the bodies of living persons. We have also learned much more about the human brain, its role in controlling not only vital bodily systems, but also as the source of personality, intelligence, emotion, and a host of other human characteristics.

It has become apparent that the traditional medical criteria for determining the fact of death have become inadequate. The question now is: Can a person whose brain function has completely and irreversibly ceased, but whose other bodily functions remain active, still be considered a living human being?

In 1975, Manitoba became the first (and so far the only) province to enact a legal definition of the moment of death. The Manitoba *Vital Statistics Act* provides that, for all civil purposes (i.e., not for the purpose of criminal law), "... the death of a person takes place at the time at which irreversible cessation of all that person's brain function occurs."[41] This definition conforms to the accepted definition of death within the modern medical community. In arriving at a new medical definition of death, a committee of the Harvard Medical School suggests that brain death is established with the cessation of all brain function, both cerebral and brain-stem, and that the cessation of such brain function must be irreversible.

With respect to human tissue donation, the laws of most of the provinces require that the death of a prospective donor be determined in this way.[42] Manitoba's legislation provides specifically that death must be determined according to the definition set out in the *Vital Statistics Act,* with bodily circulation still intact as necessary for the purposes of a successful transplant, and that such determination can only be made by at least two physicians.[43]

Further ethical and legal problems arise with respect to the removal of tissue and organs from the bodies of anencephalic neonates. Brain-stem anencephaly is demonstrated by the absence of the cerebrum, although the mid-brain cerebellum and brain stem are present and functioning. In such a newborn, there is enough lower brain function that the neonate can breathe and maintain a heartbeat for some time. It may be difficult to establish that indeed all brain function, both cerebral and brain-stem, has ceased. Furthermore, because an infant's brain cells are resistant to damage, caution must be exercised in applying brain-death criteria to children under five years of age. Specific criteria do exist for children under five, but not for infants under two weeks of age.[44]

Eventually, an anencephalic child will stop breathing. Yet, he or she can be kept on a respirator to ensure that the organs are kept healthy and viable for transplantation. There is no question that such a child will ever be able to live a meaningful life, since anencephalics are not conscious and have no mental capacity. Such a child is doomed to live in a vegetative state for the rest of its brief life, a few days at most.

The question that arises in this situation is whether or not such a child should be considered legally dead so that its organs may be removed for transplant to save another child's life. Clearly, an anencephalic is alive even by modern medical criteria, since its lower brain is still functioning and is able to sustain its breathing and circulation to a degree. The definition of death based on irreversible cessation of all brain function is of no help in this situation. Consequently, physicians and ethicists alike have recently argued for a revised definition of death that would address such a situation.

Some ethicists have argued that anencephalic donors ought to be deemed dead while respiration and circulation are maintained to keep the organs viable. Others opt for a special category of "brain absent" persons, such as anencephalics. This definition would permit removal of organs for transplant while the infant's brain was not yet dead. It is argued that this is a more utilitarian solution that preserves the donor child's humanity, spares it from further physical pain, saves the lives of recipients, prevents deterioration of the organs, and allows the parents the dignity and comfort of knowing that their child's condition and brief life were not in vain.

The Manitoba procedures for determining death in the *Human Tissue Act* do address this situation in part by permitting circulation to be maintained to ensure a successful transplant. However, even that province still relies on the complete cessation of all brain function.

Human Tissue Legislation across Canada

All provinces and both territories have enacted legislation dealing with organ donation before and after the death of the donor.[45] This legislation is remarkably uniform across Canada. The various statutes basically provide a mechanism for obtaining the consent of the donor (or others, where the donor is unable to consent) to the removal of tissue from the donor's body for transplant into the body of another, for medical education, or for purposes of scientific research.

There are two primary situations contemplated by the statutes: one where the donor is living and has consented to the removal of non-regenerative tissue[46] from his or her body for therapeutic use, such as a transplant to another person's body. This is legally referred to as an *inter vivos* gift of tissue, from the Latin meaning "among the living"; that is, the donor gives the tissue during his or her lifetime. The other situation occurs where the donor (or another, if the donor has expressed no wishes on the matter) has directed that specified body parts be removed from his or her body for transplant into another living person after the donor's death. This is legally known as a *post mortem* gift of tissue, that is, the donor (or other person authorized to consent, if the donor has not expressed any wishes on the matter) gives the tissue after he or she has died.

Legislation in all provinces and territories except Manitoba and Quebec specifically excludes such regenerative tissue as bone, blood or its constituents, skin, or other tissue that is regenerated naturally by the human body. In each of these eight provinces, an adult who is mentally competent and makes a free and informed decision may legally donate such regenerative tissue under the common law. The human tissue legislation does not apply to such a donation. For example, a person donating bone marrow in one of these provinces or territories need only be of the age of majority and mentally competent and may orally consent to giving such tissue. (In practice, most health care institutions require a signed consent to such donation for the mutual protection of all parties concerned.)

In contrast, the law in Manitoba excludes only blood or its constituents.[47] Thus, the *Human Tissue Act* of that province does not apply to a blood donation. Rather, the common law requires merely that the donor be an adult, be mentally competent, and be able to make a free and informed decision. On the other hand, a bone marrow donation, or a donation of skin for a skin graft, would have to comply with the requirements of the Act.

Similarly, the Quebec *Civil Code* allows any person in Quebec of the age of majority who is mentally capable to consent to the removal of tissue from his or her body while that person is living.[48] Since the *Civil Code* does not define "tissue," one can presume that it includes any tissue from the donor's body, including blood and other such regenerative tissue, as well as kidneys.

Consent to Transplant During Donor's Life

In a case of an inter vivos gift—for example, where the donor consents to giving a kidney for transplant into the body of a sibling—the consent is valid if it is in writing and is signed by the donor. Although the statutes are silent on this point, the consent can be revoked (cancelled) at any time thereafter, either in writing or orally.

In all provinces and territories except Ontario, Prince Edward Island, and Quebec, only a person who has reached the age of majority may legally consent to an inter vivos gift of tissue. Ontario and Prince Edward Island allow persons below the age of majority but who are at least sixteen years old to give consent without the approval of a parent or guardian.[49] In Quebec, a minor (a person who has not yet reached the age of majority) may consent to an inter vivos donation of regenerative tissue only with consent of a parent or tutor (in Quebec, the equivalent of a child's legal guardian) and with permission of the court, provided that the procedure does not result in serious risk to the health of the minor.[50] The New Brunswick[51] and Northwest Territories[52] statutes are silent on inter vivos transfers. However, the common law would likely permit such transfers where the donor was an adult, mentally competent, and making a free and fully informed decision.

Apart from being of the requisite age, a person in Ontario, Nova Scotia, Alberta, British Columbia, Newfoundland, Saskatchewan, or the Yukon Territory must be mentally competent to consent and must make a free and informed decision.[53] A "free and informed decision" (as discussed in Chapter 6) follows the same common law requirements for fully informed consent to medical treatment as set out by the Supreme Court of Canada in *Reibl v. Hughes*.[54] The physician must inform the donor of all potential and material risks inherent in the procedure that would be reasonably likely to affect the donor's decision.

For their consent to be valid, Prince Edward Islanders must specifically be able to understand the consequences and nature of transplanting tissue from their body during their lifetime.[55] If there is any doubt on this point, an independent assessment must determine whether the transplant should be carried out.[56]

Mentally Incompetent Inter Vivos Donors and Minors

Situations in which the prospective donor is a minor, or is mentally incompetent, or otherwise unable to make an informed decision through not understanding the nature and consequences of the procedure, pose a special problem. Such a situation might arise, for example, where the health risk to the donor is perfectly acceptable and minimal and the tissue is urgently required to save the life of that person's sibling. As mentioned above, the Prince Edward

Island statute provides for an independent assessment in a situation where the donor appears not to understand the nature and consequences of the transplant and yet consents to it. The assessors must consider:

(1) whether the transplant is the treatment of choice;
(2) whether the donor has been coerced or induced to give consent;
(3) whether removal of the tissue will create a substantial health or other risk to the donor; and
(4) whether the Act and its regulations have been complied with.[57]

This requirement also applies in the case of a donor under sixteen, even if he or she understands the nature and consequences of the transplant.[58] In Prince Edward Island, in the case of a minor under sixteen, parental consent is required for an inter vivos gift of regenerative tissue (e.g., bone marrow). Finally, the independent assessment must indicate that the transplant should be carried out.

The same factors must be considered in the case of a donor under sixteen, with the additional requirement that all other members of the donor's family must be eliminated as potential donors for medical or other reasons. The assessors must give written reasons for their decision. The PEI statute further provides that a person may appeal the decision to the Supreme Court of Prince Edward Island within three days.[59] The Court may confirm, vary, or quash (cancel) the assessor's decision, or return the matter to the assessors for further action. Pending the decision of the appeal, the transplant cannot proceed.

Similarly, Manitoba's *Human Tissue Act* permits persons under eighteen but at least sixteen to consent to the transplant of tissue while living. However, a physician who is not and never has been associated with the proposed recipient must certify in writing that he or she believes such person is capable of understanding and does understand the nature and effect of the transplant. Further, a parent must consent, and the donor must be a member of the recipient's immediate family.[60] The physician who makes the certificate cannot participate in the transplant operation. This provision addresses concerns over potential conflicts of interest.

In Manitoba, persons under sixteen may donate tissue only while living if these conditions are met:

(1) the proposed recipient must be a member of the donor's immediate family;
(2) only regenerative tissue may be given;
(3) the recipient would likely die without the tissue;
(4) the life and health risks to the donor must be minimal;
(5) the donor consents to the transplant;
(6) the donor's parent or legal guardian consents;
(7) the transplant is recommended by a physician who is not and never has been involved in any way with the recipient and will not be involved in the transplant; and finally,
(8) court approval must be obtained.

The term "immediate family" specifically includes the donor's mother, father, or step-father or step-mother, brother, sister, step-brother or step-sister, or half-brother or half-sister.[61]

Neither Ontario, Alberta, Nova Scotia, British Columbia, Newfoundland, Saskatchewan, nor the Yukon Territory provide for an assessment procedure in the case of a minor or mentally incompetent inter vivos donor. The statutes of all these provinces are virtually identical. However, they do provide that where the donor has given consent, and is a minor, or is mentally incompetent to consent, or is unable to give a free and informed decision, the consent is still legally valid, provided that the person acting on that consent (presumably, the physician who will perform the transplant) has no reason to believe that the donor is a minor, or is mentally incompetent, or is unable to make a free and informed decision. There is thus a requirement of good faith on the part of the person performing the transplant, and a duty upon him or her to ensure that a prospective donor is indeed a mentally competent adult who is giving a free and informed consent.

In most cases, this provision does not pose a problem. Most physicians and nurses are competent to assess the general mental capabilities of their patients. A careful review with the patient of all material risks inherent in the transplant within the criteria stated in *Reibl v. Hughes* would likely address the problem of a free and informed consent. The case of the minor poses a slightly different problem when that person appears much older than he or she actually is. The level of maturity disclosed in the conversation between the health care professional and the minor is not conclusive. This provision of the statute protects health care professionals acting in good faith in such a situation.

Apart from this, such prospective donors would presumably require some sort of court authorization according to common law. This has been the traditional route in jurisdictions lacking procedures such as those required in Prince Edward Island, or explicit provisions for court authorization such as those in the Quebec *Civil Code*. A court reviewing such a case would likely consider factors such as those mentioned in the PEI Act and further, would consider the impact of the procedure on the donor.

In the case of a minor, some courts have relied on the "competent minor" rule. This rule holds that a person under the age of majority may be sufficiently mature to comprehend fully the nature and consequences of the transplant. Since in these cases, the donor is not receiving a direct health benefit from the transplant, the courts, in some American states, have considered that the infant donor still derives an emotional benefit from the survival of his or her sibling. The family is thus relieved from the potential stress of the death of one of its members, and can provide full emotional support to the donor. Further, especially in cases where the infant donor is old enough to have expressed even a rudimentary wish to help the sibling (though not fully comprehending the nature and consequences of the transplant), that child is spared the emotional guilt that may develop later in life from not having had an opportunity to save the sibling's life.[62]

Interestingly, Prince Edward Island's *Human Tissue Donation Act* deals expressly with the question of regenerative tissue donation by an infant sibling.[63] It provides that, with the consent of the infant donor's parents, and the approval of the independent assessors, bone marrow may be removed from such a child during the child's life for implantation into the child's biological sibling. Of course, the assessors will have eliminated all other eligible family members for medical or other reasons.

Post Mortem Donations

Consent to donation of tissue after the donor's death is somewhat different. The policy behind the law in such cases is to encourage the donation of organs after death, since there is always a large pool of recipients who urgently need them. Thus, the requirements for lawful consent are more relaxed and flexible.

In all provinces and both territories, a person over the age of majority (over sixteen in Ontario and Prince Edward Island) may consent in writing to the removal of any and all tissue for either therapeutic, medical educational, or medical research purposes. Except in Quebec, the written document containing the consent may be part of a will or other testamentary instrument (e.g., organ donor card, driver's licence), regardless of whether such will is legally valid.

In Manitoba, persons under eighteen but at least sixteen years of age may consent to such removal, but only with the consent of the donor's parent or guardian, unless the parent or guardian is unavailable (e.g., dead, physically or mentally ill, or otherwise absent).[64] This provision permits flexibility and promotes the availability of organs.

Consent given by a person under sixteen is deemed valid if the person who acted on it had no reason to believe that the donor was in fact under sixteen. This mirrors the provisions of inter vivos donations in most provinces, and imposes a requirement of good faith on the part of physicians acting upon the donor's directive.

In Quebec, a minor fourteen years of age or older may authorize the removal of organs or tissue or give his or her body for medical or scientific purposes. A minor under fourteen may also do so with the written consent of a parent or guardian.[65]

Most provinces allow the consent to be made orally by the donor in the presence of two witnesses during the donor's last illness. Manitoba and Prince Edward Island do not specify whether the consent must be written or may also be made orally. The statutes of those two provinces speak of the removal of tissue "as may be specified in the consent," which implies a requirement for written consent. However, in a case where a clear, unequivocal oral consent is given in the presence of two or more witnesses, it is possible that such consent would be permissible as clear evidence of the donor's last wishes. In all cases, the donor may revoke (cancel) his or her consent at any time prior to death. The law will respect the absolute final wishes of the donor and the right to change his or her mind, even at the last possible moment.

The consent is effective upon the donor's death. The determination of death can be problematic, as discussed above. All statutes across Canada require that, in cases where organs are to be removed, death must be determined by at least two physicians. Neither may be persons associated with the intended recipient such as might influence the physician's judgement. Conversely, no physician involved in determining the death of the donor may participate in the transplant. This is to avoid potential conflicts of interest.

A valid consent may not be acted upon if the person acting on it has reason to believe that the donor has not reached the age of consent, is not mentally competent, or is not able to make a free and informed consent. Thus, physicians and nurses involved in the transplant should be alert to any such indications. If there is no reason for such suspicions, the consent will be valid even if it later turns out that the donor was under age, was mentally incompetent, or was otherwise unable to make a free and informed consent.

The consent grants complete authority to use the body, remove and use parts specified in the consent for any purpose specified, unless the person acting on it has reason to believe that consent was withdrawn by the donor before death. This is consistent with the principle permitting the donor to change his or her mind at any time. The withdrawal can be made either orally to witnesses, or in writing signed by the donor.

Post Mortem Donations Lacking Deceased's Consent

What of situations where the deceased expressed no wishes regarding donating tissues or organs after death, or was incapable of giving consent? This is different from specifically refusing consent, since the law requires that such refusal, however unfortunate for the prospective recipient, be respected. Yet, in such cases (e.g., the prospective donor has expressed no wishes, and death is imminent in the opinion of a physician), organs or tissue may be urgently needed to save the life of another. Here, the law in all jurisdictions allows other specific persons to make the decision of whether tissue or organs may be removed from the deceased's body.

There is a hierarchy of persons who may be approached to make this decision:

(1) first, the spouse of the donor;
(2) if there is no spouse, any of the donor's children over eighteen;
(3) if there are no children, either one of the donor's parents (or legal guardian, in some provinces)[66];
(4) any of the donor's siblings;
(5) the donor's next of kin; and finally, if no such persons are available,
(6) anyone who is in lawful possession of the body may give the required consent.

The statutes make clear that the sixth category excludes the coroner, medical examiner, embalmer, and funeral director. It might conceivably include the executor or administrator of the donor's estate, since such person is responsible for the proper and respectful disposal of the deceased's remains, either by burial or cremation.

Often, relatives of the deceased will differ over permitting the removal of organs or tissue. For example, the wife of a patient whose death is imminent might refuse a physician's request for removal of the man's kidneys, whereas the patient's father may favour such a request. The law in most provinces and both territories provides a resolution to such conflict: no person may act on a consent given on behalf of a dying or deceased donor if such person knows of an objection to it by anyone having the same or closer relationship to the donor than the one who gave the consent. Thus, in our case study, the wife's wishes would overrule those of the donor's father. Similarly, in a case where the donor's sister gave consent and the donor's brother objected, that objection would void the consent and this would be the end of the matter, unless another relative closer in relationship to the donor consented.

Manitoba's legislation does not provide a mechanism for resolving such disputes, but it is likely that a health care professional in that province faced with a similar conflict could resolve it in this manner. Quebec law allows the same hierarchy of persons as in the other provinces; further, the *Civil Code* permits the deceased's heirs or successors to give or refuse consent.[67] There is no mechanism for conflict resolution in the *Civil Code*. However, a person qualified to give consent to care of the donor (when living) may also consent to the removal of tissues or organs from the deceased's body.[68] In Quebec, a physician may proceed with the transplant of an organ or tissues from a deceased if two physicians certify that they were unable to obtain such consent in due time, and that the operation was urgently required to save a human life or significantly improve the quality of a life.[69]

Finally, the law, as always, respects the deceased or dying donor's wishes. If a health professional acting on the consent of a donor's spouse or other relative has reason to believe that the donor would object to the removal (or, in Manitoba,[70] that such removal would be contrary to the donor's religion), he or she cannot proceed on the basis of the consent. Similarly, if the health care professional in charge of the case believes that the deceased's death occurred in circumstances requiring an inquest by a coroner or medical examiner, that professional cannot proceed on the basis of the consent unless the coroner or medical examiner agrees. This requirement preserves the evidentiary value of a post mortem examination of the body in cases where the deceased has not died of natural causes and an inquest into the cause of death is required.

Strategies to Promote Organ Retrieval

Manitoba has made an attempt in its *Human Tissue Act* to encourage physicians and other health care professionals to identify potential organ donors. That Act requires the last physician who attended the deceased to consider, upon the death of one who has given no direction as to organ donation (or whose direction is invalid because the person was incompetent) whether it is appropriate to request permission of the donor's proxy or other relative to remove tissue or use the body for therapeutic purposes.[71] The physician must take into account the condition of the body and its tissues, the need for the use of these for therapeutic purposes, and the emotional and physical condition of the deceased's survivors. The Manitoba statute specifically provides for the removal of the pituitary gland and eyes (for corneal transplants).

Prince Edward Island requires a record to be made of whether any attending physician or other person discussed tissue donation with any of those authorized to provide consent on behalf of the patient to removal of organs or tissue. Such a case might arise in a hospital when a patient's death seems imminent. If no such discussion has taken place, the reason that it has not must be recorded.[72] This is as far as the PEI legislation goes. It does not demand that such a consultation take place.

In contrast, Ontario's *Public Hospitals Act*[73] requires the board of every public hospital in the province to pass by-laws to establish procedures encouraging organ and tissue donation. Such procedures include identifying potential donors and making them and their families aware of the opportunities for organ and tissue donation.[74]

Application to Case Study

The misconceptions and misinformation surrounding organ tissue laws in Canada are regrettable, and have contributed to a low rate of organ retrieval across the country. The case study of Mr. R. and Mr. S. raises the issue of whether the ICU team ought to have been more persuasive with Mr. R.'s family. This would have been an appropriate role for the nurses in Mr. R.'s team. With the valid organ donor card, they could have proceeded despite the parents' wishes. However, in practice, most hospitals do not contravene the wishes of the deceased's next of kin, even with a valid consent from the deceased. This is unfortunate. The reason for this practice may be that attempting to persuade the deceased's family to consent might be deemed coercive. However, if the team approaches the family in a gentle, diplomatic, and sensitive way, the request need not be coercive; in fact, it might garner more support from such families. Many more lives could be saved if this situation were expressly addressed in each province's legislation.

Further, can it be said that Mr. R.'s family made a truly informed consent, as they were not given the complete facts of the situation—namely, Mr. S.'s need? Legislative reform might focus on the extent and nature of the information to be given to those authorized to make such decisions on behalf of donors. It may be within the rights and duties of the nurse to make such information known to those making such a decision.

Ethical Issues

The current approach to organ donation in Canada, as described above, is a voluntary system of expressed consent. This is based on the principle of beneficence, doing good and avoiding harm. Because society does not oblige us to help others or to be altruistic, the system is based on the notion of voluntarism, and encourages organ donation through such mechanisms as providing individuals an opportunity to indicate on a driver's licence or organ donor card their willingness to donate organs at the time of death. Supporters of this system argue that procurement built on voluntarism promotes socially desirable virtues such as altruism and, at the same time, protects the rights of persons who might refuse to donate.[75]

Certain problems have arisen in regard to this approach:

(1) Individuals may choose not to sign a donor card, even when they support the concept.

(2) The donor card is not always available to health care professionals at the time of a patient's death.

(3) Regardless of whether a donor card is signed, families are approached and, in practice, their decision takes precedence.

(4) Health care professionals are still reluctant to approach families or to initiate a complex and time-consuming donation process.[76]

Item 4 raises some ethical issues with respect to the role of the team (especially nurses) as participants in organ donation. Some health professionals cite the grieving process of the family as the reason for not approaching them with respect to organ donation. Others claim that the cultural or religious perspectives of some patients preclude organ donation. The problem here is that when we decide not to raise the issue with the family, or fail to look for a signed organ donor card, then we are in fact making the decision for them not to donate, and this is disrespectful of the individual's autonomy. Furthermore, we cannot make assumptions about the views of various cultural and religious groups. In fact, most world religions support organ donation and transplantation. These include the Christian, Jewish, and Hindu religions. The Japanese Shinto religion and some sects of Tibetan Buddhism prohibit (or discourage) organ transplantation because of beliefs about the dead, taboos against injuring the body after death, and the extensive purifying rights required after death occurs.[77]

Nurses are in a good position to raise the issue of organ donation with patients' families. The nurse caring for the patient has the most opportunity to interact with the family throughout this difficult process. Nurses often develop a supportive relationship with family as they prepare them for the inevitable, and most have the communication skills to raise the issue of organ donation sensitively. Given the fact that families often forget about organ donation in the midst of crisis, it is important that nurses advocate to ensure that the issue is raised.

Regardless of the decision, the nurse has represented the interests and wishes of the patient and family. Taking part in this process also eases the nurse's own transition from caring for the needs of the patient to maintaining that patient's organs for the benefit of future recipients. The relationship with the patient continues, as the nurse ensures that the patient's wish to give to others is fulfilled.

The declaration of brain death remains a controversial process that continues to create emotional tension for the health professionals involved. It is difficult to accept that a patient is dead when the chest continues to rise and fall and colour and temperature seem normal. When most patients die, certain rituals take place that acknowledge its occurrence. Some settings observe a moment of silence to respect the deceased and to acknowledge the feelings of family and staff. This observance can also ease the transition to the next phase of the donation process. Such rituals are an issue particularly for nurses in the Operating Room, who may be left alone with the patient after removal of the organs.[78] Hospitals should be sensitive to the needs of staff left in such a situation and endorse the means to support them.

Low donor rates in relation to the growing number of patients who need organ transplants have raised questions about whether alternative systems for organ donation should be considered. Following is a brief overview of some possible approaches.

Recorded Consideration

This approach attempts to deal with the issue of families' not being asked.[79] It requires that health care staff routinely consider and document the appropriateness of a dying or brain-dead patient for organ donation. If the patient's organs are appropriate, then the family is to be approached. If the organs are not appropriate, or if the family refuses consent, then the staff are required to document this in the patient's chart. (This is required by law in Prince Edward Island.)[80]

Required Request

With this system, all patients are asked about their position on organ donation when admitted to the hospital or when they use the health care system in any way. Concerns have been raised about whether such questions are unduly stressful for patients, who hope to have their health care needs met in the hospital and thus may not wish to entertain the possibility of imminent organ donation.[81]

Presumed Consent

This approach is commonly referred to as "opting out." The assumption is that the dying or brain-dead patient would have donated his or her organs, unless he or she expressed otherwise beforehand. Those who favour this method reason that it would make approaching the family easier and would result in more organs being made available. They argue that autonomy is respected, since individuals still have the right to refuse. Those who disagree with this approach say that consent, particularly of the bereaved, cannot be presumed, and that it undermines the notion of altruism. It has been noted that in countries where presumed consent is the law (e.g., France, Belgium, Singapore), organ donor rates improved for awhile, then levelled off. This phenomenon was apparently related to the continuing reluctance of health care professionals to approach families.[81]

Market Strategies

Some suggest that organ donor rates would improve if there were a financial incentive involved, ranging from a lump-sum payment to covering the deceased's funeral expenses. Again, concerns arise that this approach would not only undermine the notion of altruism, but might take advantage of those compromised by poverty. As well, a coercive element would be introduced into the process of consent.[83] In Canada at present, the buying and selling of human tissue and organs is prohibited by law in every province and territory. Penalties for breach of this prohibition vary from province to province, but they include several thousands of dollars in fines and several months' imprisonment.

Education

Strategies to educate the public and health care professionals have been encouraged. Further knowledge and better communication would ensure that the notion of brain death is understood, that individuals are aware of the donation options available to them, and that health care professionals understand and are comfortable with their role in the organ donation process. It is not adequate to educate only health professionals working in hospitals. A significant role exists for nurses practising in the community to represent the interests of health care in general and to educate their clients about these specific issues.[84]

Redefinition of Death

Some health professionals have responded to the shortage of organs by suggesting that the definition of death be extended to include cortical death, as in the case of the anencephalic donor. This definition would include patients in a persistent vegetative state, who have no cortical activity although the brain stem is intact. Such persons can maintain their vital functions, and their body can live for years with appropriate nursing care. However, all that makes them a person—their ability to communicate, to relate to others, to remember—is gone. These patients may live for years, or may have treatment withdrawn and be allowed to die.

Those who seek to redefine death argue that we are losing a potential pool of organ donors who may have previously expressed, while competent, the wish to donate organs at the time of death. Those who argue against this redefinition suggest that we cannot redefine death whenever it is convenient to do so. Furthermore, they argue that these questions should be raised not in the context of organ donation, but out of a duty and responsibility to the patient in the persistent vegetative state.[85] To do otherwise would be to treat individuals, as Kant would say, as means and not as ends in and of themselves.

Redefining death to include cortical death would present procedural problems. Would this redefinition apply universally, or only in cases of organ donation or with the families' permission? In any case, when would biological life be deemed to end? Would this happen immediately after cortical death is declared? Or would it end when convenient—for example, when a transplant recipient appears? How would life be terminated?[86]

Summary

The key points introduced in this chapter include:
- the legal and ethical issues surrounding death and the process of dying
- the legal definitions of death, euthanasia, and assisted suicide
- the legal and ethical issues surrounding tissue donation and organ transplantation
- the legal and ethical implications of withdrawal of treatment
- the use and legality of advance directives (living wills)
- some possible redefinitions of death.

References

1. See *In re Quinlan*, 137 NJ Super. 227; 348 A.2d. 801 (Ch. Div. 1975), *In re Quinlan*, 70 NJ 10, 355 A.2d. 647 (SC 1976).
2. See *Rodriguez v. British Columbia* (AG), [1993] BCWLD 347; (1992), 18 WCB (2d) 279 (SC); aff'd. (1993), 76 BCLR (2d) 145; 22 BCAC 266; 38 WAC 266; 14 CRR (2d) 34; 79 CCC (3d) 1; [1993] 3 WWR 553; aff'd. [1993] 3 SCR 519.
3. See *Nancy B. v. Hôtel-Dieu de Québec et al.*, [1992] RJQ 361; (1992), 86 DLR (4th) 385; (1992) 69 CCC (3d) 450 (SC).
4. Canadian Nurses Association. (1991). *Code of ethics for nursing.* Value IV, Obligation 4 (p. 7).
5. See Law Reform Commission of Canada (1980), *Medical treatment and criminal law*, working paper no. 26, p. 71.
6. Since this was a jury trial, and juries do not deliver reasons for their verdict, this case has not appeared in a law report. However, the appeal decision, when rendered, may be reported.
7. Caralis, P.V., & Hammond, J.S. (1992). Attitudes of medical students, house staff, and faculty physicians towards euthanasia and termination of life-sustaining treatment. *Critical Care Medicine 20*, 683–690.
8. Genuis, S.J., Genuis, S.K., & Chang, W.C. (1994). Public attitudes toward the right to die. *Canadian Medical Association Journal 150*, 701–708.
9. Supra footnote 2.
10. Ibid., per Lamer C.J. (dissenting), at pp. 530-531 (SCR).
11. *Canadian Charter of Rights and Freedoms*, Part I of the *Constitution Act, 1982*, being Schedule B of the *Canada Act, 1982* (UK), 1982, c.11, section 7.
12. Ibid., section 15(1).
13. Ibid., section 12.
14. The provision in the *Criminal Code of Canada* making it an offence to commit or attempt to commit suicide was repealed in 1972. See *Criminal Law Amendment Act*, SC 1972, c. 13, section 16. Since then, it is no longer a crime to commit or attempt suicide.
15. Supra footnote 11, section 1.
16. Supra footnote 2, p. 592 (SCR).
17. Ibid., pp. 595–596.
18. [1993] 2 SCR 119. This case is discussed in detail in Chapter 6.
19. Supra footnote 3.
20. (1990), 72 OR (2d) 417 (CA). This case is discussed in detail in Chapter 6.
21. Supra footnote 2, p. 606 (SCR), citing a *Harvard Law Review* note: Physician-Assisted Suicide and the Right to Die with Assistance, (1992) 105 *Harv. L Rev.* 2021, at pp. 2030–31.
22. Law Reform Commission of Canada. (1983). *Euthanasia, aiding suicide and cessation of treatment*, report no. 20.

23. Supra footnote 2, p. 603 (SCR).
24. Ibid., p. 608.
25. Ibid., per Lamer J. (dissenting), p. 544.
26. Ibid., per Lamer J. (dissenting), pp. 530–531, and see supra footnote 14.
27. Ibid., per Lamer J. (dissenting), p. 559.
28. Ibid., pp. 566-567.
29. Ibid., p. 579.
30. Ibid., per McLachlin J. (dissenting), L'Heureux-Dubé (concurring), p. 618.
31. RSM 1993, c. 33, CCSM, c. H27.
32. RSNS 1989, c. 279.
33. SBC 1993, c. 35.
34. SO 1992, c. 30.
35. 14 CED (Ont. 3d.), Title 72, section 177, citing an unpublished article.
36. Supra footnote 34, section 46(1).
37. Supra footnote 31.
38. Supra footnote 32.
39. Supra footnote 33.
40. R v. Kitching and Adams, [1976] 6 WWR 697, at p. 711 (Man. CA), per O'Sullivan J.A.
41. RSM 1987, c. V60, section 2; CCSM, c. V60, section 2.
42. Alberta: infra footnote 45, section 7(1); British Columbia: infra footnote 45, section 7(1); Newfoundland: infra footnote 45, section 9(1); Nova Scotia: infra footnote 45, section 8(1); Prince Edward Island: infra footnote 45, section 11(1); Quebec: infra footnote 45, article 45; Saskatchewan: infra footnote 45, section 8(1); Yukon Territory: infra footnote 45, section 7(1).
43. Manitoba: infra footnote 45, section 8(1).
44. Capron, A.M. (1987). Anencephalic donors: Separate the dead from the dying. Hastings Centre Report, 17(1): 5–9.
45. See Alberta: Human Tissue Gift Act, RSA 1980, c. H-12, as amended; British Columbia: Human Tissue Gift Act, RSBC 1979, c. 187; Manitoba: The Human Tissue Act, SM 1987–88, c. 39, CCSM, c. 180, as amended; New Brunswick: Human Tissue Act, RSNB 1973, c. H-12, as amended; Newfoundland: Human Tissue Act, RSN 1990, c. H-15; Northwest Territories: Human Tissue Act, RSNWT 1988, c. H-6; Nova Scotia: Human Tissue Gift Act, RSNS 1989, c. 215, as amended; Ontario: Human Tissue Gift Act, RSO 1990, c. H.20; Prince Edward Island: Human Tissue Donation Act, SPEI 1992, c. 34; Quebec: Quebec Civil Code, articles 19, 23 to 25, 42 to 45; Saskatchewan: Human Tissue Gift Act, RSS 1978, c. H-15, as amended; Yukon Territory: Human Tissue Gift Act, RSYT 1986, c. 89.
46. This effectively means kidneys, and recently, liver lobectomies, since no person can continue to live adequately with the loss of any other non-regenerative organ.
47. Manitoba Act, supra footnote 45, section 1, "tissue" (c).
48. Quebec Civil Code, supra footnote 45, article 19, paragraph 1.
49. Ontario Act, supra footnote 45, section 3(1); Prince Edward Island Act, supra footnote 45, section 6(1).
50. Quebec Civil Code, supra footnote 45, article 19, paragraph 2.
51. New Brunswick Act, supra footnote 45, section 1. "Donor" speaks of consent that specified body part or parts be used after the donor's death.
52. Northwest Territories Act, supra footnote 45, sections 1(1) and (2) speak of specified body parts used after the donor's death.
53. Alberta Act, supra footnote 45, section 3(1); British Columbia Act, supra footnote 45, section 3(1); Newfoundland Act, supra footnote 45, section 4(1); Nova Scotia Act, supra footnote 45, section 4(1); Ontario Act, supra footnote 45, section 3(1); Saskatchewan Act, supra footnote 45, section 4(1); Yukon Territories Act, supra footnote 45, section 3(1).
54. [1980] 2 SCR 880; (1980) 14 CCLT 1; 114 DLR (3d) 1; 33 NR 361.
55. Prince Edward Island Act, supra footnote 45, section 6(1).
56. Ibid., sections 6(2) and (8).
57. Ibid., section 8(6).
58. Ibid., sections 7(1) and (4).

59. Ibid., section 9(1).
60. Manitoba Act, supra footnote 45, sections 10(1) and (2).
61. Ibid., sections 10(4) and 11(3). This applies in both the case of a child donor under sixteen and of a person between sixteen and eighteen.
62. This issue is more fully discussed in Sneiderman, B., Irvine, J.C., & Osborne, P.H. (1989), *Canadian medical law* (pp. 220–223). Toronto: Carswell.
63. Prince Edward Island Act, supra footnote 45, section 7(2).
64. Manitoba Act, supra footnote 45, sections 2(1) and (2).
65. Quebec *Civil Code*, supra footnote 45, article 43.
66. In Prince Edward Island, the person's guardian ranks above his or her spouse.
67. Quebec *Civil Code*, article 42.
68. Ibid., article 45, paragraph 1.
69. Ibid., article 45, paragraph 2.
70. Manitoba Act, supra footnote 45, section 4(3)(a).
71. Ibid., section 4(1).
72. Prince Edward Island Act, supra footnote 45, section 4.
73. RSO 1990, c. P.40.
74. O. Reg. 518/88, section 4(1), as amended by O. Reg. 34/90.
75. Task Force on Presumed Consent. (1994). *Organ procurement strategies. A review of ethical issues and challenges* (p.7). Toronto: Multiple Organ Retrieval & Exchange Program of Ontario.
76. Ibid, p.6.
77. Ibid., pp. 10–11.
78. Youngner, S.J., et al. (1985, August 1). Psychosocial and ethical implications of organ retrieval. *New England Journal of Medicine*, pp. 321–324.
79. Ibid., p. 17.
80. Supra footnote 45.
81. Supra footnote 74, p. 18.
82. Ibid., pp. 21–25.
83. Ibid., pp. 13–17.
84. Ibid., pp. 12–13.
85. Keatings, M. (1989). *The persistent vegetative state—Nursing perspectives.* Transplantation Proceedings.
86. Ibid.

CHAPTER Eight

Patient Rights

CHAPTER OBJECTIVES

The purpose of this chapter is to enable the reader to:
- define the rights of patients and obligations of health care professionals
- appreciate a patient's rights to confidentiality and the conditions under which disclosure is permitted
- understand the patient's rights to information, respect, and discharge from a health care facility.

As we have seen in Chapters 5 and 6, patients have the right to respect, privacy, and confidentiality; to be told the truth; and to give or refuse an informed consent. Furthermore, they have the right to refuse treatment (or to request it be withdrawn) and to die with dignity.

Nurses are obliged to ensure that these patient rights are respected and upheld. Further, to fulfil the role of caregiver, nurses must advocate on behalf of their patients, especially when they are unable to speak for themselves. These obligations are explicit in the Canadian Nurses Association's *Code of Ethics for Nursing.*[1]

Many agencies and health care institutions demonstrate their commitment to respect for patient rights by developing and publishing a bill of such rights, or they may express this commitment in their mission statement. Others state that they have adopted the values of a professional code such as the CNA's *Code of Ethics for Nursing.*

What Is a Right?

A *right* is a claim or privilege to which one is justly entitled, either legally or morally. *Legal rights* make explicit an individual's claim to such entitlement. For example, one explicit right under the Canadian *Charter of Rights and Freedoms* is the freedom or liberty of an individual to think, say, write, or otherwise act in accordance with his or her beliefs.[2] This suggests another aspect of rights, that is, autonomy, or the right to act on one's own, free of interference or control of the state or others. However, this right is not absolute. Our laws must also regulate the behaviour of citizens, and this somewhat limits the freedom of each citizen to do as he or she pleases.

A right carries a corresponding obligation. For example, in the context of health care, if someone has the right to care, then another person (or, more often, the state) has the corresponding obligation to provide that care. Otherwise, the right becomes meaningless.

The rights of patients are made explicit and clear through standards contained in professional codes of ethics, as discussed in Chapters 3 and 4. These impose an obligation on health care professionals to provide an adequate level of safe and competent care to patients.

Legal rights are enforced by individuals through court action, that is, through the coercive power of the state to compel individuals to act or refrain from acting in particular ways. In Chapter 2, we described the basic legal and political rights and freedoms held by Canadians under the *Charter of Rights and Freedoms* and in various statutes of Parliament and the provincial legislatures.

Moral rights include the right to be treated with respect for one's autonomy, for example, to be treated courteously. In a health care context, patients have the moral right to be informed not only of the risks of treatment (for purposes of granting or refusing an informed consent) but also to more general information as to what the institution and its caregivers can and cannot do. This might include information as to the general state of a patient's health, the treatment resources and alternatives available, the role of the health care professionals, the proposed treatment plan for the patient, and the plan of care after treatment. Of course, this also includes the patient's right to refuse or otherwise control the information he or she receives.

These rights are not all necessarily formally recognized in the law, but they are recognized as part of the societal norms of North American culture. They are based on ethical principles of the autonomy of the patient, beneficence, and non-maleficence (as discussed in Chapter 4). That is, the patient has the ultimate right to make any and all decisions respecting treatment. These rights are enforced, not necessarily through the courts, but through the maintenance of superior practice standards and the ethical values and rules practised by health professionals every day. If necessary, however, they could be enforced through court action in civil negligence or criminal proceedings, should the breach of these rights bring harm to the patient.

What Are Obligations?

As suggested earlier in this chapter, moral and legal rights carry corresponding obligations on others. An *obligation* is anything that a person must do or refrain from doing in order to permit the full exercise of the rights of another.

For example, in order for a patient to exercise the right to make an informed consent, the health practitioner charged with that person's care is obliged to ensure that all relevant information has been provided to the patient, that the patient has been told of all relevant material risks and consequences inherent in the procedure, and that the patient's questions and concerns have been answered to the best of the health practitioner's ability.

The health practitioner must also ensure that he or she act in a professional manner and observe all applicable standards of practice. These include the obligation to be informed and aware of the latest developments in his or her area of practice, to maintain up-to-date knowledge and competency, as well as the obligation to treat patients with respect, dignity, and courtesy.

CASE STUDY

Confidentiality and disclosure

Jim is a thirty-four-year-old man who is well known to the community health centre that both he and his family have attended for several years. He is married and has two young children. His wife is eight months pregnant. He is a computer salesman and spends much time away from home travelling to clients across the country.

A few weeks ago, Jim presented to the clinic complaining of generalized fatigue and lethargy. He had recently lost ten pounds and had noticed some unusual lesions on his inner thighs. As part of the blood screening done at that time, an HIV test was undertaken. This turned out to be positive. Given his clinical picture, it was likely that he had already developed AIDS.

Jim's primary care nurse was present when his physician relayed the bad news to Jim. Clearly distraught, Jim admitted that he had had sexual intercourse with a number of women during his business trips, and on many occasions had not bothered to use a condom. Fearful of the effects that this revelation would have on both his family and his business contacts, Jim pleaded with his caregivers to keep this information and his diagnosis confidential. Given his wife's pregnancy, he felt this information might cause her undue harm. He assured them that he and his wife had not had intercourse since her pregnancy. He refused any kind of treatment for his AIDS-related symptoms, since this would make the diagnosis obvious to everyone. Instead, he asked that people, including his wife, be told that he had terminal and incurable cancer. Jim's physician (who is also his friend) says that he will respect Jim's wishes for now.

ISSUES

1. Did the clinic have the right to test Jim for HIV without his knowledge or consent?
2. Should the health care team keep Jim's diagnosis confidential from his wife?

3. Should the fact that Jim's wife is also the clinic's patient influence their actions and decisions?

4. Does the team have an obligation to follow Jim's instructions and misrepresent his diagnosis to others?

5. If the primary nurse disagrees with the decision of the physician, what can she do?

DISCUSSION

Right to Be Informed

We have already discussed the right to informed consent in Chapter 6. This is not only a legal but also a moral right which is based on the ethical principles of autonomy, individual respect, respect for self-determination, and the right of individuals to make decisions about the course of their lives. In order to exercise these rights, patients must be fully informed regarding their health condition, prognosis, and treatment options, together with the consequences and risks. Lack of information, or the giving of incorrect or insufficient information, deprives the patient of the right to make a truly informed decision about the course of treatment. As we have seen in previous chapters, the giving of treatment without a fully informed consent can lead to legal liability for negligence—even battery, if no consent was given.

As discussed in Chapter 4, the *Code of Ethics* of the Canadian Nurses Association makes explicit the rights of patients "to control their own care." Nurses have a responsibility to inform patients of the nursing care available to them and to welcome patients as active participants in their own care. The patient also has the right to know the extent of the assessment that the agency is performing. In some provinces, public health laws require that a health care agency obtain consent for HIV testing.

In our case study, the nurse and the physician are faced with a challenge to the patient–professional relationship. They should consult with and support Jim, giving him time to digest and understand his situation, and clarify why his wife should be involved. If necessary, they should support him in disclosing this information to his wife. Because there is still the potential of harm to Jim's wife and their unborn child, the team has a moral and professional obligation to inform her of Jim's infection. Certainly, the clinic owes Jim's wife an equal duty of care, since she too is their patient. Further, the nurse and physician must tell Jim that, given the high risk of infection with HIV, they have a legal obligation to inform the local medical officer of health of his infection. This is required by law in all provinces and territories.

The nurse should discuss these points carefully with the physician. If he still refuses to manage this situation as required, it would be appropriate for the nurse to appeal to the next level of authority until she is satisfied that action is taken. The nurse should not simply let the matter drop.

Informed Consent

In Chapter 6, we discussed the elements and aspects of a truly informed consent. The consent must not only be informed, but it must also be free of all undue interference by others. There must be no coercion, inducement, or other pressure placed upon the patient to give the necessary consent, nor should the patient be forced to receive information that he or she does not wish to receive. Any fraud perpetrated on the patient to obtain consent would vitiate (negate) it.

As part of the obligation to provide general information the care team should, upon a patient's admission to a health facility, provide him or her with an orientation to the roles of the caregivers, their functions, the physical layout of the unit, as well as the unit's routines, procedures, and schedules. This advice would include information about promoting health and preventing disease. Such information is usually provided by primary care nurses (in a clinical setting) and community nurses (such as those in public health).

The nurse is further required to teach discharged patients how to care for themselves after they are released from hospital. Such teaching might include nutrition, the proper use and maintenance of any equipment by the patient at home, the proper administration of medication, and the changing of dressings. Nurses have an obligation to teach patients how to care for themselves to the extent that they are able to do so. Patients should also be given any assistance they require in seeking needed information.

Knowledge of how to gain access to the health care system is invaluable to all patients. Here, the nurse can provide a service to patients in informing them about the workings of the system, treatment alternatives and facilities, alternatives to traditional Western medical care, and so forth. For discharged or elderly patients, information as to available home care services is essential. Where incompetent patients are concerned, the nurse should discuss these matters and ensure a good working relationship with the patient's substitute decision maker(s). This is important, as the nurse involved in the day-to-day care of such a patient will be intimately aware of all aspects of the treatment and progress—what is and is not working—and will be able to relate this information to the proxy decision maker. This will, in turn, enable the proxy to make better-informed treatment decisions in the patient's best interests.

One challenge that may arise is a patient's request to a nurse about the diagnosis. Here, the nurse must proceed carefully. In Ontario, for example, under the *Regulated Health Professions Act, 1991*,[3] "[c]ommunicating to the individual or his or her personal representative a diagnosis identifying a disease or disorder as the cause of symptoms ... in circumstances in which it is reasonably foreseeable that the individual or his or her personal representative will rely on the diagnosis" is a controlled act. The nurse would be permitted to make a diagnosis only if authorized to do so under the *Nursing Act, 1991*[4] or if a physician delegated the making of the diagnosis to the nurse, and such delegation complied with any applicable rules and regulations governing the delegation of controlled acts. Ontario's *Nursing Act, 1991* does not include the communication of a diagnosis among those controlled acts that may lawfully be performed by nurses.[5] Other provinces may or may not legally restrict the making of a diagnosis, for example, in their medical professional statutes. Therefore, it is best for the nurse to tell the patient that he or she will request the patient's physician to provide the information.

A special problem for the nurse arises when the patient's physician refuses to communicate a diagnosis. If the nurse is sufficiently experienced and knowledgeable to know the diagnosis, should he or she inform the patient, regardless of the physician's refusal? In such a case, the nurse should endeavour to change the physician's mind on this point and advocate for the patient, stressing his or her right to be informed. If this does not work, the nurse may have to turn to the physician's superiors or higher authorities in the health care institution.

In most cases, an answer to the patient's question by the nurse need not entail the communication of a diagnosis, but simply the confirmation of what the patient sees as self-evident. For example, suppose that a woman patient has been previously told that she may have some form of breast cancer. Surgery is performed to explore the extent of the tumour and to remove it. The patient, once awake in the Recovery Room, asks the attending nurse whether a tumour was found and if so how much, if any, of her breast was removed. She already feels some pain from the incision and knows that her breast does not feel right. The patient's physician has left for the day without having a chance to talk to her about the results of the operation. Should the patient be left in suspense to await the physician's return? The nurse, by exercising common sense, could properly confirm the patient's suspicions with a few well-chosen words to ease her mind and lessen the emotional stress of not knowing. However, an outright diagnosis ("I'm sorry, Mrs. Jones, you have breast cancer") should be avoided. In short, the nurse should be prudent, exercise judgement, and consider all the alternatives.

Special challenges are also posed by "no CPR" (no cardiopulmonary resuscitation) and "DNR" (do not resuscitate) directions from a patient, which must be respected as part of the patient's autonomous right to refuse treatment.

A distinction should be made between "no CPR" and "DNR." The latter is a broader concept that includes any treatment given to sustain life (e.g., blood transfusions, artificial ventilation, dialysis, antibiotic therapy). CPR is limited to the technique of compressing the patient's chest without applying artificial ventilation. It is important to document carefully the precise nature of the patient's wishes (or those of the substitute decision maker) in this respect.[6] The order withholding CPR in no way limits the administration of other treatment to which the patient has not withheld consent.

Some caregivers may feel that honouring the patient's wishes regarding resuscitation conflicts with the principles of beneficence and non-maleficence—that is, to promote the patient's well-being and prevent harm. Certain guidelines have been developed to resolve such conflicts. These guidelines are similar to those followed in other treatment situations and outlined, for example, in Ontario's *Substitute Decisions Act, 1992*.[7]

First, the patient should be assessed to determine whether his or her life would likely be prolonged by the intervention of CPR. The results of the assessment should be disclosed to the patient, and his or her wishes obtained and respected. The course of action to be followed, and any discussions held between caregivers, the patient, and the patient's family with respect to the order, should be carefully documented in the patient's chart. The "no CPR" order should be recorded on the physician's order. Further, the reasons for the order should be documented in the progress notes and communicated directly to the health care team. The "no CPR" decision should be reviewed at regular intervals decided upon by the decision maker, either the patient or his or her substitute. The "no CPR" order should also be communicated to the care team of any other unit to which the patient is subsequently transferred.

In cases where the patient is incompetent, his or her advance directive should be respected, subject to any changes expressed by the patient after making it. Such changes should be documented and made known to the attending physician. If there is no advance directive, and no substitute decision maker appointed, the decision to implement or withhold CPR will be made by others on the basis of their knowledge of the patient's values and wishes.

The Medical Record

Does the patient have an unrestricted right to his or her medical record? What are the responsibilities of the health care institution and the nursing staff in this regard?

Any and all patient records are the property of the hospital or other health care facility or practitioner who made the records and in whose possession such records remain. Nevertheless, the patient has the right to the information contained in those records. It is usually in the hospital's or agency's best interest to allow the patient access to such information. If a patient asks to inspect his or her health records, this should be done, preferably in the presence of a health care professional who can explain and interpret the information disclosed in the records. This avoids confusion and possible misunderstandings, which might otherwise occur if the patient were left to examine the records on his or her own. In a home care setting, the nurse will usually leave the patient's records in the patient's home.

Right to Respect

The right to respect includes the right to be treated courteously, to privacy, to be addressed by one's preferred name or title, and the corresponding obligation of the nurse to introduce himself or herself by name to the patient. It is important for the nurse to listen carefully to what the patient says, to focus on his or her needs, to respect his or her culture, religion, values, and relationships with friends and family. For example, talking about the patient as if he or she were not present diminishes that person's humanity and is disrespectful. This is especially important when caring for patients who are dying.

Death is a significant process for a patient and his or her family. It is a time that requires all the nurse's powers of empathy, to imagine what it is like to be that patient. Providing as dignified a death as possible means being concerned about the patient's pain and symptom control, respecting the patient's privacy, knowing when he or she wishes to be left alone or with family and friends, and so forth. It also means being concerned with where the patient wants to die. Some patients may wish to remain in hospital or to be referred to a palliative care facility. Others may prefer to be at home, yet may not be aware of the resources available to make this choice possible. Rarely does anyone want to die alone.

As much as possible, nurses should keep the patient's family and friends informed of his or her status so that they will be available when necessary. When the patient's condition deteriorates, the family should be informed promptly. The nurse does not need permission to telephone a family member to let that person know what is happening.

Unfortunately, many patients in hospitals die during the process of cardiopulmonary resuscitation. It is common that, during this procedure, families are removed from the patient's room. This limits the patient's right to have a caring family member or friend present when death is imminent. Caregivers are uncomfortable with the idea of family members witnessing what is often a distressing experience. Nevertheless, this is the patient's right and the family's choice. When it appears to be their wish, a full description of the arrest procedure should be explained to the family, who then have the right to choose whether or not to be present. On occasion, family members have been present at arrests, sitting quietly and stroking the patient's face, apparently oblivious to the resuscitation efforts, but content to be there with the person they love. As part of their patient advocacy and leadership role, nurses might make attempts to change the systems and processes within their facility to ensure that this can happen more frequently.

Certain aspects of the right to respect find formal recognition in the law. For example, all patients have the right to equal access to health care resources and facilities without regard to sex, colour, mental or physical disabilities, ethnicity, creed, or religion. These rights are enshrined in various provincial human rights codes.

Right to Confidentiality

The primary legal rule with respect to any information that the health care professional obtains from the patient during the course of their professional relationship is that such information is confidential and may not be disclosed to anyone who has no valid purpose for requesting it. There are exceptions to this rule, both in the common law and as provided by statute. But in many provinces, the improper disclosure of confidential information respecting a patient constitutes professional misconduct.[8]

For example, it may be necessary for one health care provider to share with another selected information contained in the patient's medical records for consultative purposes. Or, a health practitioner who has become involved in a patient's treatment needs to know what treatment has been provided thus far, and the progress of the patient's recovery. This is a normal part of obtaining a history, which the patient should expect upon being admitted to hospital. No specific consent need be obtained in such a case, since it is clearly implied that all persons involved in the patient's treatment have a valid reason for inspecting that patient's records. Nevertheless, the patient always has the right to expect that any information divulged to a nurse or other health practitioner will remain confidential until and unless another professional has a valid need for the information.

Statutory Duty of Disclosure

In many provinces, statute law requires certain patient information and conditions to be disclosed. For example, many public health laws require health practitioners to disclose the identity of anyone diagnosed with certain communicable diseases or sexually transmitted diseases (such as gonorrhoea and HIV/AIDS, among others) to the local medical officer of health. This is especially important with respect to HIV/AIDS.[9]

In most provinces, the identity of the patient and the nature of the disease must be reported to the local medical officer of health (usually employed in the municipality by a local board of health or other such authority). In this way, the potential spread of such diseases can be controlled to some extent. The virulence and seriousness of these illnesses are deemed sufficient to justify the infringement on the patient's right to confidentiality. For example, in our case study, it would be unlawful for the physician at the clinic not to divulge the fact that Jim was HIV positive (and may, in fact, have full-blown AIDS) to the local medical officer of health.

Similarly, there may arise instances when a patient tells a nurse that he or she intends to hurt or kill another person. Such a remark may be a manifestation of the patient's illness; nevertheless, if the patient has a history of violent behaviour through which others have been hurt or killed, or if the patient seems likely to harm himself or herself or others, such a statement should be reported to the authorities in the institution and to the police.

The nurse's duty of confidentiality toward the patient is somewhat analagous to a lawyer's toward the client; however, there are situations when the law requires the nurse to disclose certain information about a patient. A lawyer is under a continuous duty to ensure that any information that his or her client discloses during the course of their professional relationship must remain confidential. For example, the lawyer may not divulge the fact that the client told the lawyer that he or she committed a crime. Such disclosure is unethical and may constitute professional misconduct.

The law has not recognized a corresponding privilege of confidentiality among other client–professional relationships such as doctors, psychiatrists, nurses, counsellors, accountants, or clergy. Legally, there is no obligation on a health care provider to aid police in their investigations. However, where a patient poses a threat to others, there is an ethical obligation to report this.

The *Code of Ethics for Nursing* of the Canadian Nurses Association provides some guidance. Value III[10] dealing with confidentiality states that although competent care requires that nurses have information, the professional relationship requires, and the patient expects, that such information will be held in confidence. By and large, the patient determines the boundaries of that confidentiality.

However, the right to confidentiality may be limited in cases where there is a legal obligation to divulge the information, such as in a disciplinary hearing of the health professional, a civil or criminal trial, or a coroner's inquest or other government-authorized inquiry. The right is also limited when the information must be disclosed to avoid harm to the patient or to a third party. In practice, however, most courts will not readily violate the client–professional relationship without a strong or compelling reason to do so.[11] For example, if required by a court, the health care provider must answer any and all questions put to him or her. Failure to do so would place such a person in danger of being found in contempt of court and liable to a heavy fine or possible imprisonment.

A confession of prior illegal activity made to a health professional may not have to be disclosed. But, it is possible that at some point a court may compel the professional to disclose such a fact. The only professional who would be exempt from disclosing such facts would be a lawyer (yet even a lawyer would have to guard against being an accessory to the client's crime). Although the health care provider is under no obligation to aid police, concealing the whereabouts of a fugitive could be construed as aiding and abetting such a person. This is especially likely in light of the *Criminal Code* offence of being an accessory to a crime after the fact.[12] One is an accessory when one "... knowing that a person has been a party to the offence, receives, comforts or assists that person *for the purpose of enabling that person to escape.*"[13] By not divulging the information with the intent that the patient should avoid detection by the police, the health practitioner may leave himself or herself open to possible criminal charges.

There are instances where provincial law requires disclosure, such as information concerning those having a communicable or sexually transmitted disease, or in cases of suspected child abuse. Many provinces have set up child abuse registries. The laws that establish these are intended to encourage the reporting of situations in which a child has been sexually or physically abused. Indeed, these laws require child care workers, physicians, nurses, and other health practitioners to report suspected cases of child abuse, either to the police or to the local Children's Aid Society for further action. In most cases, it is an offence punishable by fine or prison for a health practitioner to fail to report an instance of suspected child abuse that he or she encounters in the course of practice.

We have discussed, in Chapter 3, the obligation of the health practitioner in Ontario and some other provinces to disclose incidents of sexual abuse of patients by other health practitioners. Indeed, even in provinces where there is no such explicit requirement with respect to abuse by health professionals, such behaviour is a reportable criminal offence and constitutes professional misconduct.

Ensuring Confidentiality in the Treatment Setting

A nurse may inadvertently disclose confidential information in casual conversations with colleagues, friends, or relatives who have no valid interest in such details. Thus, the nurse must take care at all times not to divulge confidential patient information when engaged in casual conversation in social settings unconnected to his or her work and duties.

Likewise, the old saying "the walls have ears" applies to hospitals and other health care institutions. Great care should be taken when discussing details of a patient's condition in such places as hallways, stairways, and elevators. Even when discussing a case with a colleague, only such disclosure should be made as is absolutely necessary for that person's participation in the patient's care and treatment. This requires great caution and discretion on the part of the nurse.

There are other instances where confidential information may inadvertently be disclosed. For example, when a patient is being seen by a nurse in an Emergency Room in the presence of other people, the nurse should speak in a low voice in discussing the patient's problem so as to avoid being overheard. The best way to avoid such a situation is to segregate the patient in a private room or area where privacy can be assured. Often, simply closing a door or drawing a curtain around the patient's bed will ensure this.

Computer Records and Confidentiality

Many hospitals and other health care institutions now use a computerized system to maintain patient and other records. Consequently, there is wider access to a great deal of information by a potentially greater number of people. Access in most cases is controlled by means of magnetized cards and passwords. It is important for nurses to use their own passwords and not to use others' means of access since, in many cases, the use of the password and card is the nurse's electronic signature.

Many computer systems document the fact that a particular person gained access to a particular patient's record. The date and time of such access will also be noted in the computer record. There have been documented cases of hospital nursing staff having been disciplined for using their access cards for improper and unwarranted access to patient files simply to satisfy their own curiosity.

Disclosure of Confidential Information in Court Testimony

There will be occasions, such as in a medical malpractice action, or an inquest into a death, when the nurse must disclose information in court testimony. Most provincial nursing statutes and regulations permit such disclosure. However, the nurse should be careful even when lawfully disclosing patient information. Only that information which is relevant to the issues in the hearing, trial, or inquiry should be disclosed. The nurse should not give a "blanket" disclosure of all possible information, which may not be relevant to the issues under inquiry. Here, the nurse must use discretion and common sense.

Right to Privacy

This right goes hand in hand with the right to confidentiality. One cannot have one without the other. As we have seen in the context of consent to treatment, this implies a right to be free from control of the state or others as to the course of treatment to be followed.

But the right to privacy carries with it more practical aspects with respect to nursing. For example, when a patient is bathing, and to the extent that it is safe to leave the patient alone, he or she should be ensured complete privacy. This right extends to treatment situations and examinations. Thus, care should be taken when examining a patient to ensure that the room is not fitted with mirrored windows, that unauthorized persons are not permitted into the room, or that pictures not be taken without the patient's permission, even if this is done for educational purposes.

Similarly, in instances where the nurse feels that a consultation with clergy or a social worker may benefit the patient, he or she may request such a consultation on behalf of that patient. Nevertheless, the patient may refuse such help, in which case the patient's privacy must be respected.

Right to Be Discharged from a Health Care Facility

Can a patient be prevented from being discharged from a hospital? In many cases, a patient who wishes to leave a hospital or other health care facility against medical advice must sign a waiver acknowledging that he or she has been advised that leaving is not desirable at this time. If the patient refuses to sign the waiver, the fact that he or she is leaving against medical advice should be carefully documented in the patient's chart. Ultimately, there is nothing hospital staff can do to prevent a patient from leaving. A hospital is not a prison.

In cases involving psychiatric patients of unsound mind, the mental health statutes of most provinces may permit such persons to be prevented from leaving if they pose a threat or danger to themselves or to others.

When a patient is discharged, the hospital has an obligation to ensure that he or she arrives home safely. For example, in cases involving same-day surgery, a patient should not be sent home if the sedative has not yet worn off. Such a patient may have to be sent home by taxi or other means, as he or she would not be in a condition to drive. There have been reported cases in which patients still under the effect of sedatives have subsequently driven home and have been charged with impaired driving. In many hospitals and health agencies, patients who have been sedated are required to wait a specified period of time and to be accompanied by another person when they leave the institution.

Discharge from a Mental Health Facility

Most provinces have legislation governing the admission to and discharge from a mental institution.[14] As a rule, if a person's state of mental health is such that he or she poses a threat either to self or others, such a person may be committed to a mental health facility for treatment upon the order of an examining physician. The determination that such a state of mind exists must be made by a physician.[15] In Newfoundland, a person may be detained in such a treatment facility only if two physicians certify that the patient is a danger to self or others by reason of a mental disorder.[16]

Generally, there are two categories of patient on admission to a mental institution. The first comprises persons who may suffer from some mental disorder but who are not thereby a threat to themselves or others. These are usually voluntary patients. They cannot be detained in such an institution without their consent.

Violent patients who do pose a threat to their own or others' safety generally may be admitted to an institution on an involuntary basis and may be detained without their consent. The matter does not end there, however. There are certain procedural safeguards in place to provide for a review of the detention of involuntary patients and to ensure they are not arbitrarily detained or detained without proper grounds. If they cease to pose a danger to themselves or others, the law generally requires that they be released when they wish.

In the Yukon Territory, the recently passed *Mental Health Act* articulates and gives legal recognition to the rights of mental patients. As in many provinces, only minimal physical restraints may be used on such patients—that is, only what is reasonable and necessary, considering the physical and mental condition of that person.[17]

Other rights in the Yukon include the right to receive and make phone calls[18]; to have reasonable access to visitors[19]; to have access at any time to the patient's legal representative, guardian, or other authorized person[20]; to send and receive correspondence; to vote; to wear clothing of the person's choice; to security of his or her person; to confidentiality[21]; and to be informed (if detained) of the reasons for the detention.[22] In other jurisdictions, similar rights exist in common law, if they are not expressed in statute.

Summary

The key points introduced in this chapter include:
- the rights of patients and obligations of health care professionals
- the patient's rights to confidentiality and the conditions under which disclosure is permitted
- the patient's rights to information, respect, and discharge from a health care facility.

References

1. Canadian Nurses Association. (1991). *Code of ethics for nursing.* Values I–V (pp. 1–10); Value IX (p. 21).
2. *Canadian Charter of Rights and Freedoms,* Part I of the *Constitution Act, 1982,* being Schedule B of the *Canada Act 1982* (UK), 1982, c. 11.
3. SO 1991, c. 18, section 27(2), paragraph 1.
4. SO 1991, c. 32.
5. Ibid., section 4.
6. These guidelines and procedures are taken from the *Toronto Hospital Policy and Procedure Manual,* Policy #2.1.160, "No Cardiopulmonary Resuscitation Order" (pp. 1–3).
7. SO 1992, c. 30.
8. See Alberta: *Nursing Profession Code of Ethics,* Alta. Reg. 456/83, section 2(3); Manitoba: *Registered Nurses Act,* RSM 1987, c. R40, CCSM, c. R40, section 46(2); New Brunswick: *Nurses Act,* SNB 1984, c. 71, section 42(1); Northwest Territories: *Nursing Profession Act,* RSNWT 1988, c. N-4, section 22(e); Ontario: O. Reg. 799/93, section 1, paragraph 10; Saskatchewan: *Registered Nurses Act, 1988,* SS 1988, c. R-12.2, section 26(2)(h).
9. See, e.g., Alberta: Alta. Reg. 238/85, schedule 4 "AIDS," amended by Alta. Reg. 357/88; British Columbia: Health Act Communicable Disease Regulation, B.C. Reg. 4/83, Schedule A; Manitoba: Man. Reg. P210-R2, amended by Man. Reg. 338/88R; New Brunswick: N.B. Reg. 86-66, section 94(1)(s); Newfoundland: Nfld. Reg. 60/87; Nova Scotia: Regulation in respect of communicable diseases, N.S. Reg. 171/85; Ontario: RRO 1990, Reg. 557, as amended; Prince Edward Island: Notifiable and Communicable Diseases Regulation, E.C. 330/85; Quebec: Regulations respecting the application of the *Public Health Protection Act,* RSQ c. P-35, regulation 1; Saskatchewan: Sask. Reg. 307/69, amended by Sask. Reg. 2/88.
10. Supra footnote 1, pp. 5–6.
11. See, e.g., AG v. *Mulholland,* [1963] 2 QB 477; *Slavytych v. Baker,* [1975] 4 WWR 620 (SCC).
12. *Criminal Code of Canada,* RSC 1985, c. C-46, section 23(1), as amended.
13. Ibid.
14. See British Columbia: *Mental Health Act,* RSBC 1979, c. 256, as amended; Alberta: *Mental Health Act,* SA 1988, c. M-13.1; Yukon Territory: *Mental Health Act,* SYT 1989–90, c. 28; Northwest Territories: *Mental Health Act,* RSNWT 1988, c. M-10; Saskatchewan: *Mental Health Services Act,* SS 1984–85–86, c. M-13.1, as amended; Manitoba: *Mental Health Act,* RSM 1986, c. M110, CCSM, c. M110, as amended; Ontario: *Mental Health Act,* RSO 1990, c. M.7, as amended; Quebec: *Mental Patients Protection Act,* RSQ 1977, c. P-41, as amended; New Brunswick: *Mental Health Act,* RSNB 1973, c. M-10,. as amended; Nova Scotia: *Hospitals Act,* RSNS 1989, c. 208, as amended; Prince Edward Island: RSPEI 1988, c. M-6, as amended; Newfoundland: *Mental Health Act,* RSN 1990, c. M-9.
15. Ontario Act, ibid., section 15(1).
16. Newfoundland Act, supra footnote 14, section 5(2).
17. Yukon Act, supra footnote 14, section 18(1).
18. Ibid., section 40(2)(a).
19. Ibid., section 40(2)(b).
20. Ibid., section 40(2)(c).
21. Ibid., subsections 40(3), (4) and (5), and section 42.
22. Ibid., section 41.

Nine

Nursing Documentation

CHAPTER OBJECTIVES

The purpose of this chapter is to enable the reader to:
- clarify the legal requirements of proper nursing documentation
- appreciate the importance of accurate and complete documentation in ensuring safe and effective nursing care
- establish guidelines for timely and accurate documentation, and apply them to a hypothetical case study and real case law
- appreciate the role of nursing assessments and their importance in the nursing notes
- explain the use and significance of incident reports
- clarify how nursing notes may be used in a legal proceeding
- explain the role of expert witnesses in interpreting nursing documentation.

Careful and accurate documentation is a key component of professional nursing. The nurse's assessment and progress notes monitor, on a continuing basis, the course of a patient's treatment and the effect of interventions. From this record, a clearer picture emerges of the patient's progress toward the stated goals and outcomes, and any impending complications can be identified before they become problematic. As we have seen in the *Meyer and Thompson Estate* cases in Chapter 5, failure to document specific acts of treatment accurately and contemporaneously can have dire consequences for the health practitioner in a negligence action. This chapter will examine the legal and practical aspects of proper documentation.

CASE STUDY[1]

Documentation

An eight-month-old boy is brought into a hospital Emergency Department late one evening experiencing vomiting and diarrhoea and having a history of toxoplasmosis. On arrival, his pulse rate is 120 and respiration rate 24. He is seen by the physician on duty in the Emergency Department and then by the hospital paediatrician, who admits the child and writes treatment orders for an IV, as well as tests for haemoglobin and BUN electrolytes.

While in hospital, the child's condition deteriorates. The nurses monitoring him over the next four to five hours note that his heart rate has increased to 164 and that his respiration is 64. Nurse H., who is looking after the boy, is concerned. She speaks to the charge nurse, who confirms her concerns, then phones the child's physician at his home.

It is now the middle of the night. Nurse H. informs the physician of the child's condition, pulse rate, respiration, and of the results of the tests for haemoglobin and BUN electrolytes, which were also abnormal. In particular, the CO_2 level was at 10.9 instead of the normal range of 22 to 32. The physician replies: "Well, that's fine; just continue doing what you've been doing."

Nurse H. is not satisfied with the doctor's response. After speaking with him, she speaks again to the charge nurse, who says: "Well, you're not the doctor; he is. Whatever he says, that's fine; don't worry about it."

All these abnormal results and readings are duly recorded by Nurse H. in the boy's medical chart. Also noted is the conversation with the charge nurse and the boy's physician, and the times at which these took place. The boy dies the next morning at 06:00 hours.

ISSUES

1. What should the charge nurse have done when Nurse H. consulted her after phoning the boy's physician?
2. Should Nurse H. have taken her concerns about the boy's poor test results to a higher authority?
3. What steps should have been taken with respect to documenting the boy's vital signs and fluid intake, both in the Emergency Department and in Paediatrics?
4. Should Nurse H. have called the physician back to confirm his instructions? In speaking with the doctor, should she have placed greater emphasis on the boy's abnormal vital signs and test results?

DISCUSSION

Nursing Practice

In this case study, the critical issue is that the charge nurse should have assisted Nurse H. in getting the help of the physician. Firstly, Nurse H. should have made further attempts to contact the physician a second time to impress upon him the urgency of the situation, especially if he'd been roused from a deep sleep that might have clouded his judgement.

Secondly, Nurse H. obviously realized the seriousness of the boy's condition from the vital signs that she observed. The standard of care in this case demanded that Nurse H. by-pass her non-supportive charge nurse and find a higher authority for instructions. Lack of support from a supervisor, even if accurately documented in the medical record, would not protect a nurse from liability.

Further, a nurse, having determined the high risks of inaction, must act and cannot hide behind the excuse that "the doctor said...." The nurse cannot avoid liability for inaction by simply documenting the doctor's instructions. There was also a corresponding duty to protect the patient from harm. The appropriate standard of care demanded that the nurses should have known and understood the severe consequences of inaction when the boy was in this condition. The conduct of both nurses in this case study clearly fell below the required standard of care.

In the real-life situation on which this case study is based, a coroner's inquest was called to investigate the boy's death. (For a discussion of the coroner's function and role, see Chapter 5.) One of the issues that arose at the inquest was related to documentation of the fluid balance, particularly in the Emergency Department. It had not been totalled accurately, and it was difficult to determine how much fluid the patient had been given, both in the Emergency Department and in the Paediatrics Ward.

At the inquest, the boy's physician denied that the nurse had reported the patient's vital signs. The doctor further denied that he'd been given the results of the electrolyte tests (specifically, the CO_2 level). There were no other nurses on the floor that evening who witnessed what was going on, and thus no one to corroborate the nurse's telephone conversation with the physician. The doctor claimed he'd been roused from a deep sleep, that he had been up all the night before, that he was very tired, and that if the nurse had really had such a pressing concern, she should have phoned him back to confirm his instructions and make sure he realized the severity of the situation. In such a case, he said, he certainly would have taken the appropriate action. It was obvious that, regardless of which version of events was the correct one, the child died because of a serious breakdown in communication.

The coroner's jury found that the nurse should have documented her concerns in greater detail, and that this record should ideally have been witnessed by another nurse. She should have called the doctor back to repeat her concerns and had another nurse present to attest that she did so. Secondly, the hospital should have had procedures in place to by-pass the physician's instructions and to seek another doctor in the hospital to ensure that proper instructions were provided in the treatment of this child.

The cause of death, as determined in the autopsy, was dehydration. The IV that had been administered to the child was wholly inadequate. The inquest determined that the boy's fluid intake should have been checked more frequently and recorded systematically. In particular, the levels might have been checked and recorded by nursing staff just prior to the child's leaving the Emergency Department, and then again by the nurses in Paediatrics, immediately upon his transfer to that ward.

The jury did not accept the physician's excuse in this case, and he was found negligent for having given improper instructions. He was subsequently reported to the College of Physicians and Surgeons of Ontario and severely disciplined.

The Need for, and Uses of, Documentation

In most cases, the patient's chart, nurses' progress notes, and other medical documentation constitute the only written evidence of what care and treatment a patient has received. This record is vital during the course of treatment in that it facilitates communication between nurses and other health care providers actively involved in the patient's treatment. Without it, effective, safe, and proper nursing and other care would be impossible. In this case, as the fluid balance was inaccurately recorded, the standard of accurate and complete documentation was not met.

The record is also a useful tool in planning the course of treatment. It encourages an accurate tracing of the patient's vital signs and condition. This promotes quality control of nursing and other medical care, and permits caregivers to assess which interventions should be altered and which left in place. Thus, assessments must be complete and comprehensive. The documentation should also reflect the nurse's judgements, including identification of any problems and the focus of the action to be taken. This, in turn, permits others to follow through and to follow up on the efficacy of any action taken.

For example, suppose that an assessment of a patient notes that she is in severe pain. How adequate is such a description? Was this pain reported to the patient's physician? Was any medication given, or some other intervention tried? Did such medication or intervention work? Or, as another example, if the patient is agitated, what is the source of the agitation? Was there a review of the previous documentation? What was done before, and did it work? Accurate documentation aids in addressing such issues.

Further, a good patient record will contain information on any allergies, including allergies to medications, to which that patient may be susceptible, and some information about whom to contact in an emergency. This is especially important in cases where the patient is not capable and a substitute decision maker has been appointed to make treatment decisions on the patient's behalf. Equally important, the record should contain all previous treatment orders for the patient, plus any notes concerning follow-up of those orders.

Finally, the record is important in that it is evidence of the adequacy of any treatment administered, the appropriateness of care, and the quality of care received. This is especially important for audit purposes, in any disciplinary proceedings for alleged improper or unprofessional conduct, and in any negligence actions, criminal proceedings, or coroner's inquests in the event of the patient's death under circumstances requiring investigation.

Accuracy of Documentation

The documentation must be an accurate record of what was done, what medication was administered, and what the patient's condition was at the time the action was taken.

In the *Meyer v. Gordon*[2] case (see Chapter 5), much was made of the fact that the nurses' notes were inaccurate and inadequate. For one thing, the time of the plaintiff's arrival at the hospital was not recorded.[3] Upon her initial examination of the patient, Nurse W. noted that the foetal heart rate was "normal," that the plaintiff's labour was "good," and that her cervix had dilated three centimetres, with "strong" contractions every two minutes.[4] The duration of the contractions was not recorded, as it should have been. Nurse W. also noted that the position of the foetus was at "mid" station.

The court found that the description of the labour as "good" did not indicate the fact (later brought out in Nurse W.'s testimony) that the plaintiff was also in active labour, which would normally have required a foetal heart rate check every fifteen minutes.[5] The court was equally critical of the inexact description of the foetus' position as "mid" and of the lack of record as to the character or effacement of the cervix. This inaccuracy contributed to a poor appreciation of the extent and advanced stage of the plaintiff's labour.

In most court cases, failure to document a particular act during the course of treatment does not necessarily mean that the court will assume the act was not done. Yet, such failure undermines the "weight" of the evidence, that is, how *probative* it is (how much the testimony proves, or how convincing it is that the act was done). If the record is sketchy and incomplete, it may not be accorded much weight by the court.

In assessing the quality and accuracy of Nurse W.'s recorded observations, the court relied on the expert evidence of two nurses (presumably, with obstetrical experience) who stated that an obstetrical nurse, when assessing foetal position, looks for the height of the presenting part of the foetus in relation to the ischial spines of the mother's pelvis. One of the experts, when asked about Nurse W.'s assessment of the foetal position as "mid," commented that such a notation was not specific enough to aid in the evaluation of the labour. The other expert stated that the expression "mid" used in the record had no meaning.[6] This case thus illustrates the importance of accurate and precise observations when documenting details of patient care and treatment.

Other Standards of Documentation

There are agency and government regulations that govern how records ought to be made and organized. For example, the Canadian Council on Hospital Accreditation (CCHA) has set standards. As well, the particular health care agency's nursing department will likely have standards and policies governing proper patient documentation, for example, charting by exception. In this practice, a problem or condition is documented only if it deviates significantly from what one would normally expect in such circumstances. Otherwise, no notation is made.

Another practice is that of recording facts by means of defined checklists. For example, nurses may initial beside a listed procedure. This may mean (according to the policy manual on documentation) that the procedure was completed with no problems. If problems or changes in the patient's condition had in fact occurred, the policy would require further documentation in the progress notes.

Whatever standards are in use, these will be backed by policies of the institution and definitions of those standards. When these standards, definitions, and policies exist, such documentation falls within legally acceptable standards.

Guidelines for Proper Documentation

Some rules of thumb have evolved to ensure timely and accurate recording, from both a legal and a practice perspective, of various details of a patient's care, condition, and treatment from hour to hour.

Record contemporaneously

The record should be made at the time of occurrence of the event or action that is recorded. If not, the record or note should be made as soon as possible after the event. This makes the record more accurate and reliable, ensures safer care, and affords the record greater weight in any legal proceedings.

It is not always possible to record items, events, or actions at the time they occur, especially during emergencies. The longer the delay in documenting a fact, the more likely it is that the accuracy of the observation or detail will be questioned later, especially in a court trial. For example, in *Meyer v. Gordon,*[7] the nurses who treated the plaintiff had recorded some of their observations a considerable time after the fact, and further, had altered the record to make it appear that the observations had been recorded contemporaneously. Thus, the nurses' notes were deemed unreliable as an evidentiary source.

Another reason for contemporaneous documentation is that one's memory fades with time. A fact is more likely to be recorded accurately and completely soonest after the occurrence. Documentation of treatment is vital in court proceedings, as it is often the only source of evidence on what occurred. As considerable time may pass before a trial or hearing is convened, a well-constructed and well-maintained record serves to refresh the memory of the person who made it.

If it was not possible to record the act or event when it occurred (e.g., the nurse had other pressing obligations, or simply forgot), the late entry should still be recorded, to the nurse's best recollection, and noted as a late entry, thus:

> 12:30 hours, patient regurgitated reddish coffee-ground fluid; recorded at 13:30 hours because called away on emergency to assist in another patient's resuscitation. [*Signed*, etc.]

A late entry is clearly better than no entry at all. The nurses in the *Meyer* case attempted to cover up the fact that some of their entries had been made late rather than contemporaneously. This practice is strongly discouraged.

Record only your own actions

The nurse should record only his or her own actions. Since the notes may form the basis of testimony in any ensuing legal criminal or civil proceedings, the nurse will be permitted to testify only as to his or her own actions.

In particular, care should be taken when documenting a fact or detail on computer. The nurse should use only his or her own password or access card when gaining access to the computer record. This ensures that the computer log will accurately reflect the fact that a particular nurse made the entry.

Record in chronological order

All entries should be made in chronological order. Otherwise, a confused record would result, which could have serious repercussions in the course of treatment, especially with respect to the administration of medication. It would also make the record of limited use in any litigation and undermine the nurse's testimony.

Record clearly and concisely

Entries should be clear, concise, factual, and as objective as possible. Any evidence that leads the nurse to draw a particular conclusion should be carefully documented. A subjective entry potentially creates problems in patient care, and might leave the nurse's testimony open to challenge in a court proceeding.

Make regular entries

The nurse should make sure that the record contains regular entries throughout. If there are significant gaps in the record, the benefits of continuous monitoring of the patient are lost. Further, a lengthy gap in the record would be questioned in court (e.g., a gap of a number of hours prior to a patient's cardiac or respiratory arrest, pulmonary edema or, in a psychiatric setting, a psychotic event or suicide attempt).

Record corrections clearly

Any alterations, corrections, or deletions to the record should be carefully documented, dated (including the hour), and initialled by the nurse who makes the change. Otherwise, the nurse's credibility could be undermined in a court proceeding. No attempt should be made to cover up one's mistakes by surreptitiously altering the record to make it look complete.

In cases where a coroner's investigation is begun, the coroner usually quickly seizes nursing notes and other patient records in order to ascertain the circumstances of the patient's treatment or condition in the moments prior to death. This is especially so with the advent of computerized records. An entry in the computer is dated with the computer signature of the person making it. Because this can never be altered in most computer systems, the recorded act is "etched in time." Yet, there have been situations where nurses have attempted to alter the record upon learning of a coroner's inquest, only to learn later that the coroner had already seized the record and made copies of it. The coroner thus had an accurate version of the record at the moment of the patient's death, as well as evidence that the nurses attempted to alter the record afterward. Such situations are embarrassing. It is best to avoid them by making clear that one is documenting a fact some time after it has occurred, or that one is correcting a previous inaccuracy.

Record accurately

Vague terms, such as those used by the nurse in the *Meyer* case, should be avoided. Rather than describing the foetal position as "mid" (an imprecise and utterly useless observation), the nurse should have recorded the position by documenting the height of the presenting part relative to the ischial spines of the mother's pelvis.

Nursing assessments are key to care planning. The initial assessment when a patient enters the care process is crucial, and should therefore be thorough and comprehensive. Most agencies and hospitals require that initial assessments be made within a specified period of time from the time of admission. Inaccurate or incomplete assessments can affect the outcomes of care and raise serious questions in any ensuing legal proceedings.

The frequency of repeat assessments is based on patient need, complexity of care, and agency protocols. For example, in some settings, the initial assessment determines whether or not a patient is fall-prone. If so, this would necessitate reassessment on a regular basis. If this part of the assessment were omitted, and the patient subsequently fell, a negligence suit against the nurses and hospital could result. The trial would question why the assessment was incomplete, and would likely conclude that hospital staff were negligent in (a) failing to foresee that the plaintiff was prone to falling, and (b) failing to take appropriate precautions to prevent this.

Key aspects of the initial assessment are: whom to contact in an emergency; who is the patient's proxy (if any); what decisions have been made by the patient or proxy regarding CPR (see Chapter 8); and whether there are any advance directives made by the patient. All details from the initial assessment should be recorded in the patient's chart. Any reassessment should likewise be documented to ensure a complete record.

Thus, a notation in the patient's record: "Slept well, had a good day" is of limited use. In a court trial, the nurse who made the note could well be asked detailed questions about what he or she meant by "a good day" (e.g., any pain felt by the patient, symptoms, vital signs) in an attempt to pinpoint the patient's condition at the time when the notation was made. The nurse would probably be unable to answer such questions helpfully, as the original meaning of "had a good day" would have been forgotten.

For example, it is far better to document: "Patient reported sharp pains in chest radiating down the left arm of ten minutes' duration, relieved with rest," rather than: "Patient reported chest pain." The latter notation would not bear scrutiny in a legal proceeding. More importantly, it would be of limited use in an attempt to diagnose the patient's ailment accurately.

File incident reports

Sometimes a patient falls, or a mistake is made in administering medication. In such cases, a report should be prepared that documents and describes the incident, all relevant facts, any injuries sustained by the patient, and any action taken to remedy the situation.

Accident reports do not form a part of the medical record. They are used, firstly, to document occurrences out of the ordinary, for investigative or quality assurance purposes. For example, an insurance company might investigate a claim made against a hospital's general liability insurance policy; or, a hospital may be monitoring or auditing the rate of occurrence of certain types of incident over a specified period. Thus, such reports can contribute to the hospital's risk management by identifying possible problem areas in systems or procedures. The information gained can be used to educate staff to prevent similar occurrences in future.

Finally, in the event that a negligence action is brought against the hospital arising out of an incident, the incident report can form part of the evidentiary record at trial and assist the court in understanding the cause of the incident. Such a report is usually introduced along with the testimony of the health care provider(s) who made it.

Record legibly

The records, and any corrections, should be legible. This is especially important given the speed with which nurses sometimes are required to perform their duties.

Nursing Theories and Conceptual Frameworks

Most hospitals or agencies base their standards for nursing documentation on a nursing theory or conceptual framework. Theories and frameworks drive and guide the clinical processes used by nurses when deciding patient care. Thus, the chart should document the patient's plan of care. This would include assessment, analysis, nursing diagnosis, problems or outcome identification, nursing interventions, orders, and evaluation. Standards of care require that these processes be charted, not only to provide evidence that the plan was developed and implemented, but also to ensure effective communication among those providers involved in the patient's care.

Telephone Advice

A nurse should be very careful when giving advice over the telephone. Here, accurate and complete documentation of the patient's name, address, phone number, and symptoms is crucial. As well, any advice given to a patient over the telephone should be carefully noted, as well as the date and time of the call. If the patient seems to be experiencing a serious medical problem, he or she should be told to attend at the Emergency Department without delay.

Use of Documentation in Legal Proceedings

Evidentiary Use

In many medical malpractice cases, the trial of the action will often occur several years after the events leading up to and including the negligent acts. Memories fade with time, and the evidence given by witnesses, such as nurses and physicians, will often be hazy or incomplete. Therefore, the medical notes and records prepared by the health care team assume added value and significance, as these are often the only documentation of what occurred.

The courts wish to obtain the truth. Often, the truth lies in the medical records. Courts are impressed by meticulous, clear, legible, and well-organized records. These not only help the court (i.e., the judge and, in some cases, the jury) to determine the exact sequence of events and the circumstances of medical treatment, but also, they improve the credibility of the witnesses who made them. Thus, with a well-constructed medical record, the nurses and other health care providers who made them will be able to impart their testimony more forcefully. Therefore, that testimony will be accorded greater weight than would be the case with an inadequate record.

The court will be interested in all aspects of the record, including nursing progress notes, care plan, checklists, flow charts, hospital policies in force at the time, and so forth. These will provide a more complete picture of events. In many cases, the record will also document the thought processes and frame of mind of the health care providers at the time. For example, the patient's chart may reveal that a certain treatment or intervention was or was not warranted under the circumstances and given that patient's condition. This is a further reason for ensuring that records are made and kept according to the highest possible standards.

Expert Witnesses

As we saw in Chapter 5, assessing the conduct of nurses in a particular case in relation to the appropriate standard of care often involves drawing upon expert testimony. The court calls upon experts because the judges trying a case rarely possess the necessary expertise to make valid conclusions and draw inferences from technical data. A nursing expert, on the other hand, can interpret the medical record and assist the court in reconstructing the events and drawing inferences. Experts can also be used by the parties to a lawsuit either to support the plaintiff's position and interpretation of the evidence, or to refute these for the defence, and perhaps suggest another cause for the injury. Although such inferences are properly the function of the judge or jury, the expert, because of his or her unique knowledge and experience, is permitted to formulate and express an opinion. This is an exception to the general evidentiary rule that a witness's opinion on a matter in issue is inadmissible.

More importantly, the nurse, as an expert witness, is able to describe the appropriate standard of care in a particular case. The nurse expert is often called upon to review the medical record, and in particular, the nursing notes, in order to give an opinion on whether proper documentation and nursing procedures were followed.

Prior to giving testimony, the nurse must be qualified before the court as an expert. This means the lawyer for the party wishing to rely on the nurse's evidence must first ask the nurse questions about his or her education, experience, nursing background, and continuing education. The purpose here is to establish in the trial record that the witness has the necessary qualifications to give such testimony or opinion.

In some cases, the expert testimony may also be elicited as part of the nurse's own involvement in the care of the plaintiff. Here, the nurse may be asked questions on his or her notations in the patient's record. It is important that the nurse answer such questions truthfully and as accurately as possible. As well, it is important that he or she ensure accuracy, clarity, and objectivity when compiling those notes in the first place.

Problems may arise with respect to alterations, deletions, or additions made to the nursing notes some time after the original entries, as in the *Meyer* case. As a rule of evidence, the nurse or other person recording the note or observation will be allowed to use those notes to refresh his or her memory when testifying in court. However, the court must first be satisfied that:

(1) the notes were indeed made by that person;
(2) it was part of that nurse's duty to make such notes;
(3) the notes were made contemporaneously (or reasonably so) with the event or act that they record; and
(4) there have been no alterations, additions, or deletions to those notes since they were made.

Usually, items 1 and 2 pose no problem, as the nurse witness will have been involved in the patient's care, and will have been the one who made the notes in the first place as part of his or her normal duty.

Item 3 can pose a problem. For example, in the case of *Kolesar v. Jeffries,*[8] the court commented upon the documentation practices in the surgical unit where the plaintiff was placed post-operatively. The plaintiff was returned to

the Recovery Room shortly after 12:00 hours, sedated and unconscious, se-
cured in a supine position to a Stryker frame following surgery on his spinal
column. Although the standard of care in such a case would include rousing
the patient at frequent and regular intervals to cough to keep his lungs clear,
the plaintiff was permitted to sleep undisturbed by an overworked staff who
made one round at midnight with flashlights. At 05:00 hours the next morning,
one of the nurses discovered the plaintiff dead. He had suffered pulmonary
edema and haemorrhage secondary to the aspiration of gastric juices.

The court heard evidence that no nursing notes were made over a period of
seven hours.[9] Indeed, it was the practice in that nursing unit to record vital
signs and any other observations as to the patients' condition on scraps of paper
during the shift. Afterwards, the nurses would get together, and with the aid of
these scraps of paper, they would reconstruct the record for each patient over
the last few hours. The nurses would assist "each other to recall and record the
events of the evening." This practice does not fulfil the requirements of con-
temporaneity.

Upon discovering that no entries had been made on the plaintiff from 22:00
hours until 05:00 hours the next day, the assistant director of nursing asked
one of the nurses on duty that night to write up a report of the events. Here,
the court noted:

> One is always suspicious of records made after the event, and if any credence is to
> be attached to [the nurse's report], it shows that at all times the patient was quite
> pale, very pale, and was allowed to sleep soundly to his death.[10]

Thus, the absence of adequate nursing records served only to reinforce the
court's opinion that the standard of nursing practised in this patient's care had
been wholly inadequate. If efforts had been made to rouse the patient regularly
in order to note and record his condition and vital signs, his death could have
been avoided.

In *Meyer v. Gordon*,[11] the alteration of the records prompted Mr. Justice Legg
to remark:

> The hospital chart contains alterations and additions which compel me to view with
> suspicion the accuracy of many of the observations which are recorded. The chart
> also contains at least one entry which was discovered during this trial [in May 1980]
> to have been made after the fact. That also casts suspicion on the reliability of those
> who made the entries and undermines the accuracy of medical opinions based upon
> these entries and observations.[12]

Thus, any attempt to conceal an alteration of the medical record can effectively cast doubt on the witness' evidence, as well as any other evidence based
on the entries and observations contained in the altered medical record.

Legal Requirement to Keep Records

In all provinces, hospitals and other health care agencies are required to keep
and maintain records on all the patients they treat. For example, in Ontario, a
record of admission, diagnosis, consent forms, treatment, care plan, nursing

notes, and so forth must be kept on each patient.[13] Physicians' orders should be in writing and signed or authenticated by the physician who made the order. All entries in the patient record made by nurses and other health care providers must be initialled or signed and dated, and the exact time of the entry noted. Late entries should also be indicated.

As well, most provinces impose an obligation to obtain and record a diagnosis on an admitted patient within a specified period of time. Also, records must be kept for a specified time, for example, ten years in Ontario.[14]

Summary

The key points introduced in this chapter include:
- the legal requirements of proper nursing documentation
- the importance of accurate and complete documentation in ensuring safe and effective nursing care
- guidelines for timely and accurate documentation, and their application to a hypothetical case study and real case law
- the role of nursing assessments and their importance in the nursing notes
- the use and significance of incident reports
- how nursing notes may be used in a legal proceeding
- the role of expert witnesses in interpreting nursing documentation.

References

1. This case study is closely based upon a real situation related by Dr. Jim Cairns, Deputy Chief Coroner of Ontario, in a talk on the medical and legal aspects of charting for nurses, given at The Toronto Hospital on May 26, 1994.
2. (1981), 17 CCLT 1 (BC SC).
3. Ibid., p. 7.
4. Ibid.
5. Ibid., p. 12.
6. Ibid.
7. Ibid.
8. (1976), 9 OR (2d) 41 (HCJ); varied (1977), 12 or (2d) 142 (CA); affd. (1977), 2 CCLT 170 (SCC).
9. Ibid., p. 48.
10. Ibid.
11. Supra footnote 2.
12. Ibid., p. 15.
13. See, e.g., RRO Reg. 965, as amended, made under the *Public Hospitals Act*, RSO 1990, c. P.42.
14. Ibid.

Ten

Caregiver Rights

CHAPTER OBJECTIVES

The purpose of this chapter is to enable the reader to:
- understand the rights of Canadian nurses as citizens, professionals, and employees
- clarify when the right to a conscientious objection can be invoked
- clarify the responsibilities of nurses as employees to employers
- know the position of the law with respect to discrimination and sexual or physical abuse
- appreciate the role of labour relations and collective bargaining with respect to nursing
- understand the standards associated with occupational health and safety.

Chapters 5, 6, and 8 dealt with the rights of patients. Nurses also have rights. Along with all other Canadians, under the *Charter of Rights and Freedoms* nurses have the right to privacy and respect, and to freedom of expression—the right to think, say, write, or otherwise act in accordance with their beliefs. However, this right is not absolute. For nurses, professional rules and regulations, and ethical responsibilities to patients, may limit individual freedom. For example, when caring for a patient whose values and religious beliefs differ from the nurse's, it is not professionally or ethically appropriate to attempt to influence the patient toward the nurse's perspective.

Nurses are entitled to respect from one another, from other professionals, and from patients. As individuals, they are entitled to freedom from any form of discrimination, harassment (sexual or otherwise), and physical or sexual abuse.

Sexual harassment has received much attention in the media in recent times. It is broadly defined as unwanted sexual attention or conduct that is persistent and abusive, such as coercive sexual intercourse, unsolicited sexual contact, and more subtle behaviour such as remarks, insults, taunts, or comments of a sexual nature that may reasonably be perceived to create a negative environment for the recipient.

Further, as employees, nurses have the right to have their values respected, and to function within a work environment where risks and harm are minimized. Also, nurses have the right to collective bargaining.

Nurse Abuse by Patients

Abuse from a mentally competent patient may be grounds for charges of assault. In some situations, the nurse may be vulnerable to abuse from patients who may be confused, agitated, or mentally ill. Nurses recognize that these behaviours often result from illness and fear. Thus, nurses require the communication and management skills to defuse potentially violent or abusive situations.

Further, nurses need to be educated to identify and manage violence in confused and agitated patients. They require the skills to assess appropriately those patients who are medically or psychiatrically predisposed to violence. Then, they must be able to devise and initiate appropriate strategies for preventive management.

The nurse visiting patients in their home may seem especially vulnerable owing to isolation. Yet, abuse of nurses is more prevalent in psychiatric and emergency departments. Employers have the responsibility to ensure that all attempts are made to minimize the risk of harm to nurses regardless of where they work, and especially in high-risk environments.

Safeguards and protections to reduce the risk of harm include maintaining reasonable staffing quotas and ensuring that restraints are available (as a last resort, and as appropriate). Further, nurses should not be sent into unsafe areas alone. Nurses working in high-risk environments should be given instruction in self-defence. Many institutions now offer such training, and have implemented violence response teams for emergencies.

Rights As an Employee

As employees, nurses are under a contractual obligation to provide adequate and competent nursing care. There are times, however, when the duty to provide care will conflict with the nurse's personal values, for example, having to participate in a procedure that he or she finds objectionable on moral or religious grounds. Is the nurse still required to provide care in these circumstances?

Most such situations will not be emergencies. In an emergency, the nurse's foremost ethical obligation is to do good and not to do harm to the patient.

Refusing to act would go against these ethical principles; therefore, in an emergency, the nurse is bound to act. The following case study examines the issues surrounding conscientious objections by nurses.

The latter part of the chapter examines the larger issues of labour relations and their significance for nurses.

CASE STUDY

Abortion

Frances, a registered nurse of five years' standing, works in the Obstetrics Department of a secular public hospital in a large urban centre. She is religious and deeply opposed to abortion. Frances accepted her position with the understanding that no therapeutic abortions were performed in that department. In this hospital, abortions are usually performed in the Gynaecological Department; some such procedures involve saline injections. Frances would never be asked or required to work in this unit.

Recent cutbacks in funding to the hospital have meant staff reductions and bed closures. Consequently, when beds are tight, an abortion might occasionally be performed in Obstetrics. One afternoon, Frances discovers that she has been scheduled to assist in a second-trimester saline abortion which is to take place in the Obstetrics unit later that day. Angry and upset, she goes to her manager and says: "There's no way I'm going to assist with this! Find yourself another nurse, not me!"

ISSUES

1. What are the hospital's ethical and legal obligations to Frances and to the patient seeking the abortion?
2. How can the conflict between these interests be resolved?

DISCUSSION

The Conscientious Objector

Whenever possible, employers are obliged to respect the conscientious objections of employees who decline to participate in certain actions on moral or religious grounds. Here, we are not speaking of discrimination or indulging in the employee's prejudices. Ethically, the employee has the right not to be compelled to engage in actions to which he or she objects. In this case study, the treatment in which Frances is being asked to participate is not an emergency. If it were, she would be ethically bound to render any and all assistance needed of her. This priority would override her conscientious objections.

For example, it would be Frances's duty to render assistance if the patient were suffering complications as a result of an abortion, such as internal bleeding following a saline injection, regardless of her personal opinion of the patient's actions. While Frances could refuse to participate in the abortion, yet she might be compelled to render emergency life-saving treatment after the fact.

Further, a nurse working in a Palliative Care unit in which there was an AIDS patient could not ethically refuse to treat him on the grounds that he might be a homosexual or a drug abuser. This would be a clear case of prejudice, which an employer is not obliged to indulge.

Problem situations where there is a conscientious objection are best avoided by advising the prospective nursing employee, prior to employment, of his or her expected functions, roles, duties, and responsibilities. The nurse should be advised that, once employment is accepted, he or she will have no option but to provide the care required in the chosen area. Thus, if a prospective nursing employee applies for a position in a Gynaecological Department of a secular hospital, he or she should understand that the duties may include assisting during abortions. The nurse then has the opportunity to decline such employment without the difficulties of having to do so later.

However, if the nature of the nurse's job changes after he or she has begun employment, the agency or hospital is obligated to reassign that nurse to areas where the objectionable activities are not performed. Yet, there are no guarantees, since in emergencies, nurses are ethically obligated to provide care. They may withdraw from such situations only when it is safe to do so, or when others are available to provide the required care.

The ethical principles that apply here are justice (the patient's right to be treated fairly and equitably), beneficence (the nurse's obligation to do good for the patient), and non-maleficence (the nurse's duty to do the patient no harm). For example, if the nurse were to withdraw his or her services arbitrarily because of an objection that placed the patient in danger, the nurse would be violating the principle of non-maleficence.

The guiding rule is thus expressed in the *Code of Ethics for Nursing* of the Canadian Nurses Association:

> A nurse is not ethically obliged to provide requested care when compliance would involve a violation of her or his moral beliefs. When that request falls within recognized forms of health care, however, the client must be referred to a health care practitioner who is willing to provide the service. Nurses who have or are likely to encounter such situations are morally obligated to seek to arrange conditions of employment so that the care of clients will not be jeopardized.[1]

Professional vs. Employee Responsibility

A case that occurred in Toronto in the mid-1970s illustrates the conflict that can arise between a nurse's rights as an employee and as a union member under a collective agreement, and that nurse's duties and responsibilities as a professional. In *Re Mount Sinai Hospital* and *the Ontario Nurses Association*,[2] the staff of the Mount Sinai Intensive Care Unit (ICU) was informed one evening of the urgent need to admit a patient with cardiac problems from the Emergency Department. This occurred during the night shift, when the ICU was already working at maximum capacity. The nurses informed the Admitting Department that they could not handle another patient. They claimed, furthermore, that they were not obliged to take such an additional patient under the terms of the union's collective agreement with the hospital. The medical staff, notwithstanding the nurses' refusal to help, brought the patient to the unit. None of the nurses on the night shift agreed to render assistance to the admitting resident, and he was required to care for this very ill patient by himself for the duration of the night.

As a result of their refusal to care for the additional patient, the nurses were disciplined and suspended for three tours of duty. They grieved the matter (see Grievance Procedures, below), and the issue was passed on to an arbitrator. The arbitrator found in favour of the hospital and found the nurses guilty of insubordination, as they had refused a direct order by their supervisor to care for the patient. They were not entitled, under the collective agreement, to refuse such an order.

Quite apart from the labour aspect, this case raises interesting ethical issues. For example, the nurses had not reassessed their workload and staffing. Nor had they tried to determine whether some of the patients in their unit could have been discharged to make room for the additional patient. They had not tried to restructure their assignments to accommodate the patient. In this respect, they violated the principles of beneficence and non-maleficence. Further, they had not accorded the patient justice, fairness, or equity.

The rule that evolved from this case is now termed the "obey and grieve" rule. It states that, even if a nurse employee has a legitimate grievance under the terms of a collective agreement, or even with respect to workload or working conditions, the nurse must obey the orders of the supervisor and provide needed care, then grieve the matter to the union if he or she feels there is a legitimate complaint. There is plenty of opportunity for such complaints to be heard and adjudicated upon at a more appropriate time, using the collective agreement's grievance procedures. In the present moment, however, the rights and needs of the patient must come first, and the fact that a nurse has a complaint must not be permitted to interfere with proper patient care.

The employee is the servant of the employer and is under the employer's control. There are ample mechanisms to protect the employee's rights should these be violated by the employer, but the patient's care is paramount, especially given the fact (as seen in Chapter 5) that the health care institution is under a legal duty to provide competent and proper nursing care once a patient is admitted. This implies a corresponding right of the employer to discipline the employee, and even to terminate the employment of a nurse who repeatedly fails to work to proper nursing standards. The corresponding right of the employee in this situation is to grieve or, if not unionized, to have recourse to the courts in an action for wrongful dismissal.

Discrimination Issues in Employment

The case study also raises an employment law issue and illustrates the competing interests of employees' and employers' rights. Legally, the matter involves the application of provincial human rights legislation. This legislation is virtually identical from province to province and is essentially designed to prohibit discrimination against persons on the basis of race, sex, creed, religion, physical or mental disability, nationality, or ethnic origin. The thrust of the legislation, as it relates to employment law, is that employers are required, to the greatest extent possible, to structure work conditions and requirements such as to cause the least possible interference with the religious or cultural views, or physical or mental handicaps, of their employees. For example, the legislation requires employers to accommodate work conditions such that no employee is unduly inconvenienced by reason only of his or her sex, as in the case of providing adequate washroom facilities.

In the case study, Frances's religious views conflict with her employer's work requirements. If we alter the facts and say that she had been reassigned to the unit by a supervisor who held her religious views in contempt and merely wanted to harass her, she would have valid grounds for a complaint before the provincial Human Rights Commission. If her rights have been infringed, Frances may be awarded compensation, depending on the laws of her province or territory. She should not be forced to work in a setting to which she objects on moral or religious grounds, subject, of course, to the ethical rules and legal considerations reviewed above.

Labour Relations and Collective Bargaining

Many nurses in Canada work in public hospitals and other health care institutions in which the employees are unionized. It is thus helpful for nurses to have a basic understanding of such labour relations concepts as union formation, the collective bargaining process, grievance procedures, arbitration, and the right to strike, since they will likely come across these matters at some point in their practice.

An exhaustive study of labour law and labour relations is beyond the scope of this book. However, a brief review of these basic concepts and some of the related procedures follows in order to provide a general understanding of this subject.

Similarly, the field of occupational health and safety has grown widely in the last thirty years. Many provinces have enacted stringent occupational health and safety statutes in an effort to ensure that working conditions of all employees (whether they are unionized or not) are made as safe and healthful as possible. This impetus has arisen from growing technology and a better understanding of how the human body reacts to its environment and the hazards posed by toxic or dangerous substances or activities in the workplace. This legislation also will be briefly reviewed in this chapter as it relates to the nursing profession.

Union Formation and Certification

Union Organization

The recognition of labour unions in Canada and the rest of the industrialized world came about as a result of a long struggle fraught with labour unrest, strikes, and violence throughout the late nineteenth and early twentieth centuries. Gradually, unions and the principle of collective bargaining came to be seen as valid means to equalize the bargaining power of employees with that of the often large, wealthy, and powerful corporations who employed them. Unions were recognized as protectors of workers' interests, and ensured that they would receive fair wages and achieve better and safer working conditions. The right to unionize stems directly from the freedom of association enshrined in the Canadian *Charter of Rights and Freedoms*.[3]

A **union** is a provincially certified group of employees, in most cases having a common employer. Such employees will often work in common or related activities in the businesses or undertakings of these employers. The object of uniting is to provide bargaining influence, power, and leverage, by force of numbers, in negotiations pertaining to the terms of employment (e.g., wages, hours of work, benefits, work scheduling) affecting each employee. Thus, through their common interest in terms of their employment, the employees, through their union, negotiate the terms and conditions of the employment contract collectively for the benefit of all employees. Each employee and member thus benefits by receiving the same terms and conditions of employment as other colleagues, and is better able to obtain these than if he or she were negotiating as an individual.

Most aspects of union certification and labour relations are governed by the provinces by virtue of the jurisdiction given to them by the Constitution (see the discussion of the Canadian constitutional system in Chapter 2). All provinces have passed detailed labour relations legislation dealing with union certification, procedures for collective bargaining, procedures for strike votes (in some cases), definition of unfair labour practices, and prohibition of strike breaking, as well as the establishment of labour relations boards, their duties and powers.[4] The federal government has also passed labour legislation to deal with labour relations issues arising out of industries or activities that fall under federal legislative jurisdiction.[5] Examples include certain airline employees, postal workers, and telecommunications workers, since these activities come under federal constitutional jurisdiction. Similarly, civil servants at both the provincial and federal levels will usually be covered by separate legislation specifically applicable to such government employees.

Before it can be certified, the union must be formed. Where there is no existing union willing to apply for certification on behalf of a group of employees, those employees may themselves form a union. The question as to whether a union is properly constituted usually arises during certification proceedings before a provincial labour relations board. This body is charged, as part of its overall duties under the labour statute, with reviewing the union's application for certification and ensuring that all procedural formalities have been met.

An overview of the formalities necessary to the formation of a union was provided by the Ontario Labour Relations Board (OLRB) in one of its decisions in 1977.[6] Similar considerations would apply in other provinces. The OLRB laid down the following requirements:

(1) A constitution must be drafted wherein the purpose of the union (including the conduct of labour relations) must be stated and procedures for electing officers (i.e., president, secretary, treasurer) and calling meetings of the union must be set out.

(2) A meeting of the employees (in whose interest the union is being formed) must be held for the purposes of discussing and approving the proposed constitution.

(3) The employees attending such meeting must be admitted as members of the union. (Here, membership cards may be issued to such members.)

(4) A vote of the members at this meeting must be taken to ratify (approve) the proposed constitution.

(5) The new officers of the union should then be elected according to the procedures laid out in the newly approved constitution.

At this point, an application for certification can be prepared.

Certification

All provinces and the federal government have some form of certification process that must be passed before a union can represent the employees of a particular employer. The size and membership of the group of employees will usually be examined by the provincial labour board in order to determine whether it is appropriate for collective bargaining, that is, whether its members are truly employees and the group is of an appropriate size. Some provinces require that a specific percentage of all employees of an employer be members of the union. Others do not impose such a requirement. In some provinces, a representation vote may have to be taken to determine the union's level of support among the employees of the employer.

Once certified, the union becomes the exclusive **bargaining agent** for its employees. That union alone is then authorized to negotiate a collective agreement on behalf of the employees in the **bargaining unit** (the specific group of employees of a specific employer or group of employers whom it was certified to represent).

The labour relations statutes do not apply to managerial employees, who are seen to represent employers. To allow managers to participate in union formation, membership, and activities would create a conflict of interest, because managers are usually charged with executing the employer's administrative, disciplinary, and evaluative policies, and these activities are seen to be inconsistent with the interests of workers in collective bargaining.

For example, a nurse manager whose duties are primarily administrative and managerial will not be covered by the collective bargaining scheme and provisions of the provincial labour relations statute. Such a nurse manager is not permitted to participate in the formation of the union, nor to be listed on the certification application as a union member and thus one of the employees to be represented. In the certification process, the labour relations board may determine that nurse managers are ineligible for inclusion in the quorum of employees who will constitute the bargaining unit.

Some provinces allow employees to refuse to join a union or to refuse to pay dues to a union on religious grounds. In such cases, the statutes provide that an amount equal to the union dues be paid by the dissenter to a charitable institution mutually agreed upon by the parties. In Manitoba, Saskatchewan, Ontario, and Quebec, an employee who is eligible for membership but is not in fact a member must still pay dues to the union. Such dues are usually deducted by the employer from the employee's paycheque and paid to the union.

In some provinces, closed shops are permitted. A **closed shop** is a place of employment that requires all employees to be members of the union. This stipulation will appear among the terms of the collective agreement. Or, the contract may simply provide that, while union membership is not mandatory, preference in hiring will be given to union members over non-members.

In some provinces, certification may be automatic upon the union's demonstrating that it has achieved a certain level of membership. Not all employees of an employer need be members of the union seeking certification. But if a large majority of them are, this may be sufficient, in some provinces, for automatic certification. In Ontario, for example, it is possible for an employer to recognize a union as the bargaining agent for a group of employees without the need for certification.

Decertification

A union may also lose its right to act as bargaining agent for a group of workers, or it may be dissolved. This is usually referred to as **decertification**. For example, a union can lose its rights by failing to negotiate a collective agreement within a certain period of time. A group of the union's members can then apply for a declaration from the provincial labour board that that union no longer represents, and thus can no longer negotiate for, the employees in a given bargaining unit.

In some provinces, a minimum number of employees may have to consent to such declaration before the board may decertify the union.

The union may also lose its certification if it fails to give the employer notice within a certain period of time of its desire to begin negotiations for a new collective agreement or to renew an existing agreement.

Collective Bargaining

Collective bargaining is a process whereby workers, through their union representatives, meet with their employers in order to negotiate the terms and conditions of employment applicable to each worker. It is a right that was not recognized historically in common law and was even prohibited in past times as a conspiracy of persons in restraint of trade. Today, collective bargaining is fully recognized and promoted in the various labour relations statutes, both federal and provincial.

Under the laws of all provinces and federally, the parties to an expired collective agreement are obliged to negotiate a new contract when one of the parties serves the other with a notice to bargain for a new agreement (or, where there is no prior agreement and a union is newly certified, the first collective agreement). The notice begins the process of collective bargaining. In some provinces, a union can lose its certification and authorization to bargain for a specific bargaining unit if it does not serve such a notice and begin negotiation within a specified period of time. This will usually result in another union's being certified to represent the employees in the bargaining unit in place of the first union.

In collective bargaining, each side puts forth its desired terms and conditions for a new employment contract. Such matters may include wages, hours of work, work schedules, vacation pay, sick leave, pensions and other employee benefits, mechanisms for settling disputes that arise from the application, administration, interpretation, or alleged violation of the collective agreement (called *grievance procedures*), and perhaps representation on the joint health and safety committee set up for the workplace between the employer and employees. Often, negotiations become mired in disagreement over one or more terms. These disputes, if not settled promptly, can lead to strike action by employees or a lockout of employees by an employer. Thus, the labour relations statutes contain procedures for appointing conciliators and mediators to assist the parties in resolving such disagreements and to negotiate a contract. A conciliator may be appointed at the request of either party to resolve outstanding issues, or, in some cases, the provincial minister of labour may choose to appoint a conciliator or mediator.

In all provinces, once a notice to bargain has been given, the employer cannot change the terms or conditions of employment, including wages, unless it has the board's and the union's permission, or the provisions of the collective agreement permit it.

The Contract

The contract that emerges from the collective bargaining negotiations is called a **collective agreement**. In all provinces and at the federal level, the agreement must be for a minimum duration of one year. The agreement must be in writing, but need not be embodied in a single document. For example, an exchange of letters, notes, and memoranda may constitute the collective agreement if the parties set out the agreed-upon terms.

If the collective agreement expires before a new one is in place, the terms and conditions of the old agreement usually continue to apply provided that there is no evidence that the parties intended otherwise. Some contracts often specify that they will continue after the expiry date until and unless either party notifies the other of its desire to terminate it. In all provinces except Quebec and Nova Scotia, no employee is permitted to strike, nor may any employer lock out his or her employees during the life of the agreement. The reason for this is to preserve labour peace and maintain peaceful industrial relations. This condition applies even after the agreement has expired and until a specified period has elapsed from the time a conciliator is appointed by the minister of labour (or other authorized person) to the time a conciliator's report is released to the parties. This is colloquially known as a "cooling off" period.

Grievance Procedures and Arbitration

Since during the currency of a collective agreement workers are not permitted to strike, nor employers allowed to lock out workers, there must be a means of resolving disputes arising from the application, administration, interpretation, or alleged violation of the terms of the agreement. If not, labour tensions might build to an explosive point. The violence of past labour disputes has shown the necessity and desirability of having effective and timely dispute resolution procedures in place before matters come to a head. Indeed, all provincial labour statutes except Saskatchewan's require collective agreements to contain procedures for settling management–labour disputes. If they do not, the legislation deems such provisions to be part of the agreement.

Such grievance procedures will be negotiated as part of the terms of the collective agreement. Many agreements provide relatively informal mechanisms for the presentation of a grievance. As well, many workplaces have grievance committees with employee representatives.

For example, suppose a nurse is asked by her supervisor to work an additional hour beyond what the contract requires. The request may possibly result from a misinterpretation of the terms of the collective agreement. The nurse refuses to work and is disciplined. She may then choose to file a grievance with that supervisor.

Some hospitals have hospital-association committees comprising members of the hospital's management and non-managerial nurse employees. They meet on a regular basis to review any grievances in an attempt to resolve them in an informal, co-operative setting before they become adversarial, and part of a formal grievance process. If informal mechanisms fail, however, grievance procedures are implemented.

The following grievance procedures are not necessarily those followed across Canada, but are fairly common in many labour relations settings. They usually involve a progressive three-step process.

Step 1: Written Submission

In the event that the nurse's grievance is not settled satisfactorily after bringing it to the supervisor's attention, then, within a specified time, the grievance must be submitted in writing to the immediate supervisor for a response. Failing a settlement, it then must be filed within a specified time to the director of nursing for resolution. If it is still not settled, the procedure provides that it be submitted to the hospital administrator or other authorized hospital official within a set period of time for a meeting.

Step 2: Meeting with the Grievance Committee

The meeting is held among the administrator, the person who filed the grievance, the grievance committee, and a representative of the union. A decision by the hospital resulting from the discussions at such meeting must be made within a specified time. Thus, the procedure provides for the grievance's being submitted to a progressively higher and higher authority as long as it is not settled. (In many hospitals, this is managed through the Human Resources Department.) The collective agreement will also provide that if a settlement is reached under these procedures, then it is binding on the parties.

Step 3: Binding Arbitration

If the decision rendered by the hospital administrator does not settle the issue, then the matter is submitted to binding arbitration. If there is consensus, the collective agreement usually provides that the settlement is binding on the parties.

As we have said above, binding arbitration is a procedure mandated by the labour relations statutes of many provinces. Usually, one of the parties notifies the other within a specified time from the rendering of the hospital administrator's decision that that party wishes the matter to be submitted to binding arbitration. At the same time, it will nominate a person to be part of a three-member arbitration board.

The party to whom the notice is given then has a specified time in which to nominate a second person to that board. If such nomination is not forthcoming, the party who served the first notice may request that the minister of labour nominate a second person.

No person who has been involved in attempting to negotiate or settle the grievance prior to its submission to arbitration may sit on the arbitration board. These two persons, in turn, choose a third person to chair and complete the board. If they cannot agree, then the minister appoints a chair.

In recent years, certain issues have arisen in Ontario with respect to disputes over workloads and the right of nurses to refuse to provide services once the number of patients placed in their care exceeds their ability to provide adequate care. We have already mentioned *Re Mount Sinai Hospital* and the *Ontario Nurses Association,* in which case nurses refused to care for an additional patient who had been assigned to the unit. The nurses were disciplined, and the disciplinary measures were upheld upon arbitration under the collective agreement. The arbitration board felt that the nurses had not had just cause under the circumstances to refuse to care for the additional patient. Such a situation is now dealt with by means of the *professional responsibility* clause of the collective agreement.

Earlier in this chapter, we mentioned the "obey and grieve" rule. Under this provision, a nurse who believes that he or she is being given a workload so large as to preclude proper patient care may file a complaint in writing to the hospital-association committee within a certain period of time. The complaint, if unresolved, proceeds to an assessment committee hearing, whose members are chosen by both the hospital and the nurses' union. The committee then investigates the matter and holds a hearing to determine whether or not the complaint is well founded. It then reports its findings to the parties to the hearing and presumably makes recommendations in an attempt to resolve the situation. In this way, the professional integrity of nurses is maintained, and they are permitted some control over their workload and the number of patients under their care. Thus, their ability to deliver effective, efficient, and proper nursing care is maintained.

A matter may be submitted to arbitration only once all preliminary grievance procedures have been exhausted. A majority of the labour relations board determines the issue. All time limits for the giving of notice must be strictly adhered to and, if a notice that a party wishes the matter submitted to binding arbitration is not given within a specified time, the grievance will be deemed to have been abandoned. Alternatively, the parties may agree that the matter be settled by a single arbitrator.

Thus, through arbitration, every attempt is made to resolve disputes arising out of the collective agreement. This procedure has been referred to as the *quid pro quo,* that is, something in return for the fact that the right to strike or lockout is suspended during the life of the agreement.

Right to Strike and the Lockout

Traditionally, the common law did not recognize the right of employees to refuse to work. Today's statutes usually draw a distinction between a lawful and an unlawful strike. The same distinction applies to a **lockout,** a practice whereby an employer shuts out or refuses to continue to employ union employees as a means to pressure and influence them during negotiations for a collective agreement. It, like the strike, is a coercive tactic.

In most provinces, during the life of a collective agreement, employees may not strike, nor may an employer lock out employees. Even after the expiration of the agreement, employees and employers must wait for the passage of the "cooling off" period before a lawful strike or lockout can occur.

Once the collective agreement has expired, its terms can be continued while the parties negotiate a new agreement. However, if no agreement is reached, in some provinces, the provincial minister of labour may be requested or may decide to appoint a conciliation board to try to settle outstanding issues and effect a new collective agreement. Such board or conciliator (if one person is appointed) must file a report on the results (or lack thereof) of such conciliation efforts to the minister of labour, who then releases the report to the parties.

Once a specified period has elapsed after the report's release, or (if no conciliator has been appointed) after the minister has notified the parties that he or she considers it inappropriate to appoint a conciliator, the union may then lawfully call a strike. Similarly, the employer may lawfully lock out employees.

Certain types of union activity during the life of the collective agreement may or may not constitute a strike according to the applicable labour relations statute. Employees may vote to work to rule (i.e., to work only as much as is demanded by the terms of their employment) as a form of protest; for example, they may refuse to work overtime when requested to do so. If such conduct has the effect of stopping all work in order to pressure an employer to accede to union demands, it may be deemed a strike by the labour relations board. However, a refusal to work because of hazardous working conditions would likely not be deemed a strike, as it is not intended to affect collective bargaining but rather to avoid potentially serious injury to workers.

In most provinces, nurses and other hospital employees are not legally permitted to strike. While this provision may not affect nurses who are not employed at hospitals (which are defined in detail in the statutes), any nurse working at an institution that falls within the definition of a hospital would be prevented from going on strike.[7] Similarly, hospitals are not permitted to lock out their employees at any time. These provisions are designed to ensure that vital hospital services are not compromised, nor services to the public diminished, as a result of labour disputes. This is not to say that nurses are not permitted to form unions and to bargain collectively; however, different dispute resolution procedures may apply, and employees will not be permitted to strike to enforce collective bargaining rights.

Strike-breaking, that is, the use of strong-arm, threatening, or other such tactics by an employer in an effort to pressure striking employees to abandon a lawful strike or to give in on contract negotiations, is prohibited in all provinces. In Ontario, employers are also forbidden to employ replacement workers (known colloquially as "scab labour") when regular employees are on a lawful strike.[8]

The exception to this is in cases where replacement workers are needed to avoid the threat of serious bodily injury or possible death to patients.[9] This would also apply in cases where replacement workers are needed to do work normally done by striking employees that involves providing home care and assistance to disabled persons. In cases where nurses have gone on strike, unions have provided for emergency nursing care. There is also an exception for work done by emergency dispatch services and communications for ambulances.

Depending on the province, a strike vote among employees may be required before a strike can begin. If a strike vote is held, all employees in the bargaining unit may vote. Voting is usually by secret ballot. A vote may also be held to ratify an agreement concluded between management and the union's negotiators.

Unfair Labour Practices

All provinces have prohibited unfair management tactics, which in previous times were used by employers to pressure workers into returning to work or to induce employees to accept certain terms and conditions of employment.

For example, it is illegal for an employer to discipline a worker for taking part in a lawful strike or in lawful union activities, such as encouraging new members to join the union. Similarly, employers are prohibited from participating in or funding the creation of a union. Such prohibition is intended to avoid conflict of interest.

It is likewise illegal for an employer to discriminate in any way against employees because they either are or are not members of a union; to discipline them for exercising their rights under a labour relations statute; to use any form of intimidation against them for participating in union activity; or to induce them to join a particular union. Another example of an illegal labour practice is the "yellow dog" contract, by which it is made a condition of a person's employment that he or she will not join a union or participate in any union activities.

If an employee alleges that an employer has engaged in an unfair labour practice, the employee can bring the matter to the attention of the union representative. The matter may be taken up as a grievance by the union or, if it is serious enough, it may be reported to a labour inspector appointed by the provincial labour relations board. The labour boards of most provinces are given wide powers to order employers to cease and desist from engaging in such practices.

Occupational Health and Safety

In an effort to ensure that working conditions are as safe and healthy as possible, all provinces have enacted occupational health and safety legislation.[10] These statutes mandate the establishment of health and safety committees comprising representatives of non-managerial employees and management itself. The object of these committees is to identify and recommend solutions to potentially hazardous conditions in the workplace. Further, many provinces' statutes provide for the selection of health and safety representatives to inquire into and inspect hazardous working conditions, materials, substances, or unsafe equipment.

In some provinces, workers have the right to refuse to work under unsafe or unhealthy conditions. However, some provinces exempt nurses from this right. We have already discussed the "obey and grieve" rule. Nurses, who must often work in potentially dangerous situations, are exempt at the outset from the right to refuse to work. Yet, it would not be unethical for a nurse to refuse to work under unsafe working conditions. Nurses may or may not have legal protection, however, if they are disciplined for refusing such work.

Many occupational health and safety statutes also include obligations on employers to label hazardous substances that are present in the workplace and to provide safety equipment and instructions to employees on the proper use of such equipment. Further, they include regulations for the handling of hazardous waste and other toxic or harmful substances. This is especially important in a health care setting, with the ever-present dangers posed by biomedical waste. Nurses, as any other health care professionals working with or around such materials, have the right to learn of any and all applicable handling procedures and methods as well as the right to maximum safety in the workplace. Employers have a corresponding obligation to provide a safe and healthy workplace.

Summary

The key points introduced in this chapter include:
- the rights of Canadian nurses as citizens, professionals, and employees
- when the right to a conscientious objection can be invoked
- the responsibilities of nurses as employees to employers
- the position of the law with respect to discrimination and sexual or physical abuse
- the role of labour relations and collective bargaining with respect to nursing
- the standards associated with occupational health and safety.

References

1. Canadian Nurses Association. (1991). *Code of ethics for nursing.* Value V, "Limitations" (p. 10).
2. (1978), 17 LAC (2d) 242 (arbitrator).
3. *Canadian Charter of Rights and Freedoms,* Part 1 of the *Constitution Act, 1982,* being Schedule B of the *Canada Act 1982* (UK), 1982, c. 11, section 2(d).
4. See British Columbia: *Labour Relations Code,* SBC 1992, c. 82; Alberta: *Labour Relations Code,* SA 1988, c. L-12, as amended; Saskatchewan: *Trade Union Act,* RSS 1978, c. T-17, as amended; Manitoba: *Labour Relations Act,* RSM 1987, c. L10, as amended; Ontario: *Labour Relations Act,* RSO 1990, c. L.2, as amended; Quebec: *Labour Code,* RSQ 1977, c. C-27, as amended; New Brunswick: *Industrial Relations Act,* RSNB 1973, c. I-4, as amended; Nova Scotia: *Trade Union Act,* RSNS 1989, c. 475, as amended; Prince Edward Island: *Labour Act,* RSPEI 1988, c. L-1, as amended; Newfoundland: *Labour Relations Act,* RSN 1990, c. L-1, as amended.
5. See *Canada Labour Code,* RSC 1985, c. L-2, as amended.
6. *Local 199 UAW Building Corp.,* [1977] OLRB Rep. July, 472, at p. 473.
7. See, e.g., Ontario: *Hospital Labour Disputes Arbitration Act,* RSO 1990, c. H.14, section 11(1), as amended; *Alberta: Hospitals Act,* RSA 1980, c. H-11.
8. Supra footnote 4 (Ontario Act), section 73.1(5), added by SO 1992, c. 21, section 32.
9. Ibid., section 73.2(3).
10. See Alberta: *Occupational Health and Safety Act,* RSA 1980, c. O-2, as amended; British Columbia: *Workplace Act,* SBC 1985, c. 34, as amended; Manitoba: *Workplace Safety and Health Act,* RSM 1987, c. W210, CCSM, c. W210, as amended; New Brunswick: *Occupational Health and*

Safety Act, SNB 1983, c. O-0.2, as amended; Newfoundland: *Occupational Health and Safety Act,* RSN 1990, c. O-3, as amended; Northwest Territories: *Safety Act,* RSNWT 1988, c. S-1, as amended; Nova Scotia: *Occupational Health and Safety Act,* RSNS 1989, c. 320, as amended; Ontario: *Occupational Health and Safety Act,* RSO 1990, c. O.1, as amended; Prince Edward Island: *Occupational Health and Safety Act,* RSPEI 1988, c. O-1; Quebec: *Occupational Health and Safety Act,* RSQ 1977, c. S-2.1, as amended; Saskatchewan: *Occupational Health and Safety Act, 1993,* SS 1993, c. O-1.1.

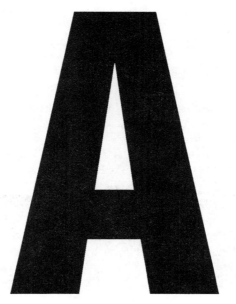

A

Canadian
Nurses
Association
Code of Ethics
for Nursing

Contents

Preamble

Nursing practice can be defined generally as a "dynamic, caring, helping relationship in which the nurse assists the client to achieve and maintain optimal health."[1] Nurses in clinical practice, education, administration and research share the common goal of maintaining competent care and improving nursing practice. "Nurses direct their energies toward the promotion, maintenance and restoration of health, the prevention of illness, the alleviation of suffering and the ensuring of a peaceful death when life can no longer be sustained."[2]

The nurse, by entering the profession, is committed to moral norms of conduct and assumes a professional commitment to health and the well-being of clients. As citizens, nurses continue to be bound by the moral and legal norms shared by all other participants in society. As individuals, nurses have a right to choose to live by their own values (their personal ethics) as long as those values do not compromise care of their clients.

This Code deals with the ethics rather than the laws governing nursing practice. Laws and ethics of health care necessarily overlap considerably, since both share the concern that the conduct of health care professionals reflects respect for the well-being, dignity and liberty of patients. An ideal system of law would be compatible with ethics, in that adherence to the law ought never require the violation of ethics. Still, the two domains, law and ethics, remain distinct, and this Code, while prepared with awareness of the law, is addressed solely to ethical obligations. The adoption of this Code represents a conscious undertaking on the part of the Canadian Nurses Association and its members to be responsible for upholding the following statements (values, obligations, and limitations). This Code expresses and seeks to clarify the obligations of nurses to use their knowledge and skills for the benefit of others, to minimize harm, to respect client autonomy and to provide fair and just care for their clients. For those entering the profession, this Code identifies the basic moral commitments of nursing and may serve as a source for education and reflection. For those within the profession, the Code also serves as a basis for self-evaluation and for peer review. For those outside the profession, this Code may serve to establish expectations for the ethical conduct of nurses.

Ethical Problems

Situations often arise that present ethical problems for nurses in their practice. These situations tend to fall into three categories:

(a) **Ethical violations** involve the neglect of moral obligation; for example, a nurse who neglects to provide competent care to a client because of personal inconvenience has ethically failed the client.

1. Canadian Nurses Association. *A Definition of Nursing Practice, Standards for Nursing Practice.* Ottawa: CNA, 1987, p. iii.
2. Ibid., p. ii

(b) **Ethical dilemmas** arise where ethical reasons both for and against a particular course of action are present and one option must be selected. For example, a client who is likely to refuse some appropriate form of health care presents the nurse with an ethical dilemma. In this case, substantial moral reasons may be offered on behalf of several opposing options.

(c) **Ethical distress** occurs when nurses experience the imposition of practices that provoke feelings of guilt, concern or distaste. Such feelings may occur when nurses are ethically obliged to provide particular types of care despite their personal disagreement or discomfort with the course of treatment prescribed. For example, a nurse may think that continuing to tube feed an irreversibly unresponsive person is contrary to that client's well-being, but nonetheless is required to do so because that view is not shared by other caregivers.

This Code provides clear direction for avoiding ethical violations. When a course of action is mandated by the Code, and there exists no opposing ethical principle, ethical conduct requires that course of action.

The Code cannot serve the same function for all ethical dilemmas or for ethical distress. There is room within the profession of nursing for conscientious disagreement among nurses. The resolution of any dilemma often depends upon the specific circumstances of the case in question, and no particular resolution may be definitive of good nursing practice. Resolution may also depend upon the relative weight of the opposing principles, a matter about which reasonable people may disagree.

The Code cannot relieve ethical distress but it may serve as a guide for nurses to weigh and consider their responsibilities in the particular situation. Inevitably, nurses must reconcile their actions with their consciences in caring for clients.

The Code tries to provide guidance for those nurses who face ethical problems. Proper consideration of the Code should lead to better decision-making when ethical problems are encountered.

It should be noted that many problems or situations seen as ethical in nature are problems of miscommunication, failure of trust or management dilemmas in disguise. There is, therefore, a distinct need to clarify whether the problem is an ethical one or one of another sort.

Elements of the Code

This Code contains different elements designed to help the nurse in its interpretation. The values and obligations are presented by topic and not in order of importance. There is intentional variation in the normative terminology used in the Code (the nurse **should** or **must**) to indicate differences in the moral force of the statements; the term **should** indicates a moral preference, while **must** indicates an obligation. A number of distinctions between ethics and morals may be found in the literature. Since no distinction has been uniformly adopted by writers on ethics, these terms are used interchangeably in this Code.

- **Values** express broad ideals of nursing. They establish correct directions for nursing. In the absence of a conflict of ethics, the fact that a particular action promotes a **value** of nursing may be decisive in some specific instances. Nursing behaviour can always be appraised in terms of values: How closely did the behaviour approach the value? How widely did it deviate from the value? The values expressed in this Code must be adhered to by all nurses in their practice. Because they are so broad, however, values may not give specific guidance in difficult instances.

- **Obligations** are moral norms that have their basis in nursing values. However, obligations provide more specific direction for conduct than do values; obligations spell out what a value requires under particular circumstances.

- **Limitations** describe exceptional circumstances in which a value or obligation cannot be applied. Limitations have been included separately to emphasize that, in the ordinary run of events, the values and obligations will be decisive.

It is also important to emphasize that even when a value or obligation must be limited, it nonetheless carries moral weight. For example, a nurse who is compelled to testify in a court of law on confidential matters is still subject to the values and obligations of confidentiality. While the requirement to testify is a justified limitation upon confidentiality, in other respects confidentiality must be observed. The nurse must only reveal that confidential information that is pertinent to the case at hand, and such revelation must take place within the appropriate context. The general obligation to preserve the client's confidences remains despite particular limiting circumstances.

Rights and Responsibilities

Clients possess both legal and moral rights. These serve as one foundation for the responsibilities of nurses. However, for several reasons this Code emphasizes the obligations of nurses, rather than the rights of clients. Because the rights of clients do not depend upon professional acceptance of those rights, it would be presumptuous for a profession to claim to define the rights of clients. Emphasizing the rights of clients may also seem unduly legalistic and restrictive, ignoring the fact that sometimes ethics require nurses to go beyond the letter of the law. (For one example, see Value II, Obligation 3). Finally, because it is sometimes beyond the power of a nurse to **secure** the rights of a client— an achievement that requires the cooperative and scrupulous efforts of all members of the health care team—it is better for a professional code of nursing to emphasize the responsibilities of nurses rather than to detail the entitlements of clients.

Nurses, too, possess legal and moral rights, as persons and as professionals. It is beyond the scope of this Code to address the personal rights of nurses. However, to the extent that conditions of employment have an impact on the establishment of ethical nursing, this Code must deal with that issue.

The satisfaction of some ethical responsibilities requires action taken by the nursing profession as a whole. The fourth section of the Code contains values and obligations concerned with those collective responsibilities of nursing; this section is particularly addressed to professional associations. Ethical reflection must be ongoing and its facilitation is a continuing responsibility of the Canadian Nurses Association.

The body of the Code is divided into sections corresponding to the sources of nursing obligations:

- **Clients**
- **Nursing Roles and Relationships**
- **Nursing Ethics and Society**
- **The Nursing Profession**

Clients

VALUE I
Respect for Needs and Values of Clients

Value

A nurse treats clients with respect for their individual needs and values.

Obligations

1. The client's perceived best interest must be a prime concern of the nurse.
2. Factors such as the client's race, religion or absence thereof, ethnic origin, social or marital status, sex or sexual orientation, age, or health status must not be permitted to compromise the nurse's commitment to that client's care.
3. The expectation and normal life patterns of clients are acknowledged. Individualized programs of nursing care are designed to accommodate the psychological, social, cultural and spiritual needs of clients, as well as their biological needs.
4. The nurse does more than respond to the requests of clients; the nurse accepts an affirmative obligation within the context of health care to aid clients in their expression of needs and values, including their right to live at risk.
5. Recognizing the client's membership in a family and a community, the nurse, with the client's consent, should attempt to facilitate the participation of significant others in the care of the client.

VALUE II
Respect for Client Choice

Value

Based upon respect for clients and regard for their right to control their own care, nursing care reflects respect for the right of choice held by clients.

Obligations

1. The competent client's consent is an essential precondition to the provision of health care. Nurses bear the primary responsibility to inform clients about the nursing care available to them.
2. Consent may be signified in many different ways. Verbal permission and knowledgeable cooperation are the usual forms by which clients consent to nursing care. In each case, however, a valid consent represents the free choice of the competent client to undergo that care.
3. Consent, properly understood, is the process by which a client becomes an active participant in care. All clients should be aided in becoming active participants in their care to the maximum extent that circumstances permit. Professional ethics may require of the nurse actions that exceed the legal requirements of consent. For example, although a child may be legally incompetent to consent, nurses should nevertheless attempt to inform and involve the child.
4. Force, coercion and manipulative tactics must not be employed in the obtaining of consent.
5. Illness or other factors may compromise the client's capacity for self-direction. Nurses have a continuing obligation to value autonomy in such clients; for example, by creatively providing clients with opportunities for choices within their capabilities, the nurse helps them to maintain or regain some degree of autonomy.
6. Whenever information is provided to a client, this must be done in a truthful, understandable and sensitive way. The nurse must proceed with an awareness of the individual client's needs, interests and values.
7. Nurses have a responsibility to assess the understanding of clients about their care and to provide information and explanation when in possession of the knowledge required to respond accurately. When the client's questions require information beyond that known to the nurse, the client must be informed of that fact and assisted to obtain the information from a health care practitioner who is in possession of the required facts.

VALUE III
Confidentiality

Values

The nurse holds confidential all information about a client learned in the health care setting.

Obligations

1. The rights of persons to control the amount of personal information revealed applies with special force in the health care setting. It is, broadly speaking, up to clients to determine who shall be told of their condition, and in what detail.

2. In describing professional confidentiality to a client, its boundaries should be revealed:

    (a) Competent care requires that other members of a team of health personnel have access to or be provided with the relevant details of a client's condition.

    (b) In addition, discussions of the client's care may be required for the purpose of teaching or quality assurance. In this case, special care must be taken to protect the client's anonymity.

    Wherever possible, the client should be informed of these necessities at the onset of care.

3. An affirmative duty exists to institute and maintain practices that protect client confidentiality—for example, by limiting access to records or by choosing the most secure method of communicating client information.

4. Nurses have a responsibility to intervene if other participants in the health care delivery system fail to respect the confidentiality of client information.

Limitations

The nurse is not morally obligated to maintain confidentiality when the failure to disclose information will place the client or third parties in danger. Generally, legal requirements or privileges to disclose are morally justified by these same criteria. In facing such a situation, the first concern of the nurse must be the safety of the client or the third party.

Even when the nurse is confronted with the necessity to disclose, confidentiality should be preserved to the maximum possible extent. Both the amount of information disclosed and the number of people to whom disclosure is made should be restricted to the minimum necessary to prevent the feared harm.

VALUE IV
Dignity of Clients

Value

The nurse is guided by consideration for the dignity of clients.

Obligations

1. Nursing care must be done with consideration for the personal modesty of clients.
2. A nurse's conduct at all times should acknowledge the client as a person. For example, discussion of care in the presence of the client should actively involve or include that client.
3. Nurses have a responsibility to intervene when other participants in the health delivery system fail to respect any aspect of client dignity.
4. As ways of dealing with death and the dying process change, nursing is challenged to find new ways to preserve human values, autonomy and dignity. In assisting the dying client, measures must be taken to afford the client as much comfort, dignity and freedom from anxiety and pain as possible. Special consideration must be given to the need of the client's family or significant others to cope with their loss.

VALUE V
Competent Nursing Care

Value

The nurse provides competent care to clients.

Obligations

1. Nurses should engage in continuing education and in the upgrading of knowledge and skills relevant to their area of practice, that is, clinical practice, education, research or administration.
2. In seeking or accepting employment, nurses must accurately state their areas of competence as well as limitations.
3. Nurses assigned to work outside an area of present competence must seek to do what, under the circumstances, is in the best interests of their clients. The nurse manager on duty, or others, must be informed of the situation at the earliest possible moment so that protective measures can be instituted. As a temporary measure, the safety and welfare of clients may be better served by the best efforts of the nurse under the circumstances than by no nursing care at all. Nurse managers are obligated to support nurses who are placed in such difficult situations and to make every effort to remedy the problem.

4. When called upon outside an employment setting to provide emergency care, nurses fulfil their obligations by providing the best care that circumstances, experience and education permit.

Limitations

A nurse is not ethically obliged to provide requested care when compliance would involve a violation of her or his moral beliefs. When that request falls within recognized forms of health care, however, the client must be referred to a health care practitioner who is willing to provide the service. Nurses who have or are likely to encounter such situations are morally obligated to seek to arrange conditions of employment so that the care of clients will not be jeopardized.

Nursing Roles and Relationships

VALUE VI
Nursing Practice, Education, Research and Administration

Value

The nurse maintains trust in nurses and nursing.

Obligations

1. Nurses accepting professional employment must ascertain to the best of their ability that conditions will permit the provision of care consistent with the values and obligations of the Code. Prospective employers should be informed of the provisions of the Code so that realistic and ethical expectations may be established at the beginning of the nurse–employer relationship.

2. Nurse managers, educators and peers are morally obligated to provide timely and accurate feedback to nurses, nurse managers, students of nursing and nurse educators. Objective performance appraisal is essential to the growth of nurses and is required by a concern for present and future clients.

3. Nurse managers bear special ethical responsibilities that flow from a concern for present and future clients. The nurse manager must seek to ensure that the competencies of personnel are used efficiently. Working within available resources, the nurse manager must seek to ensure the welfare of clients. When competent care is threatened due to inadequate

resources or for some other reason, the nurse manager must act to minimize the present danger and to prevent future harm.

4. Student–teacher and student–client encounters are essential elements of nursing education. These encounters must be conducted in accordance with ethical nursing practices. The nurse educator is obligated to treat students of nursing with respect and honesty and to provide fair guidance in developing nursing competence. The nurse educator should ensure that students of nursing are acquainted with and comply with the provisions of the Code. Student–client encounters must be conducted with client consent and require special attention to the dignity of the client.

5. Research is necessary to the development of the profession of nursing. Nurses should be acquainted with advances in research, so that established results may be incorporated into clinical practice, education and administration. The individual nurse's competencies may also be used to promote, to engage in or to assist health care research designed to enhance the health and welfare of clients.

The conduct of research must conform to ethical practice. The self-direction of clients takes on added importance in this context. Further direction is provided in the Canadian Nurses Association publication *Ethical Guidelines for Nursing Research Involving Human Subjects.*[1]

VALUE VII
Cooperation in Health Care

Value

The nurse recognizes the contribution and expertise of colleagues from nursing and other disciplines as essential to excellent health care.

Obligations

1. The nurse functions as a member of the health care team.
2. The nurse should participate in the assessment, planning, implementation and evaluation of comprehensive programs of care for individual clients and client groups. The scope of a nurse's responsibility should be based upon education and experience, as well as legal considerations of licensure or registration.
3. The nurse accepts responsibility to work with colleagues and other health care professionals, with nursing interest groups and through professional nurses' associations to secure excellent care for clients.

---

1. Canadian Nurses Association. *Ethical Guidelines for Nursing Research Involving Human Subjects.* Ottawa: CNA, 1983.

VALUE VIII
Protecting Clients from Incompetence

Value

The nurse takes steps to ensure that the client receives competent and ethical care.

Obligations

1. The first consideration of the nurse who suspects incompetence or unethical conduct must be the welfare of present clients or potential harm to future clients. Subject to that principle, the following must be considered:
   (a) The nurse is obliged to ascertain the facts of the situation before deciding upon the appropriate course of action.
   (b) Relationships in the health care team should not be disrupted unnecessarily. If a situation can be resolved without peril to present or future clients by direct discussion with the colleague suspected of providing incompetent or unethical care, that discussion should be done.
   (c) Institutional mechanisms for reporting incidents or risks of incompetent or unethical care must be followed.
   (d) The nurse must report any reportable offence stipulated in provincial or territorial professional nursing legislation.
   (e) It is unethical for a nurse to participate in efforts to deceive or mislead clients about the cause of alleged harm or injury resulting from unethical or incompetent conduct.
2. Guidance on activities that may be delegated by nurses to assistants and other health care workers is found in legislation and policy statements. When functions are delegated, the nurse should be satisfied about the competence of those who will be fulfilling these functions. The nurse has a duty to provide continuing supervision in such a case.
3. The nurse who attempts to protect clients or colleagues threatened by incompetent or unethical conduct may be placed in a difficult position. Colleagues and professional associations are morally obliged to support nurses who fulfil their ethical obligations under the Code.

VALUE IX
Conditions of Employment

Value

Conditions of employment should contribute in a positive way to client care and the professional satisfaction of nurses.

Obligations

1. Nurses accepting professional employment must ascertain, to the best of their ability, that employment conditions will permit provision of care consistent with the values and obligations of the Code.
2. Nurse managers must seek to ensure that the agencies where they are employed comply with all pertinent provincial or territorial legislation.
3. Nurse managers must seek to ensure the welfare of clients and nurses. When competent care is threatened due to inadequate resources or for some other reason, the nurse manager should act to minimize the present danger and to prevent future harm.
4. Nurse managers must seek to foster environments and conditions of employment that promote excellent care for clients and a good worklife for nurses.
5. Structures should exist in the work environment that provide nurses with means of recourse if conditions that promote a good worklife are absent.

VALUE X
Job Action

Value

Job action by nurses is directed toward securing conditions of employment that enable safe and appropriate care for clients and contribute to the professional satisfaction of nurses.

Obligations

1. In the final analysis, the improvement of conditions of nursing employment is often to the advantage of clients. Over the short term, however, there is a danger that action directed toward this goal could work to the detriment of clients. In view of their ethical responsibility to current as well as future clients, nurses must respect the following principles:
   (a) The safety of clients is the first concern in planning and implementing any job action.
   (b) Individuals and groups of nurses participating in job actions share the ethical commitment to the safety of clients. However, their responsibilities may lead them to express this commitment in different but equally appropriate ways.
   (c) Clients whose safety requires ongoing or emergency nursing care are entitled to have those needs satisfied throughout the duration of any job action. Individuals and groups of nurses participating in job actions have a duty through coordination and communication to take steps to ensure the safety of clients.
   (d) Members of the public are entitled to know of the steps taken to ensure the safety of clients.

Nursing Ethics and Society

VALUE XI
Advocacy of the Interests of Clients, the Community and Society

Value

The nurse advocates the interests of clients.

Obligations

1. Advocating the interests of individual clients and groups of clients includes helping them to gain access to good health care. For example, by providing information to clients privately or publicly, the nurse enables them to satisfy their rights to health care.
2. When speaking in a public forum or in court, the nurse owes the public the same duties of accurate and relevant information as are owed to clients within the employment setting.

VALUE XII
Representing Nursing Values and Ethics

Value

The nurse represents the values and ethics of nursing before colleagues and others.

Obligations

1. Nurses serving on committees concerned with health care or research should see their role as including the vigorous representation of nursing's professional ethics.
2. Many public issues include health as a major component. Involvement in public activities may give the nurse the opportunity to further the objectives of nursing as well as to fulfil the duties of a citizen.

The Nursing Profession

VALUE XII
Responsibilities of Professional Nurses' Associations

Value

Professional nurses' organization are responsible for clarifying, securing and sustaining ethical nursing conduct. The fulfilment of these tasks requires that professional nurses' organizations remain responsive to the rights, needs and legitimate interests of clients and nurses.

Obligations

1. Sustained communication and cooperation between the Canadian Nurses Association, provincial or territorial associations and other organizations of nurses are essential steps toward securing ethical nursing conduct.
2. Activities of professional nurses' associations must at all times reflect a prime concern for excellent client care.
3. Professional nurses' associations should represent nursing interests and perspectives before non-nursing bodies, including legislatures, employers, the professional organizations of other health disciplines and the public communication media.
4. Professional nurses' associations should provide and encourage organizational structures that facilitate ethical nursing conduct.
   (a) Education in the ethical aspects of nursing should be available to nurses throughout their careers. Nurses' associations should actively support or develop structures to enhance sensitivity to, and application of, norms of ethical nursing conduct. Associations should also promote the development and dissemination of knowledge about ethical decision-making through nursing research.
   (b) Changing circumstances call for ongoing review of this Code. Supplementation of the Code may be necessary to address special situations. Professional associations should consider the ethics of nursing on a regular and continuing basis and be prepared to provide assistance to those concerned with its implementation.

Appendix

1954   CNA adopted the ICN Code as its first Code of Ethics
1980   CNA Code of Ethics: an Ethical Basis for Nursing in Canada adopted
1985   Code of Ethics for Nursing adopted
1991   Code of Ethics for Nursing revised

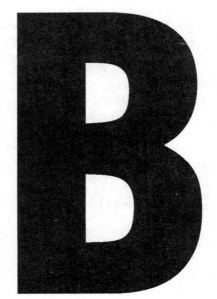

University of Toronto Centre for Bioethics Living Will

The Centre for Bioethics Living Will was developed by Dr. Peter A. Singer. It is a guide to help you think about and express your wishes about life-sustaining treatment. The Living Will is not intended to be used in the absence of specific medical or legal advice. The Centre for Bioethics and Dr. Singer assume no liability for any reliance by any person on the information contained herein. The University of Toronto makes no representations regarding the technical quality, accuracy or lawfulness of the material presented herein. Many people have provided helpful comments about previous versions of this living will. Colleagues who reviewed this version and suggested improvements include: Ms. Iris Allen, Dr. Jaques Belik, Dr. Ed Etchells, Prof. Eike-Henner W. Kluge, Mr. James Lavery, Dr. Heather MacDonald, Prof. Eric Meslin, Mr. Jeffrey Schnoor, and Mr. Gilbert Sharpe. If you have any suggestions for improving this living will, please send them to Dr. Singer at the Centre for Bioethics, University of Toronto, 88 College Street, Toronto, Ontario M5G 1L4 (tel. 416-978-2709; fax 416-978-1911).

What Is a Living Will?

A living will is a written document containing your wishes about life-sustaining treatment. You make a living will when you can understand treatment choices and appreciate their consequences (i.e., when you are "capable"). A living will only takes effect when you can no longer understand and appreciate treatment choices (i.e., when you are "incapable"). Various types of living wills are also called "advance directives", "health care directives", and "powers of attorney for personal care". There are two parts to a living will: an *instruction directive* and a *proxy directive.*

What Is an Instruction Directive?

An *instruction directive* specifies what life-sustaining treatments you would or would not want in various situations. Some common health situations and life-sustaining treatments are described in this pamphlet. Your doctors would determine whether you were in one of the situations described, and whether it was likely to be permanent, before following your instructions.

What Is a Proxy Directive?

A *proxy directive* specifies who you want to make treatment decisions on your behalf if you no longer can do so. The proxy should be someone you know and trust, like a spouse, partner, family member, or close friend. This person should be capable him/herself to make health care decisions and willing to be your proxy. Because the proxy is responsible for carrying out your wishes, it is important that you discuss your wishes with your proxy. Otherwise, it may be difficult for your proxy to guess what your wishes might be. You may name more than one person to act as your proxy, but you should state what will be done if they disagree with each other.

What Type of Living Will Should You Complete?

Because instruction and proxy directives are complementary, if possible, your living will should contain both of these directives. However, if you do not have someone you trust to make treatment decisions on your behalf, then you may want to complete only the instruction directive. If you find that making treatment decisions for a possible future illness is too difficult, then you may want to complete only the proxy directive. In your living will, you may want to say whether you would want your doctors to follow the treatment decisions of your proxy or your wishes as expressed in the instruction directive if these two appear to be in conflict.

What Should You Do with Your Living Will?

Since a living will speaks for you when you are no longer able to speak for yourself, other people must know that it exists. You should give copies of your living will to your proxy, doctor(s), lawyer, and family members. If you review your wishes with these people and give them the opportunity to discuss your living will with you, they will be more likely to understand and follow your wishes. The Centre for Bioethics Living Will is designed for easy photocopying onto legal size (8 1/2" x 14") paper.

When Should You Update Your Living Will?

You can change your mind about your treatment decisions or your proxy at any time. If you change your mind, you should change your living will. Review your living will at regular intervals, such as once a year, and when there are important changes in your life, for example: if your medical conditions changes, if you are admitted to hospital, if you marry or divorce, or if your proxy dies. If you change your living will, destroy all copies of the old one, and replace them with copies of the new one.

Who Should Complete a Living Will?

People who want to maintain control over future life-sustaining treatments should consider making a living will. However, to make a living will, you must consider the prospect of your own sickness and death. Some people might find this distressing. Each person should decide for him/herself whether completing a living will is right for them. Remember, a person may choose to complete an instruction directive, a proxy directive, both, or perhaps neither.

Is a Living Will "Legal" in Canada?

The provinces of Nova Scotia and Quebec have laws recognizing the use of proxy directives. In 1992, Manitoba and Ontario passed laws recognizing both proxy and instruction directives.

The Manitoba law came into force on July 26, 1993. In Manitoba, a living will is called a "Health Care Directive." People who are 16 years of age or older are presumed capable to make a health care directive. The person appointed to be the proxy must be at least 18 years old. To be valid, a health care directive must be in writing, signed by the person making it, and dated. The health care directive does not need to be witnessed if the person making it can sign for himself. The legislation does not require that a particular form be used.

The Ontario law is expected to come into force in 1994. In Ontario, a living will is called a "power of attorney for personal care." The person making the power of attorney for personal care, as well as the person appointed to be the proxy, must be at least 16 years old. The power of attorney for personal care must be witnessed by two people. The witnesses must have no reason to believe the person making it is incapable of giving a power of attorney for personal care. The following people cannot act as witnesses: the proxy; the spouse of the patient or proxy; a child of the patient; anyone who himself or herself has a legal guardian; and anyone who is less than 18 years old. The legislation does not require that a particular form be used.

It is reasonable to expect that other provinces will pass laws about living wills in the future. There are also court cases in Canada that would support the use of living wills. As well, the Canadian Medical Association has published a policy supporting the use of living wills.

You do not need a lawyer to complete your living will. However, some people might feel more comfortable if they review their living will with a lawyer. If there is some question about whether you are capable to make a living will, or if you anticipate conflict about who will make decisions for you or what decisions will be made, you probably should review your living will with a lawyer. A lawyer can also give you more specific and current information about the laws regarding living wills in your province.

Individuals interested in obtaining copies of the University of Toronto Centre for Bioethics Living Will may send requests to the Centre for Bioethics, University of Toronto, 88 College Street, Toronto, Ontario M5G 1L4 (tel. 416-978-2709; fax 416-978-1911).

CENTRE FOR BIOETHICS
Living Will

Patient Information

I have read and understood all sections of this living will. All previous living wills made by me are to be disregarded and this directive followed according to my wishes stated here.

Name: _____

Address: _____

Signature: _____

Date: _____

Witness Information

We have witnessed the signature above and have no reason to believe the person making this living will is incapable of making a living will.

Witness 1:

Name: _____

Address: _____

Signature: _____

Witness 2:

Name: _____

Address: _____

Signature: _____

Instruction Directive

DIRECTIONS: Refer to "Health Situations" and "Life-Sustaining Treatments" [p. 256] for the definitions of terms used in this directive. Write your treatment decision (yes, no, or undecided) in the boxes below for each combination of health situation and treatment. For example, if you want tube feeding in severe dementia you would write "yes" in the bottom right hand box; if you do not want tube feeding in severe dementia, you would write "no"; and if you are undecided, you would write "undecided". Under "Further Instructions" [p. 258], you may express in your own words the situations in which you would or would not want various life-sustaining treatments.

	CPR	RESPIRATOR	DIALYSIS	LIFE-SAVING SURGERY	BLOOD TRANSFUSION	LIFE-SAVING ANTIBIOTICS	TUBE FEEDING
CURRENT HEALTH	yes	yes	yes	yes	yes	yes	yes
PERMANENT COMA	no	no	no	no	no	no	no
TERMINAL ILLNESS	no	no	no	undecided	yes	yes	undecided
MILD STROKE	undecided	temporarily	temporarily	yes	yes	yes	temporarily
MODERATE STROKE	no	no	no	no	no	no	no
SEVERE STROKE	no	no	no	no	no	no	no
MILD DEMENTIA	yes	yes	yes	yes	yes	yes	yes
MODERATE DEMENTIA	no	no	no	no	no	no	no
SEVERE DEMENTIA	no	no	no	no	no	no	no

Health Situations

In order to make an instruction directive, you need to imagine yourself becoming very ill or nearing death. It is not easy to imagine these situations or to decide upon treatments for them. To help you with this, we describe in detail some health situations in which a living will might be needed.

Current health

This describes the way your health is now.

Permanent coma

This means you would be permanently unconscious. Permanent coma is usually caused by decreased blood flow to the brain, for example, from the heart stopping. You would be unable to eat or drink and would need a feeding tube for nourishment. You would not have bowel or bladder control. You would need to be in bed and you would never regain consciousness. You could live at home with someone caring for you all day and night; otherwise you would probably need to be cared for in a chronic care hospital.

Terminal illness

This means you would have an illness for which there is no known cure, such as some types of cancer. It is likely that you would die within six months even if you received treatment.

Stroke

This means you would have damage to the brain causing permanent physical disability such as paralysis. You might also have trouble communicating because of impaired speech. These problems stay the same for the rest of your life. They do not get worse with time unless there is another injury to the brain, such as another stroke. Stroke can be described as:

• **Mild:** You would have mild paralysis on one side of the body. You could walk with a cane or walker. You would be able to have meaningful conversations, but might have trouble finding words. You could carry out most routine daily activities, such as work and household duties, dressing, eating, bathing, and using the toilet. You would have bowel and bladder control. You could live at home with someone caring for you for a few hours a day.

• **Moderate:** You would have moderate paralysis on one side of the body. You would be unable to walk and would need a wheelchair. You could carry out conversations, but you might not always make sense. You would need help with routine daily activities. You may have bowel and bladder control. You could live at home with someone caring for you throughout the daytime; otherwise you would probably need to live in a nursing home.

• **Severe:** You would have severe paralysis on one side of the body. You would be unable to walk, and would need to be in a chair or bed. You would not have meaningful conversations. You would be unable to carry out routine daily activities. You would need a feeding tube for nourishment. You would not have bowel or bladder control. You could live at home with someone caring for you all day and night; otherwise you would probably need to be cared for in a chronic care hospital.

Dementia

This means you would have a progressive and irreversible deterioration in brain function. You would be awake and aware but you would have trouble thinking clearly, recognizing people, and communicating. The most common cause of dementia is Alzheimer's disease. Dementia gradually gets worse over months or years. Dementia can be described as:

• **Mild:** You could have meaningful conversations, but would be forgetful and have poor short term memory. You could carry out most routine daily activities, such as work and household duties, dressing, eating, bathing, and using the toilet. You would have bowel and bladder control. You could live at home with someone caring for you for a few hours each day.

• **Moderate:** You would not always recognize family and friends. You could carry out conversations but you might not always make sense. You would need help with routine daily activities. You may have bowel and bladder control. You could live at home with someone caring for you throughout the daytime; otherwise you would probably need to live in a nursing home.

• **Severe:** You would not recognize family and friends, and would be unable to have meaningful conversations. You would be unable to carry out routine daily activities. You would need a feeding tube for nourishment. You would not have bowel and bladder control. You could live at home with someone caring for you all day and night; otherwise you would probably need to be cared for in a chronic care hospital.

Life-Sustaining Treatments

In each of the health situations described above, you might need one or more of the follow life-sustaining treatments.

• **Cardiopulmonary resuscitation** (CPR) is used to try to restart the heart if it has stopped beating. CPR involves applying pressure and electrical shocks to the chest, assisted breathing with a respirator (breathing machine) through a tube inserted down the throat and into the lungs, and giving drugs through a needle into a vein. It is usually followed by unconsciousness and several days of treatment in an intensive care unit. Without CPR, immediate death is certain. On average when hospitalized patients are given CPR, it is successful at restarting the heart in about 41% of patients (41 patients out of 100). However, about 14% (14 patients out of 100) will live to be discharged from hospital. Patients whose hearts are successfully restarted but who do not survive to hospital discharge spend several days in an intensive care unit before death. The chance that a person will live depends on the cause of the heart stopping and the seriousness of the person's other illnesses.

• **Respirator** (breathing machine) is used when a person cannot breathe; for example, because of emphysema or a serious pneumonia. A tube is put down the person's throat into the lungs. The respirator is needed as long as the person's lungs are not working. Without the respirator, a person with respiratory failure will probably die within minutes to hours. With the respirator, the chance that a person will live depends on the cause of the respiratory failure, and the seriousness of the person's other illnesses.

• Dialysis (kidney machine) replaces the normal functions of the kidney. Dialysis removes excess potassium, water, and other waste products from the blood. Without dialysis, the potassium in the blood would build up and cause the heart to stop. Dialysis is needed as long as the person's kidneys are not working. Without dialysis, a person with kidney failure will die within 7 to 14 days. With dialysis, the chance that a person will live depends on the cause of the kidney failure and the seriousness of the person's other illnesses.

• **Life-saving surgery** may involve a wide range of procedures, for example, removal of an inflamed gall bladder or appendix. Without surgery, a person with a serious illness may die within hours to days. With surgery, the chance that a person will live depends on why the person needed surgery and the seriousness of the person's other injuries or illnesses.

• **Blood transfusion** refers to blood given through a needle inserted in a person's vein. A person who is bleeding very heavily from a car accident, a stomach ulcer, or during major surgery, needs a blood transfusion. Without a blood transfusion, a person who is bleeding very heavily will probably die within hours. With a blood transfusion, the chance that a person will live depends on the seriousness of the person's other injuries or illnesses.

• **Life-saving antibiotics** refers to the drugs needed to treat life-threatening infections; for example, pneumonia or meningitis. These drugs usually are given through a needle inserted in a person's vein. Without antibiotics, a person with a life-threatening infection will likely die in hours to days. With antibiotics, the chance that a person will live depends on the seriousness of the infection and the seriousness of the person's other illnesses.

• **Tube feeding** involves putting a tube into a person's stomach (through the nose, or through a small hole in the abdomen). A person who cannot eat (e.g., someone in a coma) needs a feeding tube. Tube feeding is needed as long as the person cannot eat. Without tube feeding, a person who cannot eat or drink will die within days to weeks. With tube feeding, the chance that a person will live depends on the seriousness of the person's other injuries or illnesses.

Further Instructions

In the space below, you may express in your own words the situations in which you would or would not want various life-sustaining treatments.

_____

_____

_____

_____

_____

_____

_____

_____

_____

_____

_____

_____

_____

_____

_____

_____

_____

_____

_____

Proxy Directive

I request that in accordance with current standards of the province, the following person(s) be appointed to make treatment decisions on my behalf if I am no longer capable of making them myself:

Name: _____

Relationship: _____

Address: _____

Telephone: _____

If there is disagreement between the people I have named as my proxy, I want my doctors to follow the decisions of (check one):

    ☐ the person named above

    ☐ a majority of my proxies

If you want more than one person to be your proxy, add the additional name(s) below:

Name: _____

Relationship: _____

Address: _____

Telephone: _____

Name: _____

Relationship: _____

Address: _____

Telephone: _____

If there is disagreement between my instructions about treatment and the treatment decisions of my proxy, I want my doctors to follow (check one):

    ☐ my instructions

    ☐ decisions of my proxy

GLOSSARY

Actus Reus. The physical element of a criminal offence, i.e., the voluntary performance of a prohibited act that results in physical or other harm (e.g., assault causing bodily harm).

Administrative Tribunals. Government boards, agencies, councils, and commissions charged with administration of a particular area (e.g., property taxes, human rights complaints, energy rates, transport licences). These often operate like courts in that they decide claims before them, grant licences, etc.

Advance Directive. A document made and signed by a mentally competent adult detailing specific medical treatments that are to be administered or withheld in the event that the maker later becomes incapable of expressing such wishes owing to mental or physical illness (e.g., Alzheimer's disease, coma).

Affidavit. A written statement of facts made under oath or solemn affirmation.

Appellant. The party to a court action (usually the party who loses at trial or against whom an unfavourable judgement is made) who brings an appeal of a trial decision in an appellate court.

Assault. Conduct (such as a physical or verbal threat) that creates in another person an apprehension or fear of imminent harmful or offensive contact.

Bargaining Agent. In labour relations, a union certified by provincial statute and authorized to negotiate collectively on behalf of a group of employees.

Bargaining Unit. In labour relations, a group of employees who are members of a union and who are bound by the terms of a collective agreement (employment contract) negotiated by the union on their behalf with their employer.

Battery. Harmful or offensive and non-consensual contact with the person or clothing of another.

Bill. A draft or proposed law that is not yet passed and must be voted upon by Parliament or a legislature. Usually introduced by the government party, but any member of Parliament may introduce a bill.

Burden of Proof. The obligation on a party to litigation (i.e., a criminal or civil suit) to prove a certain fact or facts and to persuade the judge or jury of the existence of such fact or facts.

Case Law. The law as set forth in decided cases. This is called *jurisprudence* in civil law systems.

Civil Code. A central written and formal source of civil law principles and rules organized by subject.

Civil Law. A system of law based on Roman law prevalent in most European countries and the Province of Quebec in which legal principles and rules are codified or written in organized fashion into a central statute or code.

Closed Shop. In labour relations, a place of employment in which, as a condition of employment, a worker is required to belong to the union representing the employees.

Codification. The process of formally arranging legal rules and principles on any area into a central source of law known as a code.

Collective Agreement. In labour relations, a written contract of employment between an employer or group of employers and a unionized group of non-managerial employees. It binds all employees, lasts for a term of at least one year, and sets out the conditions of employment (e.g., wages, hours of work, benefits, sick leave, pension, layoffs, termination, disciplinary action, arbitration of grievances).

Collective Bargaining. In labour relations, the process by which a union (the bargaining agent) negotiates the conditions of employment of a group of non-managerial employees (the bargaining unit) with an employer or group of employers.

Common Law. English system of law dating back to the eleventh century, based on unwritten principles derived from judicial precedents.

Complainant. In professional disciplinary matters, a person who complains, through a formal disciplinary procedure, about the treatment accorded him or her by a member of a self-governing profession (e.g., a physician, nurse, dentist, lawyer).

Constitution. A written law that sets forth the fundamental rules and principles defining how a country is organized and its laws passed, and the extent of the government's powers and the powers of its courts.

Contributory Negligence. A situation in which a plaintiff, who has sued another for damages for negligence, is held partly responsible for the damage or injury sustained because the plaintiff is partly at fault.

Controlled Act. In Ontario (under the *Regulated Health Professions Act 1991,* so 1991, c. 18, section 27), a specific medical act or procedure that may be performed only by a person who is a member of a health profession (e.g., a nurse, doctor, dentist, etc.) and who is authorized by a health profession Act (e.g., the *Nursing Act, 1991,* so 1991, c. 32) to perform such an act. (See Chapter 5 for a list of controlled acts.)

Coroner's Inquest. An inquiry convened under the authority of a coroner to look into the circumstances of a death when that person has died in suspicious circumstances, as a result of wrongdoing, possible negligence, or accident (i.e., not through natural causes). The inquest is presided over by a deputy coroner, and determinations of fact and recommendations are made by a jury.

Criminal Negligence. Conduct in which the actor (the accused) has acted intentionally in a reckless or wanton manner, showing disregard for the rights or safety of others who might reasonably be expected to suffer harm or damage as a result of such conduct, and where damage or harm ensues.

Custom. Practice or rules of a particular trade or industry given force of law by the courts in the absence of specific statute law, case law, or doctrine governing the particular area.

Damages. A sum of money awarded by a court at the end of a civil trial and claimed by the plaintiff against the defendant as compensation for an injury to person or property caused by the defendant.

Decertification. In labour relations, the process whereby a union, as bargaining agent for a group of employees, loses its right to represent those employees and to bargain collectively on their behalf, either through its failure to take steps to negotiate a collective agreement, or through a vote of the employees in the bargaining unit.

Defendant. A person or party against whom a lawsuit is brought; the party sought to be made responsible for the plaintiff's damages.

Deposition. In Quebec, under the *Professional Code,* a written complaint of a complainant given under oath according to the procedures in such code.

Disclosure. The obligation of each party to a lawsuit under the rules of civil procedure to reveal to the other party or parties all evidence, documents, reports, records, etc. that will be relied upon at trial.

Doctrine. Texts, journal articles, treatises, restatements of the law, and other writings of legal scholars on any legal subject; used by lawyers and judges as an aid in interpreting or developing existing law.

Documentary Discovery. The right of each party in a lawsuit to obtain copies of all relevant documents possessed by or in the control of the opponent(s), and upon which the opponent(s) will rely at trial.

Dual Procedure Offence. A criminal offence that may be tried either as a summary offence or an indictable one at the option of the Crown attorney. The choice usually depends on the seriousness of the facts surrounding the laying of charges.

Due Process. The right of every citizen, regardless of race, sex, colour, creed, or religion, to receive fair treatment according to established rules and procedures and rules of natural justice.

Duty of Care. A legal obligation imposed on an individual to act or refrain from acting in a way such as to avoid causing harm to the person or property of another who might reasonably be affected by that conduct and who ought to be in the actor's contemplation.

Evidence. Information gathered through documents, photographs, physical objects, or oral testimony, tending to prove a fact or set of facts.

Examination for Discovery. A preliminary oral examination at which the lawyer for each party in a trial has the opportunity to ask relevant questions of the other party or parties, under oath, to obtain full disclosure of all evidence and facts that will be relied upon at trial.

Garnishment. A court-ordered procedure by which individuals or corporations owing money to a defendant debtor are required to pay a portion or all of it to the sheriff for distribution among the defendant's creditors, including the plaintiff.

Guardian of the Person. In Ontario, under the *Substitute Decisions Act, 1992,* so 1992, c. 30, a person appointed by court order to make decisions with respect to the care, feeding, housing, clothing, medical treatment, and hygiene of another person who has been found incapable of making such decisions by reason of physical or mental illness or infirmity.

Indictable Offences. Generally the most serious of criminal offences triable by jury, but only after a preliminary hearing at which the accused is ordered to stand trial. Punishment ranges from several years to life imprisonment and/or heavy fines.

Inferior Court. A lower level of court that is judicially subordinate to a superior one. Usually a trial court, which is bound by previous decisions of an appeal court.

Informed Consent. In health care, a legally capable patient's consent to a specific medical treatment, in which the patient is informed by the health care practitioner of the nature and purpose of the treatment, all material risks and benefits of such treatment, as well as the material risks of not proceeding with the treatment. A *material risk* is one that a patient would reasonably wish to know prior to making the decision of whether to undergo or forgo the proposed treatment.

Judgement Debtor Examination. An oral examination at which the defendant gives answers under oath to questions by the plaintiff's lawyer concerning his or her finances, sources of income, property, and ability to pay the judgement against him or her.

Jurisdiction. The authority that a court has over a given area, category of legal dispute (e.g., civil or criminal), or particular territory, as well as the types of orders and judgements it may make.

Jurisprudence. Judges' written decisions in past court cases, which serve as precedents for future decisions in civil law systems; not binding, but seen as evidence of how past courts have interpreted a civil code provision or legal principle.

Legislative Assembly. A provincial parliament consisting of only one house, called the legislature.

Liability. The legal responsibility owed by a party at fault to another for damages incurred or injury suffered by that other.

Litigant. A person or corporation who is a party to a lawsuit.

Living Will. A written document signed by a mentally competent person setting forth specific instructions regarding medical treatments to be applied or withheld in the event that the maker later becomes incapable of expressing those wishes. For example, the document might indicate whether resuscitation should or should not be attempted in the event of a cardiac arrest.

Lockout. In labour relations, the employer's equivalent of the strike in which the employer locks out its unionized employees from the workplace, or refuses to continue to employ them in an effort to pressure them to concede during contract negotiations or in labour disputes. In most provinces, a lockout, like a strike, may occur only after the expiry of a collective agreement and only after a "cooling off" period has elapsed under the applicable provincial labour statute.

Malfeasance. Doing an act that is one's duty to perform but doing it poorly, incorrectly, or negligently.

Mens Rea. The mental element of a criminal offence, that is, the accused's state of mind when he or she is alleged to have committed a crime; the requirement that he or she was aware and intended willfully to commit it, knew that the action was wrong, or was reckless as to the consequences of the action.

Negligence. The non-intentional category of tort law wherein one person has, through carelessness, failed in a duty of care toward another such that that other has sustained injury to person or property.

Non-feasance. Failing to do that which is one's duty to do.

Original Jurisdiction. The first court to hear a criminal or civil case, i.e., the court in which the litigation process begins.

Parliament. A body of elected lawmakers (Members of Parliament) entrusted with the power to make laws for the country or a province. It consists of two houses (the Senate and the House of Commons) and the Queen (the Head of State).

Plaintiff. The party who brings a lawsuit and seeks damages against another for breach of contract or other wrong done to that party.

Pleadings. The court documents filed by each party to the lawsuit outlining the nature of the claim, of the defence to the claim, and the issues to be tried in the action.

Power of Attorney. Generally in Canada, a document in which a legally capable person appoints another to manage the maker's financial affairs and make decisions on the maker's behalf in the maker's absence or unavailability. In Ontario, under the *Substitute Decisions Act, 1992,* so 1992, c. 30, two types of powers of attorney are recognized in law: a power of attorney for property (as above), and a power of attorney for personal care. In the latter, the maker of the document appoints someone to make decisions on his or her behalf regarding medical treatment, care, feeding, clothing, shelter, hygiene, etc., in the event that the maker becomes incapable owing to physical or mental illness. Unlike the guardian of the person, the attorney for personal care exercises authority pursuant to the document made by the maker, not by virtue of a court order.

Precedent. A previous judge's decision that serves as a guide or basis for deciding future cases having similar facts or legal issues. A higher-court precedent is usually binding on an inferior court.

Preliminary Inquiry. A hearing held before a provincial court judge at which the Crown prosecutor is required to show that the evidence presented is such that a reasonable jury properly instructed could convict the accused. If the evidence is found insufficient in this regard, the accused must be discharged.

Presumption of Innocence. The presumption that a person charged with a criminal offence is not guilty until and unless proven guilty of the offence at trial. The Crown (i.e., the prosecution) is obliged to prove that the accused committed the offence beyond a reasonable doubt; the accused need not prove that he or she did not commit the offence.

Pre-trial Conference. A conference of all parties and their lawyers held a few weeks before trial in the presence of a judge other than the one who will hear the trial. The judge reviews the facts of the case and the positions of each party, as well as the strengths and weaknesses of each party's case.

Then the judge advises the litigants how the case might be decided. This is a last attempt to reach a settlement without a lengthy and expensive trial.

Procedural Law. Law that regulates how individual rights are asserted and enforced in the judicial system, such as which court hears the matter, what documents must be filed and when, etc.

Proximate Cause. A concept of causation wherein damage, injury, or other resulting event must not be too remote or unforeseeable a consequence of a particular act or omission.

Proxy. In health care, a person appointed or otherwise authorized by law to give consent to a specified medical treatment or procedure on behalf of another where the patient is unable to give such consent owing to physical or mental incapacity.

Proxy Consent. In health care, the person legally authorized or appointed to give consent to medical treatment on behalf of an incapable patient.

Regulations. Detailed secondary laws passed by federal or provincial cabinet pursuant to a specific statute. The statute usually gives the cabinet the power to make detailed rules to carry out the intent and purpose of the Act but which are too detailed and time-consuming for parliament to enact.

Remedies. The judgements and orders that a court may grant under the law in favour of a plaintiff to correct a wrong done to his or her person or property by a liable defendant. These include damages, an order that the defendant do or refrain from doing a particular action, an order reversing a transaction or contract, etc.

Respondent. The party to a court action (usually the successful party) against whom an appeal of a trial decision is brought in an appellate court.

Rules of Civil Procedure. Detailed rules and regulations that govern procedure in the commencement and conduct of court actions, trials, the gathering of evidence, documentation, and the enforcement of court orders and judgements. They are essentially the rules of litigation and have the force of law.

Sheriff. An officer of the court in a particular county or judicial district who is responsible for enforcing court orders, carrying out judicial sales of real estate or other property, and serving court documents on witnesses.

Standard of Care. Legal yardstick against which a person's conduct is measured to determine whether that person has been negligent.

Stare Decisis. Rule of English common law whereby courts are legally bound to follow previous court decisions, which have the force of law. Usually courts will follow precedents whose facts and legal issues are similar or identical to the case they are deciding.

Statement of Claim. A document prepared and filed by the plaintiff which initiates the court action. It sets forth the damages and other relief sought from the court and the bare facts (but not the evidence) upon which the plaintiff relies to support a claim against the defendant.

Statement of Defence. A document prepared and filed by the defendant in a lawsuit. It sets forth the defendant's version of the facts (but not the evidence) giving rise to the action and the legal grounds or reasons why the defendant is not liable for the plaintiff's damages.

Statute Law. A formal written law passed by Parliament or a provincial legislature, which takes precedence over and supersedes common law case law. Also found in civil law systems.

Substantive Law. Law that sets out detailed rights and obligations of citizens in private dealings with one another and with society in general.

Summary Conviction Offences. Criminal offences of a less serious nature which are tried without a jury in a fairly rapid, straightforward way and for which the maximum punishment is six months' imprisonment or a fine of up to $2000, or both.

Tort. An intentional or non-intentional (i.e., negligent) wrongful act that causes damage or injury to another's person, reputation, or property.

Union. In labour relations, a group of non-managerial employees in a common trade or industry organized in association with a constitution and membership for the purpose of advancing the common interests of its members and regulating employment relations with a common employer or group of employers.

Vicarious Liability. In negligence law, the liability of a principal (an employer) for the negligent or tortious acts of the principal's agent (an employee) done within the scope of the agent's authority or employment.

TO THE OWNER OF THIS BOOK

We are interested in your reaction to *Ethical and Legal Issues in Canadian Nursing*. With your comments, we can improve this book in future editions. Please help us by completing this questionnaire.

1. If you are a student, please identify your school and the course in which you used this book.

   _____

   SCHOOL _____

   PROGRAM _____

2. In what way did this book assist you in your course?

   _____

   _____

   _____

3. What did you like best and least about this book?

   _____

   _____

   _____

4. Please add any comments or suggestions:

   _____

   _____

   _____

☐ May we contact you for further information?

☐ Do you wish to receive information on Saunders Reference Books?

NAME _____

_____

ADDRESS _____

_____

POSTAL CODE _____ PHONE _____

(fold here and tape shut)

0116873899-M8Z4X6-BR01

WB SAUNDERS CANADA
c/o Heather McWhinney
PO BOX 35211 STN BRM B
TORONTO ON M7Y 6E1